Hysteria: The Rise of an Enigma

Frontiers of Neurology and Neuroscience

Vol. 35

Series Editor

J. Bogousslavsky Montreux

Hysteria: The Rise of an Enigma

Volume Editor

J. Bogousslavsky Montreux

59 figures, 3 in color, and 2 tables, 2014

KARGER

Basel · Freiburg · Paris · London · New York · Chennai · New Delhi · Bangkok · Beijing · Shanghai · Tokyo · Kuala Lumpur · Singapore · Sydney

Frontiers of Neurology and Neuroscience
Vols. 1–18 were published as Monographs in Clinical Neuroscience

Julien Bogousslavsky, MD
Center for Brain and Nervous System Diseases
GSMN Neurocenter, Clinique Valmont
CH-1823 Glion/Montreux (Switzerland)

Library of Congress Cataloging-in-Publication Data

Hysteria (Bogousslavsky)
Hysteria : the rise of an enigma / volume editor, J. Bogousslavsky.
p. ; cm. -- (Frontiers of neurology and neuroscience, ISSN 1660-4431 ; vol. 35)
Includes bibliographical references and indexes.
ISBN 978-3-318-02646-7 (hard cover : alk. paper) -- ISBN 978-3-318-02647-4 (e-ISBN)
I. Bogousslavsky, Julien, editor. II. Title. III. Series: Frontiers of neurology and neuroscience ; v. 35. 1660-4431
[DNLM: 1. Hysteria--history. 2. History, 19th Century. 3. History, 20th Century. 4. Mental Disorders--history. W1 MO568C v.35 2014 / WM 11.1]
RC532
616.85'24--dc23
2014013484

Bibliographic Indices. This publication is listed in bibliographic services, including Current Contents® and Index Medicus.

www.karger.com
Printed in Germany on acid-free and non-aging paper (ISO 9706) by Kraft Druck, Ettlingen
ISSN 1660–4431
e-ISSN 1662–2804
ISBN 978–3–318–02646–7
e-ISBN 978–3–318–02647–4

Contents

VII **Foreword**
Boller, F. (Bethesda Md.)

IX **Preface**
Bogousslavsky, J. (Montreux)

1 **Before Charcot**
Pearce, J.M.S. (Hull)

11 **Socioeconomic Background of Hysteria's Metamorphosis from the 18th Century to World War I**
Edelman, N. (Nanterre); Walusinski, O. (Brou)

20 **'Fin-de-Siècle' Epidemiology of Hysteria**
Luauté, J.-P. (Romans)

28 **Clinical Manifestations of Hysteria: An Epistemological Perspective or How Historical Dynamics Illuminate Current Practice**
Medeiros De Bustos, E.; Galli, S.; Haffen, E.; Moulin, T. (Besançon)

44 **Jean-Martin Charcot and His Legacy**
Bogousslavsky, J. (Montreux)

56 **Hypnosis and the Nancy Quarrel**
Piechowski-Jozwiak, B. (London/Warsaw); Bogousslavsky, J. (Montreux)

65 **The Girls of La Salpêtrière**
Walusinski, O. (Brou)

78 **Public Medical Shows**
Walusinski, O. (Brou)

90 **Emma Bovary, Hedda Gabler, and Harold Brodkey Would Not Have Lived without Charcot: Hysteria in Novels**
Kaptein, A.A. (Leiden)

99 **Traces of Hysteria in Novels**
Haan, J. (Leiderdorp/Leiden); Koehler, P.J. (Heerlen)

109 **Sigmund Freud and Hysteria: The Etiology of Psychoanalysis?**
Bogousslavsky, J. (Montreux); Dieguez, S. (Fribourg)

126 **Paul Sollier, Pierre Janet, and Their Vicinity**
Walusinski, O. (Brou)

139 **Criticism of Pithiatism: Eulogy of Babinski**
Poirier, J.; Derouesné, C. (Paris)

149 **The Borderland with Neurasthenia ('Functional Syndromes')**
Paciaroni, M. (Perugia); Bogousslavsky, J. (Montreux)

157 **World War I Psychoneuroses: Hysteria Goes to War**
Tatu, L. (Besançon); Bogousslavsky, J. (Montreux)

169 **Hysteria around the World**
Carota, A. (Genolier/Basel); Calabrese, P. (Basel)

181 **History of Physical and 'Moral' Treatment of Hysteria**
Broussolle, E.; Gobert, F.; Danaila, T.; Thobois, S. (Lyon); Walusinski, O. (Brou); Bogousslavsky, J. (Montreux)

198 **'Hysteria' Today and Tomorrow**
LaFrance, W.C., Jr. (Providence, R.I.)

205 **Author Index**

206 **Subject Index**

Foreword

Hysteria is undoubtedly a fascinating subject. It has inspired a large number of books, films, paintings, and even poetry. However, when it comes to clinicians and researchers, opinions and reactions tend to vary widely. Many of us are uneasy when seeing patients supposed to suffer from it or when trying to write about the condition. A number of problems arise. For a start the origin of the word and its heavy uterus-related gender connotation, besides being politically incorrect, grossly contradicts the clinical reality that males also demonstrate these symptoms, even though less frequently than females. Yet there is hardly another fully agreed upon term to label it. Freud introduced the label 'conversion disorders', but it is not universally recognized nowadays. The terms 'psychogenic' or 'functional' disorders have the supposed advantage of being compatible with our inability to demonstrate a tangible 'lesion' of the nervous system. However, psychogenic implies a psychiatric background which in many cases is hard to demonstrate. As for the term 'functional', it was probably chosen by the authors of the new DSM-5 because it implies that we are confronted with a system which is malfunctioning even though we do not know why. Use of the word, however, contradicts the dictionary definition of the term ('having a special purpose; practical, necessary'). Frankly, it strikes me mainly as a euphemism which has become part of medical slang so as not to offend the laypersons who hear it.

Several sources indicate that the condition is inversely correlated to socioeconomic status and in many cases, it is clearly related to stress. The poor Salpêtrière women described by Charcot probably had many reasons for being stressed. Also, there is a massive recrudescence of 'hysteria' during wars. We have in mind the shell shock occurring so frequently during the incredibly anxiogenic conditions of trench warfare during World War I. We all remember General Patton's gesture so vividly represented by George C. Scott in Franklin Shaffner's 1970 film. In August 1943, at the height of the battle of Sicily, the General found out that two soldiers were in evacuation hospitals without apparent physical injuries and 'battle fatigue' as the only reason for being away from the front. That infuriated him to the extent that he struck and insulted them, a gesture which almost cost him his subsequent career and which forced him to apologize in front of the troops. Much closer to us, there seems to be an increase in cases of hysteria in war-torn Iraq [1].

Have current laboratory techniques much improved our understanding of hysteria? Not a lot – probably in part because of the heterogeneity of the disorder. Both structural and functional imaging data confirm the absence of consistent and reproducible structural lesions. Available data, however, are compatible with dysfunction of a network. This may lead to the erroneous cognitive processing of adverse events which in turn appears to be associated with the physical symptoms of hysteria.

A recent editorial in the *Journal of Neurology, Neurosurgery and Psychiatry* [2] is provocatively entitled 'Don't know what they are, but treatable?' It accompanies an article by McCormack et al. [3] showing good response of severe motor conversion disorders to inpatient psychiatric treatment. These two articles correctly point to one element that most patients with hysteria have in common: they tend to improve with nonpharmacological therapies ranging from psychoeducation to randomized clinical trials of controlled behavioral therapy. Patients with psychogenic nonepileptic seizures have benefitted the most, but a moderate effect has been found in other cases of hysteria. This allows reasoning based on response to treatment, 'ex juvantibus' as the old saying goes, corroborating the theory of a cause unrelated to physical factors.

In conclusion, the precise nosology and pathophysiology of hysteria remain elusive. Yet, although we may be ill at ease seeing these patients, we all also like enigmas. That is why I am convinced that many people, whether health-related professionals or not will derive great pleasure from reading this work by Julien Bogousslavsky and his exceptional consortium of authors.

François Boller, Bethesda Md., USA

References

1 Najim H, Al-Habbo DJ, Sultan KO: Trends of admissions of conversion disorder in Mosul Iraq. Psychiatr Danub 2011;23(Suppl 1):S29–S31.

2 Rickards H, Silver J: Don't know what they are, but treatable? Therapies for conversion disorders. J Neurol Neurosurg Psychiatry 2013, DOI: 10.1136/jnnp-2013-306061.

3 McCormack R, Moriarty J, Mellers JD, Shotbolt P, Pastena R, Landes N, Goldstein L, Fleminger S, David AS: Specialist inpatient treatment for severe motor conversion disorder: a retrospective comparative study. J Neurol Neurosurg Psychiatry 2013, DOI: 10.1136/jnnp-2013-305716.

Preface

Hysteria and enigma: a nice rhyme! Hysteria is perhaps the condition which best illustrates the tight connections between neurology and psychiatry. While this link has recently renewed interest in hysteria, it has in fact been present since early studies in the 19th century, mainly through the work of Jean-Martin Charcot and his collaborators at La Salpêtrière. Indeed, the great names of neurology and psychiatry studied hysteria with Charcot, which include Pierre Janet, Joseph Babinski, Paul Richer, Georges Gilles de la Tourette, and Sigmund Freud. At the time, the border between psychism and the brain was more permeable than what it would become in the 20th century, during which, unfortunately, hysteria commonly was considered as a neurological condition by psychiatrists and as a psychiatric condition by neurologists. This grotesque paradox probably reflected the fear, sometimes even repulsion, that hysteria generated in many people, including doctors. Nobody wanted to deal with it. The fact that the term 'hysterical' has a negative meaning in popular language is a good example of the reputation of the condition, which was systematically associated with demoniac possession until the 18th century. Part of Freud's legacy is to have been able to replace this devilish flavor by the gross concept of 'conversion', indeed another religious term, but which suggests a (presumably more tolerable) somatic problem rather than a psychological one. 'Conversion' has had such a fortune that it even colonized textbooks and insurance classifications made by people who would be horrified to realize that they are just pure Freudian zealots.

The present developments in the 21st century seem to correspond to a reductionist brain-centric approach to the *psyche*, which may not necessarily lead to significant advances in the understanding of hysteria and psychological conditions. Functional magnetic resonance imaging is now progressively being considered as the new truth about the brain, despite its technical limitations, its wide tendency to be overinterpreted, and its philosophical paradigm which a priori implies that psychism and the mind are selectively located within the brain. We now have a new generation of Gall-type scientists, who pretend to localize love, faith, or crime in specific areas of the brain. Moreover, it is most comical to see that the finding of brain areas being activated or deactivated during certain thoughts and feelings, as shown by such a technique, indeed came up as a major discovery, as if there had been doubt about it. These findings have inevitably led to new beliefs and dogmas, such as the fact that thoughts would exclusively take place in the brain. Perhaps one should re-read the Nobel prize winner and great philosopher Henri Bergson, who claimed that neither perception nor memory were located in the brain. For him, the issue of 'location' was a wrong problem for such functions, a problem which only reflected the preeminence of space coordinates in modern-day science. I am pretty sure that the actual new positivists of brain research would diagnose madness here! We should nevertheless remember that with whatever technique, including functional magnetic resonance imaging, we can only measure the presence or absence of activity in an organ, without addressing the more interesting issue of whether what we measure is a cause or a consequence of the function we study. Perhaps the future of a better understanding of hysteria lies beyond these organ-centered approaches?

I am very grateful to the international panel of experts who made this book possible, in which we review the origins and developments of the concepts of hysteria: an ever-changing enigma.

Julien Bogousslavsky, Montreux

Bogousslavsky J (ed): Hysteria: The Rise of an Enigma. Front Neurol Neurosci. Basel, Karger, 2014, vol 35, pp 1–10
DOI: 10.1159/000359985

Before Charcot

J.M.S. Pearce
Department of Neurology, Hull Royal Infirmary, Hull, UK

Abstract
From the time of Greco-Roman Medicine, the uncertain nature of hysterical illness was a fertile source of controversy. Because there were no testable objective signs of disease, the diverse ideas relating hysteria to the uterus and to psychological and physiological causes generated persisting polemics. Theories fluctuated chaotically, influenced by social changes of prosperity or deprivation, current attitudes, and issues of gender. Faced with a large number of patients with such illnesses as well as many with epilepsy, mental illnesses, and organic nervous disorders, Charcot set about investigating hysterics to determine what neurological abnormalities might explain them. His many predecessors, from Sydenham and Willis in the 17th century to Briquet and Bourneville in the 19th century, whose views are outlined in this chapter, both conditioned and influenced his efforts. Charcot succeeded in promoting his work at Salpêtrière, which for a time was respected throughout the world.

> [Hysteria] ... symptoms of almost every other disease of the nervous system, since there is scarcely one which may not be simulated by this Protean malady.
> *W. Gowers* [1]

While no one has yet framed a satisfactory definition of hysteria, most physicians claim they can recognize it [2]. The term derives from the Greek ('hysterikos') and Latin ('hystera') terms for the uterus. Gowers [1] called it 'that strange disease', but also remarked, 'Hysteria... seems to be a product of the cerebral development that accompanies the process of civilization...'. Johnson [3] referred to it as the 'mocking-bird of nosology'. Of those with neurological hysterical symptoms, about 20% have Briquet's hysteria, though many eventually show an underlying physical disease [2]. Many have a recognizable psychiatric illness, particularly depression; hysteria often is subtly conjoined with physical disease [4].

Before Charcot (1825–1893), the varied symptoms were known, but there was no analysis of present ideas of conversion, dissociation, and somatoform (DSM-IV) disorders. At Salpêtrière, between 1872 and 1878, Charcot demonstrated to awestruck audiences a bewildering spectrum of hysterical manifestations. He showed dramatic, much publicized representations of female hysterical attacks like the ones in *Iconographie photographique de la Salpêtrière* [5]. By 1895, Freud and Breuer published their *Studien über hystérie*

(Studies on Hysteria), in which Breuer supported a neurophysiologic cause, while Freud supported a psychological one.

The murky story of hysteria, however, begins much earlier. Historically, theories of hysteria can be simplified:

- Antiquity marked the 'wandering womb'
- In the Middle ages it was caused by demonic possession
- The 17th century favored a neurological disorder
- The Enlightenment saw the recurrence of uterine causes in the 'furies' of the womb
- In the late 19th century Charcot resurrected ideas of a brain disorder, but its delineation was incomplete

In Greco-Roman literature, hysteria became apparent when the female reproductive system was inactive or ungratified. It has been alleged that the Hippocratic corpus refers to a variety of illness symptoms, such as suffocation of the womb (hysterika); however, a common interpretation of this as psychogenic hysteria has been debated [6]. An instance is Aretaeus [7], who differentiated epilepsy from hysterical suffocation by lack of convulsions in the latter. Generally, hysteria was supposedly caused by migration of the uterus to other body sites if it became dried up from lack of fluids. Pregnancy might alleviate the disorder, which became known as 'the wandering womb': an idea arguably mooted in ancient Egyptian papyri [8]. In *Timaeus* (circa 360 BC), Plato speculated about the transmigration of the uterus inside women's bodies, causing symptoms as it moved. Certain Hippocratic texts give graphic descriptions of the uterus as a restless animal, furiously raging through the female owing to prolonged continence, which produced bizarre symptoms including a sensation of suffocation, palpitations, and aphonia. In keeping with these beliefs, prescribed treatments included massage of the pelvic area, ovarian pressure, drugs applied to entice the uterus back into place, and of course sexual intercourse. Classical theories [9] were immensely influential. For centuries hysteria was defined as an illness confined to women, 'the quintessential female malady' [8, 10].

The symptoms of hysteria have also long been ascribed to 'demonic possession and witchcraft'. From the fall of the Roman Empire to the Enlightenment, many illnesses and cures were attributed to sorcery, witchcraft, and saints, and little distinction was made between medical, neurological, and psychological disorders. Much human suffering was the result of a 'Divine', who inflicted disease as punishment for malefaction or sins, or of witches and warlocks doing the Devil's work. Charlemagne (742–814 AD) sentenced those suspected of practising witchcraft to death. Such beliefs led to the infamous witch trials, the organized persecution, torture, and murder of thousands of people who were psychologically or neurologically ill. During the Middle Ages, although it had not yet acquired a respectable name, physicians studying 'hysteria' started to dispel the ideas of witchcraft. Much later, as the 'dark ages' of science receded, the 17th century saw the emergence of an organic basis for mental illness [11].

The word 'hystérique' did not develop in French until 1568; the adjective 'hysterical' appeared in English in 1615 (Crooke): 'Hysterical women, that is, such as are in fits of the mother'. In 1801 the noun 'hysteria' emerged: 'Account of Diseases in an Eastern District of London... Chronic Diseases... Hysteria'. And French 'hystérie' appeared in 1812. The anatomical site moved from the uterus to the head, i.e. brain, the mind, and the nervous system, allowing the possibility of hysteria in men.

In 1603 Edward Jorden (1569–1632) wrote an important discourse [12] which dispelled supernatural and demonic agencies (fig. 1): 'Affections of the mind doe beare such rule in this disease, seeing we doe observe that most commonly besides the indisposition of the bodie…'. The notion of a disordered womb also persists in his book. He described 'perturbations of the mind': 'Melancho-

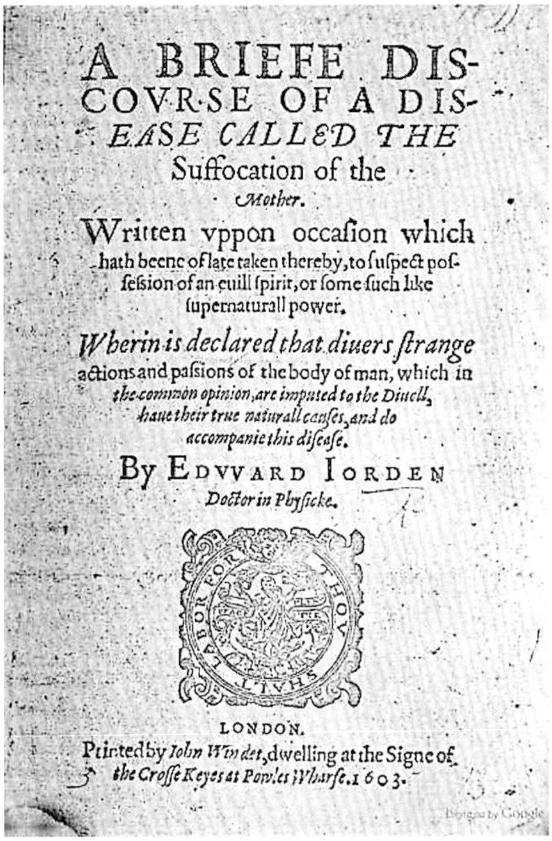
A BRIEFE DIS-
COVRSE OF A DIS-
EASE CALLED THE
Suffocation of the
Mother.
Written vppon occasion which
hath beene of late taken thereby, to suspect pos-
session of an euill spirit, or some such like
supernaturall power.
Wherein is declared that diuers strange
actions and passions of the body of man, which in
the common opinion, are imputed to the Diuell,
haue their true naturall causes, and do
accompanie this disease.
By EDVVARD IORDEN
Doctor in Physicke.
LONDON.
Printed by Iohn Windet, dwelling at the Signe of
the Crosse Keyes at Powles Wharfe. 1603.

Fig. 1. Jorden E. A Briefe Discourse of a Disease called the Suffocation of the Mother. 1603 [38].

like or capricious conceit joined withal of love, feare, hatred, jealousie… which being by policie or good instruction and perswasions removed, the disease is easily overcome.' Jorden reported:

> This disease is called: Passio Hysterica, Suffocatio, Proefocatio, and Strangulatus uteri, Calculus matricis, &c. In English the Mother, or the Suffocation of the Mother, because most commonly it takes them with choaking in the throat: and it is an affect of the Mother or wombe wherein the principal parts of the bodie by consent do suffer diversely according to the diversitie of the causes and diseases wherewith the matrix is offended.

He imputed 'true natural causes' and advocated release of the psychological stresses thought to have determined the symptoms [13]. By the end of the 17th century a cascade of socially acceptable labels had joined melancholia and hysteria: vapors, swooning, attacks of the spleen, and hypochondria. In J. Harris's *Lexicon Technicum.* (1704), vapors were 'the Disease called otherwise Hysterick, or Hypochondriack Fits, or Melancholy'. As in Charcot's cases, bizarre fits, spasms, contractures, and sensory impairments figured prominently.

In the 17th century, the concept of hysterical manifestations of disordered brain function started to replace hysterogenic theories [14]. In England, Thomas Willis (1622–1675; fig. 2) and Thomas Sydenham (1624–1689) posited the notion of a 'nervous distemper' or 'animal spirits' which afflicted certain susceptible patients. The uterine nature was questioned and regarded as a cloak to conceal physicians' ignorance. Willis dismissed ideas of a wandering womb: 'tyed by neighbouring parts that it cannot of itself be moved, or ascend…'. For instance, in the chapter 'The passions commonly called hysterical or fits of the mother' of his *Practice of physic* [15], he found hindbrain abnormalities and noted:

> When at any time a sickness happens in a Woman's body, of an unusual manner, or more occult original, so that its causes lie hid, and the Curatory indication is altogether uncertain, presently we accuse the evill influence of the womb (which for the most part is innocent) and in every unusual Symptom, we declare it to be something hysterical, and so to this Scope, which oftentimes is only a subterfuge of ignorance and medical intentions, and use of Remedies are directed… .

He went on to further explain that: '… I have opened some women…very obnoxious to Hysterical passions, in whom the Womb being very well, I have found in the hinder parts of the head, the beginnings of the nerves moistened and wholly drowned with a sharp serum…'. Willis also reported hysterical symptoms in men.

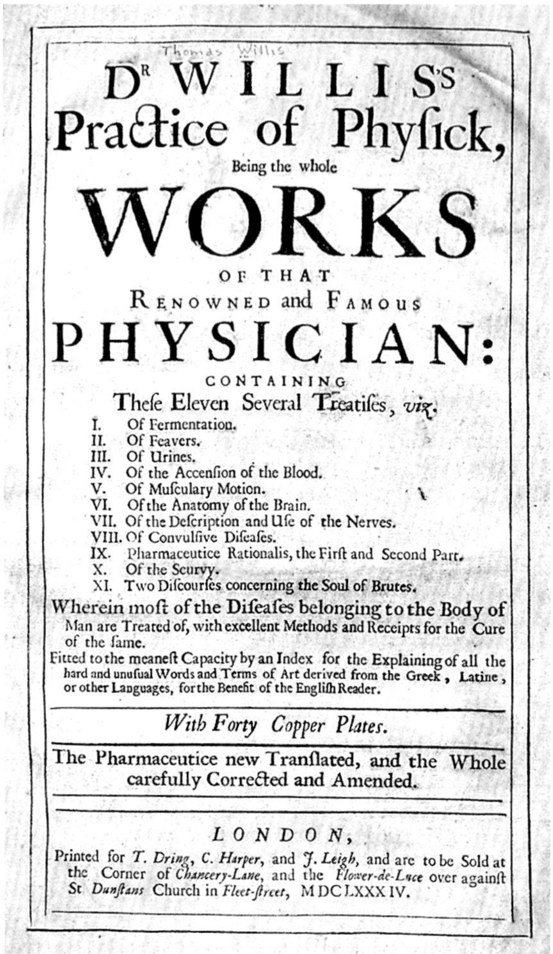

DR WILLIS'S Practice of Phyſick,
Being the whole
WORKS
OF THAT
Renowned and Famous
PHYSICIAN:
CONTAINING
Theſe Eleven Several Treatiſes, *viz.*

I. Of Fermentation.
II. Of Feavers.
III. Of Urines.
IV. Of the Accenſion of the Blood.
V. Of Muſculary Motion.
VI. Of the Anatomy of the Brain.
VII. Of the Deſcription and Uſe of the Nerves.
VIII. Of Convulſive Diſeaſes.
IX. Pharmaceutice Rationalis, the Firſt and Second Part.
X. Of the Scurvy.
XI. Two Diſcourſes concerning the Soul of Brutes.

Wherein moſt of the Diſeaſes belonging to the Body of Man are Treated of, with excellent Methods and Receipts for the Cure of the ſame.
Fitted to the meaneſt Capacity by an Index for the Explaining of all the hard and unuſual Words and Terms of Art derived from the Greek, Latine, or other Languages, for the Benefit of the Engliſh Reader.

With Forty Copper Plates.

The Pharmaceutice new Tranſlated, and the Whole carefully Corrected and Amended.

LONDON,
Printed for *T. Dring*, *C. Harper*, and *J. Leigh*, and are to be Sold at the Corner of *Chancery-Lane*, and the *Flower-de-Luce* over againſt St *Dunſtans* Church in *Fleet-ſtreet*, MDCLXXXIV.

Fig. 2. Willis T. Practice of Physick. 1684 [39].

For Sydenham, it was 'an affliction of the mind' with protean physical symptoms, yet a cause of great suffering. It manifested as hysteria in women and hypochondriasis in men. Anger, fear, love, or grief could induce symptoms, which included copious urine discharge after a 'fit', visceral, muscular, and articular pains, and clavus hystericus (the feeling of a nail driven through the skull). Sydenham expressed his ideas in his epistolary dissertation, dated January 20, 1682 written to Dr. William Cole, where he commented [16, 17]:

> Of all chronic diseases, hysteria – unless I err – is the commonest... . As to females, if we except those who lead a hard and hardy life, there is rarely one who is wholly free from them [hysterical complaints]... . Then, again, such males as lead a sedentary or studious life, and grow pale over their books and papers, are similarly afflicted... . The frequency of hysteria is no less remarkable than the multiformity of the shapes it puts on... .

Robert Whytt (1714–1766; fig. 3) thought that the disorder was caused by 'an uncommon delicacy or unnatural sensibility of the nerves... this sentient and sympathetic power of the nerves.' He too equated male hypochondria with female hysteria, but anticipated Slater [2], warning: 'symptoms commonly calculated hysteric, are less frequently owing to the unsound state of the womb than to faults somewhere else in the body' [18].

In 1733, George Cheyne (1671–1743; fig. 4) composed a famous work, *The English Malady* [19].

> The Title I have chosen for this Treatise, is a Reproach universally thrown on this Island by Foreigners, and all our Neighbours on the Continent, by whom Nervous Distempers, Spleen, Vapours, and Lowness of Spirits, are, in Derision, call'd the ENGLISH MALADY. [...] These nervous disorders... make almost one third of the complaints of the People of Condition in England.

Cheyne believed that the moist climate, rich food, and luxury of 18th-century Britain contributed to the malady which plagued many of the wealthy; women suffered from a type of melancholic hysteria. Fainting or swooning indicated the frailty of the nervous system and became a fashionable way for women to behave. But when symptoms were severe it was usually diagnosed as hysteria; in accord with Sydenham, hypochondria was preferred for men. William Cullen (1710–1790) proposed a variety of hysteria joined with nymphomania, which he termed 'hysteria libidinosa' [20].

For the psychiatric reformer, Philippe Pinel (1745–1826) wrote in his *Nosographie philos-*

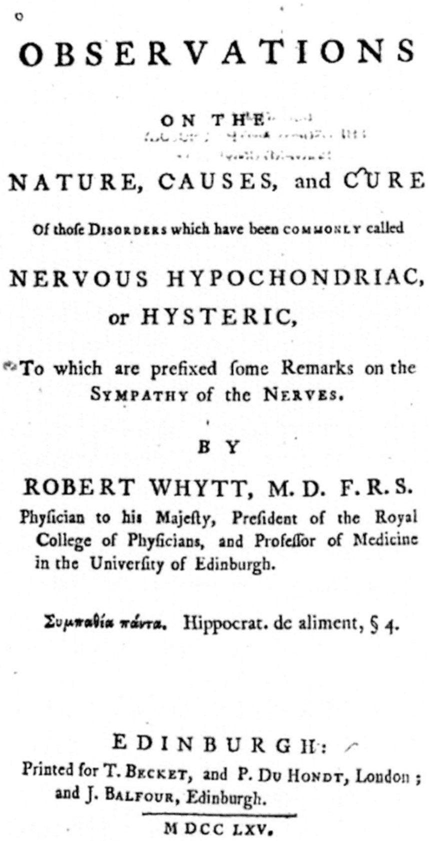

OBSERVATIONS

ON THE

NATURE, CAUSES, and CURE

Of thoſe DISORDERS which have been COMMONLY called

NERVOUS HYPOCHONDRIAC,

or HYSTERIC,

To which are prefixed ſome Remarks on the SYMPATHY of the NERVES.

B Y

ROBERT WHYTT, M. D. F. R. S.

Phyſician to his Majeſty, Preſident of the Royal College of Phyſicians, and Profeſſor of Medicine in the Univerſity of Edinburgh.

Συμπαθία πάντα. Hippocrat. de aliment, § 4.

EDINBURGH:

Printed for T. BECKET, and P. DU HONDT, London; and J. BALFOUR, Edinburgh.

M DCC LXV.

Fig. 3. Whytt R. Observations on the Nature, causes, and Cure of Those Disorders Commonly Called Nervous Hypochondriac, or Hysteric. 1765 [40].

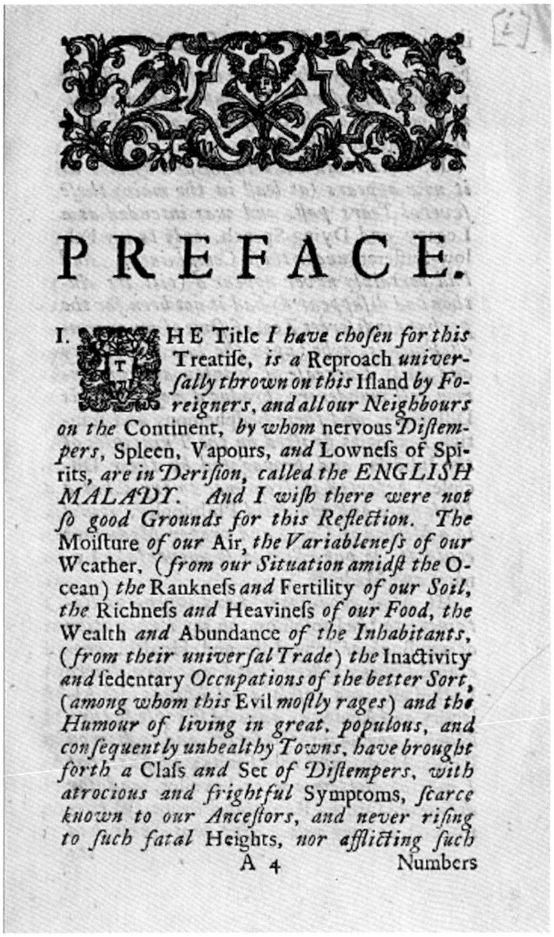

PREFACE.

I. THE Title *I have choſen for this* Treatiſe, *is a* Reproach *univerſally thrown on this* Iſland *by Foreigners, and all our Neighbours on the* Continent, *by whom* nervous *Diſtempers*, Spleen, Vapours, *and* Lowneſs of Spirits, *are in Deriſion, called the ENGLISH MALADY. And I wiſh there were not ſo good Grounds for this Reflection. The* Moiſture *of our* Air, *the Variableneſs of our* Weather, (*from our Situation amidſt the* Ocean) *the* Rankneſs *and* Fertility *of our Soil, the* Richneſs *and* Heavineſs *of our Food, the* Wealth *and* Abundance *of the Inhabitants,* (*from their univerſal Trade*) *the* Inactivity *and* ſedentary *Occupations of the better Sort,* (*among whom this* Evil *moſtly rages*) *and the Humour of living in great, populous, and conſequently unhealthy Towns, have brought forth a* Claſs *and* Set *of Diſtempers, with atrocious and frightful* Symptoms, *ſcarce known to our Anceſtors, and never riſing to ſuch fatal* Heights, *nor afflicting ſuch*

A 4 Numbers

Fig. 4. Cheyne G. The English Malady or a Treatise of Nervous Diseases. 1733 [41].

ophique [21] that hysteria was one of the 'genital neuroses of women'. He mentioned the difficulty in treating 'insanity from religious enthusiasm', and denounced demoniacal possession. Although ideas of the wandering womb had long been discredited, its remnants still appeared in some accounts.

'Fashions, after all, are only induced epidemics', said George Bernard Shaw – how well that applies to fashionable ideas about hysteria. Despite the 17th century 'neurological' theory, subsequent centuries brought a resurgence of hysterogenic etiology. Many examples are present in novels, most famously in Gustave Flaubert's bourgeois narcissist, Madame Bovary (1857), and her dreamy, illusory visions of happiness. Throughout history, hysteria appears as a puzzling 'entente' between passions of the mind and the constitution of the body [22].

Social factors and gender were also recognized. In the 18th century it was widely held that hysteria affected only the 'upper classes' of women. The 'lower class' and 'working women' were believed to be 'insufficiently impressionable and of too coarse a sensibility' to fall victim to the disorder. A hundred years later Charcot stressed it as a disorder of lower classes. The disease was most likely to affect young women, when she and her womb were most impressionable. There were many epidemics of hysteria that are well documented: the dancing mania of Strasbourg (1518), the legendary Camelford water pollution accident, the phantom anesthetist of Mattoon, the invasion from Mars, and the Royal Free epidemic of benign myalgic encephalomyelitis are well documented. In modern times, epidemic dizziness, fainting, vomiting, and screaming of school children have been recorded [23].

A landmark was the monograph in 1816, *Traite des maladies nerveuses ou vapeurs et particulièrement de l hystérie et de l'hypochondrie* by Louyer-Villermay (1776–1837), a French alienist. This reverted to a uterine cause which involved the nervous system. He stated that the nerves of the uterus spread through the body to cause all nervous and mental maladies in women [24]. The onset was between puberty and menopause. For Louyer-Villermay, hysteria was a 'uteromania'. He rejected male hysteria: 'Man cannot be hysterical, he has no uterus.' Dubois d'Amiens, Landouzy, and Moritz Romberg supported this view. Five years later the independent Étienne-Jean Georget (1795–1828) stridently denounced as 'absurd and ridiculous' uterine theories in his *De la physiologie du systeme nerveux et specialement du cerveau* (1821) which marked a return to a cerebral origin for hysteria.

The Victorians recognized psychological and social stress as well as inherent vulnerabilities; they identified both precipitating factors and constitutional predispositions. Excitement, overwork, or lascivious behavior might trigger attacks; susceptible individuals, i.e. those with hysterical constitutions, were manipulative and prone to volatile behavior, flirtatiousness, impulsiveness, emotional outbursts, and hypersexuality.

The prevailing alienist view was that organic lesions did not cause symptoms of madness; this opinion was countered in 1822 by Antoine Laurent Bayle (1799–1858) and Louis Florentin Calmeil (1798–1895). In 1840, Thomas Laycock (1812–1876), a physician in York and teacher of Hughlings Jackson and Jonathan Hutchinson, stressed the rarity in men, but again focused on the nervous system. Laycock worked with Daniel Hack Tuke, a psychiatrist at the York Retreat. A variety of pseudoepileptiform fits, and paroxysms could be manifest in either sex. In his chapter 'Hysteria is peculiar to females', Laycock noted:

> ...cases have occurred occasionally in the male sex, presenting the phenomena of convulsive hysteria; but so rarely, and under such circumstances, that even if their exact similarity to the hysterical paroxysm of the female be admitted, like other exceptions, they but serve to prove the rule, namely, that it is the nervous system of the woman which is implicated in these affections. [...] Indeed, the general fact is so universally acknowledged, and so constantly corroborated by daily observation, that anything in the shape of proof is unnecessary.

Laycock believed that the entire nervous system was the seat of reflex function in which the mind played no part. This revolutionary idea paved the way for the experiments of Sechenov, Pavlov, Ferrier, and Sherrington. Laycock published this notion in *Mind and Brain* in 1860. His role in this fundamental aspect of the study of the mind and brain has been understated [25]. In 1855, he became Professor of Medicine in Edinburgh, where he pointed the young David Ferrier towards Neurology.

Against these background controversies, Pierre Briquet's (1796–1881)[1] *Traité clinique et thérapeutique de l'hystérie* of 1859 (fig. 5), an epidemiological study of 430 patients with hysteria seen over a 10-year period, appeared. 'If one takes

[1] *Index Biographique de l'Academie de Médicine* and the *Biographische Lexikon* gave his first name as Paul. The *Dictionaire de Biographie Française* and his gravestone are marked Pierre.

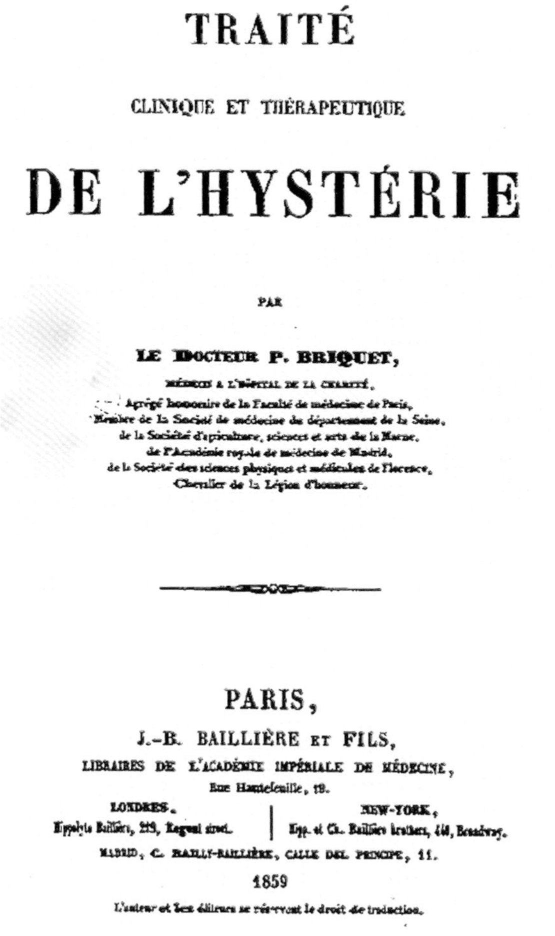
TRAITÉ

CLINIQUE ET THÉRAPEUTIQUE

DE L'HYSTÉRIE

PAR

LE DOCTEUR P. BRIQUET,

MÉDECIN À L'HÔPITAL DE LA CHARITÉ,
Agrégé honoraire de la Faculté de médecine de Paris,
Membre de la Société de médecine du département de la Seine,
de la Société d'agriculture, sciences et arts de la Marne,
de l'Académie royale de médecine de Madrid,
de la Société des sciences physiques et médicales de Florence,
Chevalier de la Légion d'honneur.

PARIS,
J.-B. BAILLIÈRE ET FILS,
LIBRAIRES DE L'ACADÉMIE IMPÉRIALE DE MÉDECINE,
Rue Hautefeuille, 19.

LONDRES. Hippolyte Baillière, 219, Regent street. | NEW-YORK, Hipp. et Ch. Baillière brothers, 440, Broadway.

MADRID, C. BAILLY-BAILLIÈRE, CALLE DEL PRINCIPE, 11.

1859

L'auteur et les éditeurs se réservent le droit de traduction.

Fig. 5. Briquet P. Traité clinique et thérapeutique de l'hystérie. 1859 [42].

any hysterical symptom, one will find always its model in an act that constitutes… painful sentiments, and emotions that are sad or violent' [26]. The predisposing factors included: female sex, affective and impressionable temperament, family history, low social class, and situational difficulties. He considered 'une névrose de l'encéphale' as the final common pathway that mediated these causative agents. Briquet tried to remedy adverse social circumstances and environmental problems [27, 28].

Briquet dismissed previous opinions (especially Louyer-Villermay's) centered on the uterus. Multiple, ill-defined physical symptoms in women with no organic basis were of a hysterical nature. 'Briquet's hysteria' is now equivalent to 'somatization disorder'.

His broadly neurological concept was crucial to Charcot's later experiments and demonstrations of 'hystérie simple', 'grande hystérie', 'hystéro-epilepsie', and 'hystéro-neurasthenie'. For Briquet, hysterical illness conformed to regular laws ascertained by clinical analysis, an inherited illness, predominantly of women but unrelated to the uterus. However, hysterogenic models of hysteria continued: Briquet, though acknowledged by Charcot as his predecessor in hysteria, had failed to sway contemporary views.

'Consistency is the last refuge of the unimaginative', said Oscar Wilde, a comment which pertains to opinions about hysteria. The next swing of opinion came in 1861 with the second edition of Wilhelm Griesinger's (1817–1868) influential textbook *Die Pathologie und Therapie der psychischen Krankheiten*, which incorporated ideas about hysteria. He believed that phenomena with no objective signs were presumed imaginary. Authentic hysteria involved 'morbid action of… the brain'. Generally linked to genital erotic sensations, female hysteria was either the product of genital disease or a work of art (implying artifice). But Griesinger related cases in both sexes to precipitating factors of local genitourinary diseases or to puberty, menstruation, pregnancy, or parturition.

At this time, there developed an ovarian theory that irregularities or congestion of the ovaries were caused hysterical symptoms, notably iliac fossa pain. Charcot repeatedly demonstrated hysterical signs resulting from ovarian compression, which he thought confirmed this theory. An irritation of the ovaries precipitated a pelvic neuralgia, which through nervous reflexes caused hysteria. He then explored 'hysterical' manifestations (motor, sensory, and visual), as well as seeking elements of hysteria in tics, migraines, epileptiform attacks, somnambulism, and mutism [29].

Charles Lasègue's paper *De la toux hysterique* (1854) reported the fluctuating, elusive, and conceptual chaos of hysteria. Briquet (1859) and Russell Reynolds (1869), Thomas Laycock, and Robert Bentley Todd in England were all acknowledged by Charcot as his predecessors who revived interest and triggered experiments in hysteria. Desiré Magloire Bourneville (1840–1909) also stimulated Charcot's work. The publication (under Bourneville's editorship) of the *Iconographie photographique de la Salpêtrière* (1876–1877) was a vital element in the Paris hysteria cult [30]. This mixed art and technology with clinical description, became widely advertised, and was a source of fascination for its lurid accounts of the hysterics' 'délire erotique' and its photographs of hypnotized females in varied stages of hystero-epilepsy, paralysis, contractures, somnambulism, and opisthotonus, as well as willing, flamboyant subjects of ovarian compression and hypnosis [31].

Opinions just before Charcot's investigations were crystallized in 1869 by John Russell Reynolds, a London neurologist at the British Medical Association meeting in Leeds [29]:

> The object of this paper is to show (1) That some of the most serious disorders of the nervous system, such as paralysis, spasm, pain, and otherwise altered sensations, may depend upon a morbid condition of emotion, of idea and emotion, or of idea alone; (2) That such symptoms often… appearing as complicated diseases of the brain or spinal cord; (3) That they resist many different kinds of treatment, … but that they disappear entirely upon the removal of the erroneous idea; (4) That they occur independently of a… insanity of mind, hysteria, hypochondriasis, or malingering; (5) That they are often … associated with some bodily weakness or general debility; (6) That they sometimes associate themselves with distinct and definite diseases of the nervous centres, so that it becomes very important to know how much of a given case is due to organic lesion, and how much to morbid ideation….

Charcot attended this meeting and frequently praised this paper as an important contribution to his work; thereafter, he received Reynolds as an honored visitor at Salpêtrière. Weir Mitchell (1829–1914) [32], recognized 'psychic' varieties of blindness, anesthesia for touch, anosmia, blindness, and 'true and false palsies'. Like Robert Carter [33] he also saw conscious deception, i.e. malingering as a possible mechanism. Charcot, however, generally resisted this inference, insisting there was a 'functional' or 'dynamic' mechanism, but on occasion Charcot appeared ambivalent, commenting '… about malingering. It is found in every phase of hysteria… the ruse, the sagacity and the unyielding tenacity… women display in order to deceive…' [34].

Conclusion

Because of the uncertain status of hysteria in the medical corpus, its many proponents predating Charcot undoubtedly influenced his investigations [35]. Was the brain, mind, or uterus the origin of the malady? Another outstanding issue was the nature of dissociation, conscious, or subconscious, i.e. the confusion between hysteria and malingering, which had not been systematically studied, and which remains an unresolved area of uncertainty. The physiological and particularly the psychological determinants of hysterical manifestations were largely obscure before Charcot's numerous detailed case histories in which hypnosis and suggestion played a large part. The possible coexistence of hysteria with organic disease [18], and the simulation of hysteria by physical disease [36] had been inadequately explored.

Charcot was the inspirational if highly controversial [29] leader whose vision was to encompass hysteria within the somatic framework of observable scientific medicine. He tried to reduce the widespread confusion surrounding hysteria by including it in an ordered categorization of brain disorders. His lucid, meticulous descriptions were principally organically orientated, serving as exemplary if theatrical clinical teachings. Yet precise definition eluded him (Bogousslavsky [this vol., pp. 44–55]).

The subject of hysteria has reflected attitudes about health, religion, class, and gender [8]. Investigations to unravel its knotted psychological and physiological complexities are likely to occupy doctors for years to come.

Two classic papers illuminate the unsolved dilemmas. Eliot Slater (1904–1983) [2] rejected it as an entity, concluding 'the diagnosis of "hysteria" is a disguise for ignorance and a fertile source of clinical error. It is in fact not only a delusion but also a snare.' Sir Francis Walshe's (1885–1973) elegant critique [37] of Slater's position stated: 'Nevertheless, Slater's nihilism in regard to hysteria is a challenge to neurologists once again to justify the concept of hysteria as a nosological entity in its own right… . Its essential difference from somatic disease is that it constitutes a behavior disorder, a human act, on the psychological level.'

References

1 Gowers W: A Manual of Diseases of the Nervous System, ed 1. London, Churchill, 1888, vol 2, p 935.
2 Slater E: Diagnosis of 'hysteria'. Br Med J 1965;1:1395–1399.
3 Johnson W: An Essay on the Diseases of Young Women. London, Simpkin & Marshall, 1849, p 5.
4 Marsden CD: Hysteria – a neurologist's view. Psychol Med 1986;16:277–288.
5 Bourneville D-M, Régnard P: Iconographie photographique de la Salpêtrière (3 vols). Paris, Bureaux du Progres Medical, Delahaye & Lecrosnier, 1876–1880.
6 King H: Once upon a text: hysteria from Hippocrates; in Gilman SL (ed): Hysteria Beyond Freud. Berkeley, University of California Press, 1993, pp 3–64.
7 Adams F (ed and transl): On the paroxysm of epileptics; in Aretaeus the Cappadocian: The Extant Works. Book I. London, Sydenham Society, 1856.
8 Veith I: Hysteria: The History of a Disease. Chicago, University of Chicago Press, 1965.
9 Micale MS: Hysteria and its historiography: a review of past and present writings. Hist Sci 1989;27:223–261, 317–351.
10 Wesley GR: A History of Hysteria. Washington, University Press of America, 1979.
11 Pearce JMS: Brain disease leading to mental illness: a concept initiated by the discovery of general paralysis of the insane. Eur Neurol 2012;67:272–278.
12 Jorden E: A briefe discourse of a disease called the suffocation of the mother, 1603; in Lord Brain: Doctors Past and Present. London, Pitman, 1964, pp 29 et seq.
13 Micale MS: Approaching Hysteria: Disease and Its Interpretations. Princeton, Princeton University Press, 1995.
14 Micale MS: Charcot and the idea of hysteria in the male: gender, mental science, and medical diagnosis in late nineteenth-century France. Med Hist 1990; 34:363–411.
15 Willis T: Practice of physic. Being the whole works of that renowned and famous physician (English transl by S. Pordage). London, 1684, p 69; cited in Spillane JD: Doctrine of the Nerves. Oxford, Oxford University Press, 1981, p 72.
16 Latham RG: The works of Thomas Sydenham, MD. London, Sydenham Society, 1850, vol 2, pp 85–99.
17 Dewhirst K: Dr. Thomas Sydenham (1624–1689): His Life and Original Writings. Berkeley, University of California Press, 1966.
18 Whytt R: Observations on the Nature, Causes, and Cure of Those Disorders Commonly Called Nervous Hypochondriac, or Hysteric. Edinburgh, Becket, 1765, pp 85–111. http://books.google.co.uk/books?id=0P8TAAAAYAAJ&q=nature#v=onepage&q=hysteric&f=false.
19 Cheyne G: The English Malady or a Treatise of Nervous Diseases of All Kinds as Spleen, Vapours, Lowness of Spirits, Hypochondriacal, and Hysterical Distempers, Etc. (London, G. Strahan and J. Leake, 1733); in Porter R (ed): London, Routledge, 1990.
20 Cullen William: Of hysteria or the hysteric disease; in First Lines of the Practice of Physic, new ed. Edinburgh, Elliot, 1788, vol 4, p 98.
21 Pinel Philippe: Nosographie philosophique, rev ed 3. Paris, Brasson, 1807, vol 2, pp 279–286.
22 Porter R: The Body and the mind, the doctor and the patient: negotiating hysteria; in Gilman SL: Hysteria Beyond Freud. Berkeley, University of California Press, 1993, pp 235–236.
23 Leading article. Epidemic hysteria. Br Med J 1979;2:408–409.
24 Louyer-Villermay J-B: Traité des maladies nerveuses ou vapeurs, et particulièrement de l'hystérie et de l'hypochondrie. Paris, Baillière, 1816, vol 1, pp 1–217.
25 Pearce JMS: Thomas Laycock (1812–1876). J Neurol Neurosurg Psychiatry 2002;73:303.
26 Micale MS: Hysterical Men: The Hidden History of Male Nervous Illness. Cambridge, Harvard University Press, 2008, pp 93–98.
27 Briquet P: Traite clinique et therapeutique de l'hystérie. Paris, Baillière, 1859, pp 11–12.

28 Mai FM, Merskey H: Briquet's treatise on hysteria. A synopsis and commentary. Arch Gen Psychiatry 1980;37: 1401–1405.
29 Russell Reynolds J: Paralysis and other disorders of motion and sensation dependent on idea. BMJ 1869;2:483–485.
30 Bourneville DM, Régnard P: Iconographie photographique de la Salpêtrière, Service de M. Charcot. Paris, Bureau du Progrès Médical, V. Adrien Delahay et Cie, 1877.
31 Hustvedt Asti: Medical Muses, Hysteria in 19th-century Paris. London, Bloomsbury, 2011.
32 Mitchell SW: Lectures on Diseases of the Nervous System: Especially in Women, ed 2. Philadelphia, Lea Brothers & Co., 1885.
33 Carter RB: On the Pathology and Treatment of Hysteria. London, Churchill, 1853.
34 Georges Guillain: J-M Charcot (1825–1893). Sa vie, son oeuvre. Paris, Masson et Cie, 1955, pp 138–139.
35 Rousseau GS: 'A strange pathology': hysteria in the early modern world, 1500–1800; in Gilman SL (ed): Hysteria Beyond Freud. Berkeley, University of California Press, 1993.
36 Buzzard T: On the Simulation of Hysteria by Organic Disease of the Nervous System. London, Churchill, 1891, pp 91–186.
37 Walshe F: Diagnosis of hysteria. Brit Med J 1965;2:1451–1454.
38 http://books.google.co.uk/books?id=6Z1PAQAAIAAJ&printsec=frontcover&source = gbs_ge_summary_r&cad = 0#v = onepage&q&f=false.
39 http://mulibraries.missouri.edu/specialcollections/exhibits/anatomy/images/willis.jpg.
40 http://www.heritagebookshop.com/photos/images/65812_2.jpg.
41 http://p2.la-img.com/199/9043/1780562_1_l.jpg.
42 https://archive.org/details/traitcliniquee00briq.

J.M.S. Pearce
304 Beverley Road
Anlaby, East Yorks, HU10 7BG (UK)
E-Mail jms.pearce@me.com

Bogousslavsky J (ed): Hysteria: The Rise of an Enigma. Front Neurol Neurosci. Basel, Karger, 2014, vol 35, pp 11–19
DOI: 10.1159/000359988

Socioeconomic Background of Hysteria's Metamorphosis from the 18th Century to World War I

Nicole Edelman[a] · Olivier Walusinski[b]

[a]Professor of Contemporary History, Université Paris Ouest, Nanterre, and [b]Family Physician, Private Practice, Brou, France

Abstract

The many changes in the etiopathogenic theories of hysteria, developed from the end of the 18th century to the end of World War I, can only be understood by studying the social, political, economic, and cultural transformations of the Western world during the same period. These transformations, presented below along with concurrent medical discoveries, make it possible to explain the ongoing metamorphosis of both hysteria and the image of the hysteric patient.

Despite incessant changes in its etiological interpretation, hysteria has for millennia maintained the same name, which derives from the Greek and refers to the uterus. The illness has been attributed to several causes: the uterus understood as a small living animal within women's bodies that moves around when unsatisfied, clogging or poisoning of the uterus by feminine seed, vapors from fermentation in the womb that rise to the brain, and satanic possession. And though hysteria has remained largely linked to the uterus, certain physicians, notably the English doctors Thomas Willis (1621–1675) and especially Thomas Sydenham (1624–1689) at the end of the 17th century, believed that men could suffer from hysteria as well. The metamorphosis of hysteria and the hysteric patient is historically bound to the social, political, economic, and cultural transformations of the Western world. This metamorphosis was particularly rapid from the end of the 18th century to the beginning of the 20th century [1–3].

A Paradoxical Continuity: From the End of the 18th Century to the Beginning of the 19th Century

The end of the 18th century brought two revolutions to the Western world: the revolution that gave rise to the USA and the French Revolution.

Although in different ways, both led to a redefinition of the individual's status. In France, during the first months of the Revolution, female revolutionaries thought they would gain the social and political status of their male counterparts. This turned out to be far from true. Women were barred from political bodies as well as clubs and armies (at least in the capacity of soldiers), and in 1804, wives were considered immune from liability, along with the insane and children, under the newly promulgated Napoleonic Civil Code, which would become a model for Western societies. However, these measures were not sufficient to form a coherent social category for women. To justify their exclusion and inferiorization, political leaders drew support from medical science, which was also undergoing a clinical revolution and appeared to offer a form of truth. This reliance on medicine gave women a single identity, based on specific, natural characteristics. Women were 'sex', and were totally dominated by it. They were intrinsically different than men, as their sole purpose was procreation. Their being was made to love, attend to, and serve their children, husbands, and parents. However, women were always vulnerable to disturbances of their sex, of the uterus, and thus to hysteria. The image of the hysteric nonetheless remained acceptable for a few decades in the early 19th century. The illness was still strongly characterized by vapors, as the physicians under the 'old regime' (i.e. the royalty) conceived of them. These vapors and the fainting spells they produced were considered part of a social code used by the aristocracy and the high bourgeoisie [4, 5]. The illness was thus linked to the delicate sensibility and natural weakness of women, and their role as mothers, since most French physicians viewed hysteria as a condition of the uterus pending pregnancy (a 'future mother's lack'), with a few exceptions such as Etienne-Jean Georget (1795–1828) or Charles Humbert Antoine Despine (1777–1852). In 1815, Jean Baptiste Louyer-Villermay (1775–1837) attributed hysteria to a sort of uterine clogging. In 1830, Frédéric Dubois d'Amiens (1799–1873; fig. 1) asserted that an overexcitation of the womb was involved. Consequently, the main treatment for hysteria was marriage, sexual relations, and pregnancy [6–8].

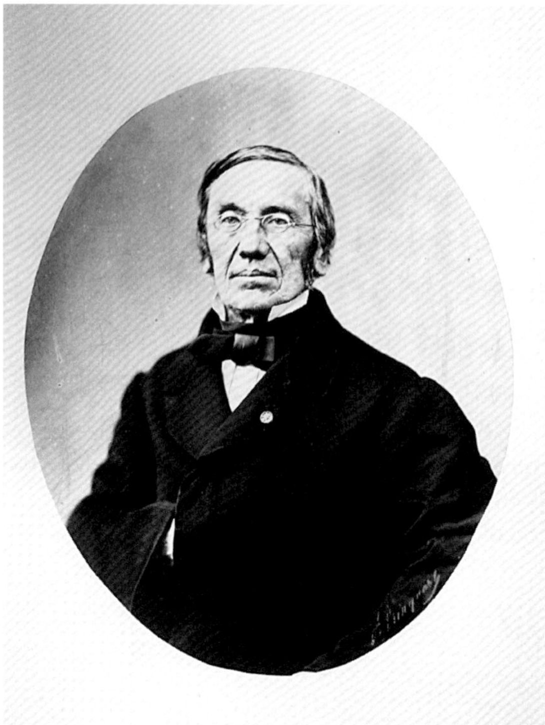

Fig. 1. Frédéric Dubois d'Amiens (1799–1873). Private collection of the author.

Basis for Change: The 1830s

European society underwent rapid transformation during the first decades of the 19th century: new economic activities emerged along with technological innovations (steam engines) that changed manufacturing structures (textile, metallurgy) and work organization, with important differences from country to country. France remained largely rural with production taking place in workshops, whereas Great Britain moved rapidly towards factories and urbanization. Many women worked, even in France. They were primarily involved in agriculture, i.e. wives of landowners, maids, and day laborers, but many worked at home for various industries. Others worked in workshops, or in small factories (tobacco, lace, weaving), as well as in mines. Those with hysteria no longer suffered from the aristocratic vapors, but rather from insanity or satanic possession. In the political arena, a liberal ideology was spreading across Europe, as evidenced by the revolutions of 1830. In France, the July Revolution put an end to the Restoration and brought Louis Philippe d'Orléans (1773–1850) to the throne. The main concern of governments everywhere was social order. To this end, those in power returned the family to its nodal position or strengthened it [9]:

> Body of fundamental regulation [...] as the atom of civil society, [the family] must manage 'private interests', which need to be in good order for the proper functioning of States. As the cornerstone of production, the family brings forth children and provides their initial education. The family is also responsible for the purity and health of the race. As the crucible of the national conscience, the family transmits symbolic values and fundamental memory. The 'good family' is the foundation of the State.

François Guizot (1787–1874), a professor of history and a politician, went further, remarking that marriage allows social order because the family lays the ground for each person to accept their subordination: mother to father, children to parents – to their father primarily, then to their mother. With the changes in society, the status of women was once again thrown into question. While the main model remained based on bourgeoisie practices, with women remaining at home, the number of female workers began to grow, and gradually other models took shape. For example, socialist theories offered new ideas on social organization and economy: the Saint-Simonians [inspired by the philosophy of the economist Claude-Henri de Rouvroy de Saint-Simon (1760–1825)] opened for women the possibility of emancipation, which some of them seized. Similarly, Charles Fourier (1772–1837), a French philosopher involved with 'critical-utopian socialism', believed that as a general hypothesis, social progress happened through the advancement of women towards liberty, whereas social decline resulted from a decrease in their freedoms. Hence, he saw the extension of privileges to women as a principle for all social progress. In addition to these political, economic, and social foundations, medical work on the nervous system and brain advanced during the early decades of the 19th century, and there was also the discovery of mammalian ovulation in 1827 – all of which had an impact on the evolving image of the hysteric. Hysteria involving vapors could no longer be part of a social code. In keeping with family decorum, the hysteric could not be perturbed by the sexual needs of her uterus, given that procreation was henceforth understood to be ensured by the involuntary and natural production of eggs. The illness therefore became associated with an etiology involving the nervous system, with either a genital or cerebral origin [3, 4, 9].

In 1830, the Royal Academy of Medical Sciences of Bordeaux (l'Académie royale de médecine de Bordeaux) as part of a competition to test doctors' knowledge on the comparative etiology of hysteria and hypochondria, awarded the gold medal to Dubois d'Amiens (fig. 1), who highlighted an excessive sensibility specific to women characterized by sacrifice and devotion. In 1845, the Royal Academy of Medical Sciences of Paris (Académie royale de médecine de Paris) added a question on hysteria to its competition. The first prize was shared by two physicians whose hypotheses were not identical, but both believed the nervous system played a role in causing hysteria. Jean-Louis Brachet (1789–1858; fig. 2) argued in favor of a neurocerebral etiology, while Hector Landouzy (1812–1864; fig. 3) argued in favor of neurouterine causes. The representation of the

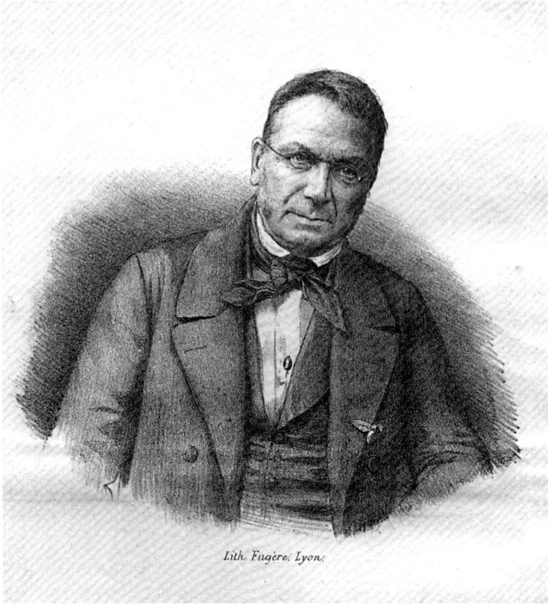

Fig. 2. Jean-Louis Brachet (1789–1858). Private collection of the author.

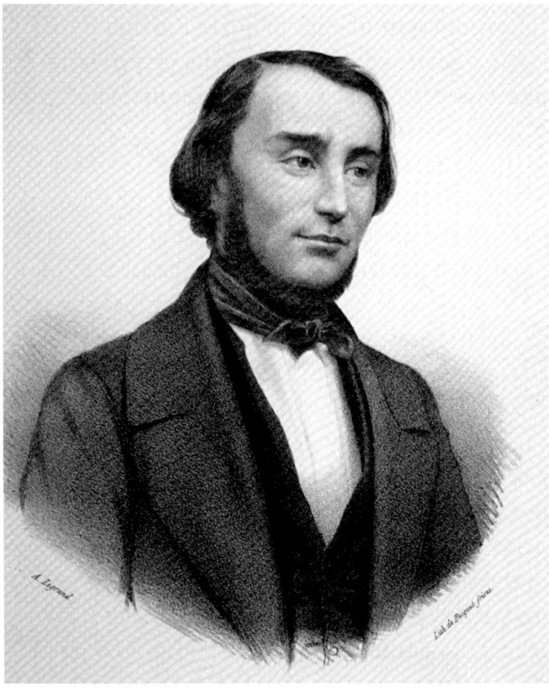

Fig. 3. Hector Landouzy (1812–1864). Private collection of the author.

hysteric by the medical community was extended to men; however, male hysterics were always 'inverts' (homosexuals) who had a feminine sensibility. The neurogenital interpretation continued to see the hysteric as immersed in genitality, in what might lead to a reproductive frenzy. The neurocerebral hypothesis did not involve this risk. This latter theory made rapid advances from the end of the 1830s to the beginning of the 1850s. The resulting turn towards the cerebral neurologization of hysteria, which was evident by the early 1850s, led to the conceptual breakthroughs in the second half of the century [10–14].

Upheaval: 1848–1850

A very serious economic crisis shook Europe at the end of the 1840s, influencing agriculture, industry, and finance. The railroad boom had inspired hope in a radiant future for big industry. These hopes went unrealized and European populations were severely affected. Revolution broke out in multiple locations, starting in 1848, but these uprisings would be short-lived. A conservative social order was rapidly restored throughout Europe, even in France, where the Second Empire replaced the Second Republic in 1851. Those in power once again promoted large families and their patriarchal form, as governed by the Civil Code. The family remained the basis for social and political order. Men in power affirmed that marital and paternal authority should not in any way be diminished, whereas the wife and mother, who was 'muse and Madonna', was praised to the skies. These proclamations were strengthened by the influence of Christianity (Catholicism more than Protestantism), which tightened its grip on girls and women with little education, leading to a proliferation of Marian apparitions. In Catholic countries, the figure of the Virgin triumphed when Pope Pius IX defined the dogma of the Immaculate Conception in 1854. The model for women was a sinless virgin and martyr. As a re-

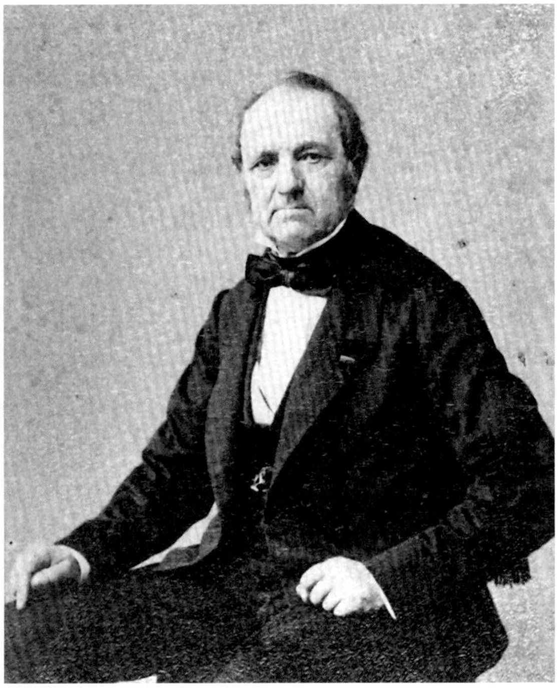

Fig. 4. Pierre Briquet (1796–1881). Private collection of the author.

sult, theorization on the natural place and role of women in society was strengthened in the 1850s. Because of the need to control hysterics, physicians found themselves with unprecedented power to assign men and women their place in society based on the characteristics of normality, which they became responsible for establishing [3, 4, 9].

With the recovery of the European economy, women were obligated to work in ever larger numbers. These proletarians found jobs in cities, either in households or workshops, as feather workers, embroideresses, seamstresses, linen maids, day laborers, cooks, florists, house servants, stitchers, hat makers, and corsetieres. They often worked more than 14 h a day for starvation wages (always half those earned by men). Many fell ill and went to hospitals, which in France were intended for the poor. This led Pierre Briquet (1796–1881; fig. 4), a physician at the Paris hospital La Charité, to call attention to hysteria in these women from the poor working classes. He believed that more than 1 in 3 city-dwelling women were hysterics, challenging the idea that most patients came from affluent classes that did not work. He focused on the sadness of his hysteric patients and framed the illness by their daily unhappiness and suffering. He painted a new picture of the hysteric, whose disease was sorrowful and related to her role as a mother; however, he continued to believe that all women are possible hysterics because of their particular sensibility. His *Traité clinique et thérapeutique de l'hystérie*, published in 1859, was an important step in the interpretation of hysteria, which became a 'neurosis of the brain' and nothing else. Briquet made the unprecedented statement that there was no link of any kind between a woman's reproductive system and hysteria. Men could thus be hysterics, but had to possess a feminine sensibility, which amounted to breaking 'the constitutive laws of society'. These conclusions would undergo a major shift with the work of Jean-Martin Charcot (1825–1893), who carried out neurological investigations from his appointment in 1860 at La Salpêtrière Hospital. He began integrating his work on hysteria in 1870 [14–17].

The Charcot Era (1870–1893): 'Hysteria Is One and Undivided'

The circumstances under which Charcot came to treat hysterics and the theories he went on to develop are detailed in this book and elsewhere (see Bogousslavsky [this vol., pp. 44–55] and Medeiros De Bustos et al. [this vol., pp. 28–43]) [17, 18]. It is surprising that Charcot did not listen to his patients or study their delirious states relative to their socially disadvantaged backgrounds (see Walusinski [this vol., pp. 65–77]). His apparent ambivalence regarding the socioeconomic context (divided as he was between his progressive Republican ideals and his ambitious desire to succeed in the eyes of high society) might explain his purely clinical symptomatology, free of any economic or emotional etiopathogenic aspects: 'By breaking down the hysterical crisis into four phases, he aligned the last phase, involving passionate attitudes, with the three others, thereby cutting it off from any expression of the passions; the reference to passion is only to allow clinicians to identify the final phase' [19].

Charcot described a single, fundamental type of hysteria, affecting both genders. The 'male hysteric' is a virile man rather than an invert, which in 1886 led Charcot to ask whether 'hysterical neurosis is really, as has been claimed until now, more frequent in women than in men' [20]. Paradoxically, Charcot highlighted sociological circumstances to explain masculine hysteria, an approach he did not take with women. This led him to examine the consequences of occupational accidents, especially railroad accidents, which were increasingly becoming frequent in the USA, Great Britain, and Germany, and later in France. Railroad workers sought out medical assessments to receive compensation (social legislation was more developed in Germany under Bismarck than it was in France). Charcot believed that the nervous shock of the accident caused the hysteria. Logically, male hysterics belonged mainly to the working and craftsmen classes, although there was a minority of cases in the bourgeoisie. At any rate, Charcot did not want to emphasize these male cases, however many there were [17, 19–21].

After 1890, his analysis evolved very quickly, causing him to further reduce the social scope of the danger posed by masculine hysteria. This entailed putting forward a new profile centered on a pathology of movement: that of the vagabond, the irrepressible traveler, the wanderer. The vagabond was a social figure specific to the end of the 19th century; in France, vagabonds were subject to a prison sentence of 3–6 months. Vagabonds were men having no trade, profession, fixed address, or means of subsistence. They were sometimes grouped together with those whom alienists called 'irrepressible travelers'. During these years, the number of such wanderers increased. Men and women were forced to leave rural areas by the major economic crisis that hit Europe in the 1870s. Wars and other political and sociological crises such as the pogroms in Russia and Poland made the situation worse. Wandering male Jews became stigmatized figures throughout Europe; Charcot viewed them as hysteric-neurasthenics [20–24].

The initial representation of the male hysteric, within the strict limits outlined above, was not only socially and politically acceptable, but also validated the widely accepted representations of men at the end of the 19th century. The shift from the male hysteric as a craftsman or railroad worker, towards the wanderer, whom most at the time viewed as a deviant, resulted in a counter-model of the normal, healthy man. At a time when the working classes had to remain in one spot to meet the demands of industrialization, the male hysteric who wandered from place to place was the antithesis of the reasonable and obedient family man. The creation of pathologies around certain workers, then around vagabonds, situated their problems outside politics and within a strategy of assistance (occupational accidents, retirement) developed in France by 'opportunistic' Republicans.

Regarding women, Charcot's social and cultural approach changed very little relative to that of his predecessors. All women were possible hysterics; they had to be monitored and protected both by their physicians and their husbands. Their natural fragility made the family the best place for them, as it protected them from the public world. They were to be educated carefully, but differently from boys. The aim was a healthy woman who would not only bear healthy babies, but who was also intelligent and capable of conversation with her husband and children, within the family, this role naturally complementing that of her spouse. The resulting harmony between the illness' interpretation and political power was nonetheless short-lived (and perhaps specifically French!) [23, 24].

Radical Changes at the End of the Century

When Charcot died in 1893, hysteria was rapidly reinterpreted and became a psychic illness. Joseph Babinski (1857–1932), Charcot's disciple for many years, reduced it to suggestion. Jules Déjerine (1849–1917) reduced it to emotion, while Hippolyte Bernheim (1840–1919) denied its existence. In contrast, Pierre Janet (1859–1947), Paul Sollier (1861–1933), and Sigmund Freud (1856–1939) gave hysteria a psychic dimension relating to the subconscious or unconscious, which was accessible by hypnosis. From that point forward, hysterics spoke not only with their bodies, though their bodies continued to manifest symptoms. While a physical signifier remained essential to hysteria, hysterics could express their suffering in words and be heard. Attacks of 'grande hystérie' disappeared once physicians began to listen to patients [21, 25, 26].

For this change to take place, not only did physicians have to begin listening to these women (and men), but the patients also had to break taboos and find the words to describe their disease. This shift was only made possible by a transformation of the entire society and its scientific, political, and cultural ways of thinking. In 1893, when Charcot died, Europe had not yet emerged from the long recession that had started in the 1870s. In addition to monetary problems, there was competition from 'new' countries, and each nation had their own difficulties as well. France experienced a long viticultural crisis after its vines were attacked by phylloxera. The country was also ravaged by the moral, territorial, and financial consequences of the Franco-Prussian War of 1870, which France lost to Germany. The major depression at the end of the century, however, did not prevent European states from building vast colonial empires and dominating what were considered 'inferior races'. Urbanization continued to expand in step with agricultural difficulties. Male and female salaried workers also continued their evolution with the appearance of new sectors of activity in banking, industry, and services. New types of transport and energy emerged, shortening travel time and improving domestic comfort. Political thought and protest took on new forms across Europe: socialism diversified, Marxism progressed, and anarchism took action. In France, the anarchist attacks in 1892–1893 fascinated and worried the population; political struggles along with strikes and protests gave rise to fear of large groups, which in turn led to an analogy with hysteria. The Dreyfus Affair, colonization, and new more violent forms of nationalism made people fear the 'other'. Understanding human beings with their strengths and weaknesses, as well as exploring the self, became a political and medical concern, which the study of hysteria made possible and encouraged [26, 27]. Moreover, in the span of a few decades, several essential scientific discoveries were made. For example, Darwin's theories affected all human sciences, particularly psychiatry and psychology [*The Descent of Man, and Selection in Relation to Sex* (1871) but also *On the Origin of Species* (1859)]. A number of studies explored the brain's neurological function, bringing new data to light [27]:

> The British scientists Laycock and Carpenter, [...] Griesinger in Germany, assert that like the spinal cord, the brain, classically considered as the seat of voluntary activity, may have a 'reflex' function. This new model allowed practitioners of nervous system medicine to promote a theory of automatic action by the brain, at work in magnetism, hysterical manifestations, somnambulism and dreaming.

Théodule Ribot (1839–1916), who founded pathological psychology in France, proposed in 1884 that the unconscious was based solely on physiology. Considering the dominant position of this learned man, the extension of the unconscious to the psyche would be all the more difficult. However, research into madness by those who had come to be called psychiatrists seemed to open new avenues for understanding the insane, with whom hysterics were sometimes grouped. In all psychotherapies, including Déjerine's methods and those of Janet and Sollier or those of Freud (which would become psychoanalysis), the physician encouraged the hysteric to relate his/her past, which was received as it was presented. However, the emergence of this new approach was difficult, and World War I proved to be a particularly challenging step. What was referred to as 'shell shock' broke out massively amongst the soldiers, regardless of nationality or social background. This mental disturbance was the most widespread injury during the war. Hysteria was very often diagnosed, even in cases of coma. The question of its interpretation and treatment was once again posed within the medical community, and the new approaches were sometimes cruel. To the amorality and laziness attributed to the male hysteric in the early 20th century, the war added effeminacy, cowardice, and unpatriotic sentiment. For treatment, most physicians applied methods of suggestion, considered effective at the time, but often coupled with other, more or less violent techniques, such as electroshock and hydrotherapy. The final goal remained returning the soldier as rapidly as possibly to his fighting unit [28, 29].

Conclusion

The horror of the large-scale killing during World War I transformed the Western world. The difficult work on hysteria continued afterwards, based on the emergence of new hermeneutics developed by psychology, psychiatry, and psychoanalysis, but also having ties to research and discoveries in neurology. Social and cultural standards and biases have continued to play a role in defining this illness, as shown in its exclusion from DSM-IV.

References

1 Veith I: Hysteria, the History of a Disease. Chicago, University of Chicago Press, 1965.
2 Micale MS: Approching Hysteria. Disease and Its Interpretations. Princeton, Princeton University Press, 1995.
3 Edelman N: Les métamorphoses de l'hystérique du début du XIXe siècle à la Grande Guerre. Paris, La Découverte, 2003.
4 Arnaud S: L'invention de l'hystérie au temps des lumières (1670–1820). Paris, Editions EHESS, 2014.
5 Georget EJ: De la physiologie du système nerveux et spécialement du cerveau. Paris, Baillière, 1821.
6 Despine CHA: De l'emploi du magnétisme animal et des eaux minérales dans le traitement des maladies nerveuses, suivi d'une observation très curieuse de guérison de névropathie. Paris, Germer-Baillière, 1840.
7 Louyer-Villermay JB: Traité des vapeurs, ou maladies nerveuses et particulièrement de l'hystérie et de l'hypocondrie. Paris, Germer-Baillière, 1832.
8 Dubois F: Histoire philosophique de l'hypochondrie et de l'hystérie. Paris, Baillière, 1837.
9 Perrot M: Les femmes ou le silence de l'histoire. Paris, Flammarion, 1998.
10 McHenry LC: Garrison's History of Neurology. Springfield, Thomas, 1969.
11 Negrier C: Pour servir à l'histoire des ovaires et des affections hystériques de la femme. Angers, Imprimerie de Cosnier et Lachèse, 1858.
12 Brachet JL: Traité de l'hystérie. Paris, Baillière, Germer-Baillière & Lyon, C. Savy jeune, 1847.
13 Landouzy H: Traité complet de l'hystérie. Paris, Baillière, 1846.
14 Bruttin JM: Différentes théories sur l'hystérie dans la première moitié du XIXe siècle. Zürich, Juris Druck & Verlag, 1969.
15 Briquet P: Traité clinique et thérapeutique de l'hystérie. Paris, Baillière et fils, 1859.
16 Charcot JM: Œuvres complètes. Paris, Bureaux du Progrès Médical, 1886–1894, vol 3.
17 Evans MN: Fits and Starts: A Genealogy of Hysteria in Modern France. Ithaca, Cornell University Press, 1991.
18 Goetz CG, Bonduelle M, Gelfand T: Charcot: Constructing Neurology. New York, Oxford University Press, 1995.
19 Trillat E: L'hystérie. Jean Martin Charcot, textes choisis et introduction. Paris, L'Harmattan, 1998.
20 Charcot JM: Leçons du mardi, 1888–1889. Paris, Progrès médical & Lecrosnier, 1889.

21 Cesbron H: Histoire critique de l'hystérie. Thèse No. 133. Paris, Asselin & Houzeau, 1909.
22 Meige H: Le Juif errant à la Salpêtrière: Etude sur certains névropathes voyageurs. Thèse de Médecine No. 315. Paris, L. Bataille, 1893.
23 Beaune JC: Le vagabond et la machine: essai sur l'automatisme ambulatoire, médecine, technique et société en France 1880–1910. Seyssel, Champ Vallon, 1983.
24 Knecht E: Le Mythe du Juif errant: essai de mythologie littéraire et de sociologie religieuse (Thèse de Lettres, Basel, 1973). Grenoble, Presses universitaires de Grenoble, 1977.
25 Bogousslavsky J: Hysteria after Charcot: back to the future. Front Neurol Neurosci 2011;29:137–161.
26 Carroy J: Hypnose, suggestion et psychologie, l'invention de sujets. Paris, Presses Universitaires de France, 1991.
27 Plas R: Naissance d'une science humaine, la psychologie. Rennes, Presses Universitaires de Rennes, 2000.
28 Audouin-Rouzeau S: 14–18, aujourd'hui No. 3, 'Choc traumatique et histoire culturelle. Paris, Noesis, 2000.
29 Bogousslavsky J, Tatu L: French neuropsychiatry in the Great War: between moral support and electricity. J Hist Neurosci 2013;22:144–154.

Dr. Olivier Walusinski
20 rue de Chartres
FR–28160 Brou (France)
E-Mail walusinski@baillement.com

Bogousslavsky J (ed): Hysteria: The Rise of an Enigma. Front Neurol Neurosci. Basel, Karger, 2014, vol 35, pp 20–27
DOI: 10.1159/000359990

'Fin-de-Siècle' Epidemiology of Hysteria

Jean-Pierre Luauté

Neuropsychiatrist, Romans, France

Abstract

An 'explanatory epidemiology' of disorders labelled 'hysteria' towards the end of the 19th century provides precious information – through the numerous statistical works of the period – about the conceptions of practitioners and the various cultural factors which made this era, in France, 'the golden age' of hysteria. The heyday of hysteria at the end of the century appears to be closely linked to the prestige of Charcot and the promotion of his ideas through the circle of his pupils. The disappearance after his death of hysteria, as he had described it in a defined and systematical manner, is a strong argument for considering it to be a transient mental illness, according to the definition of this concept by Ian Hacking. The regular appearance since then of new nonorganic diseases, avatars of hysteria, with a strong potential for contagiousness and whose causality is exterior to the person, as well as the persistence of the older, more characteristic forms, is evocative of the existence of an ancestral reactional mode taking on various clinical forms according to time and place.

The most famous candidate for a transient mental illness is hysteria, or at any rate its florid French manifestations toward the end of the nineteenth century.
Ian Hacking, 1998

When introducing the concept of a transient mental illness (TMI), Ian Hacking [1] could not avoid mentioning hysteria. Nevertheless, his inclusion of it appears limited and cautious as though hesitant in claiming that the disorder belonged to the cultural domain – as the concept of TMI directly infers – rather than a fact of nature, as claimed by Jean-Martin Charcot (1825–1893).

The epidemiology of hysteria in late 19th-century France seems so characteristic that it could serve as an example of links between the appearance of a mental illness (hysteria 'à la Charcot'), its creator's life, and his influence on the zeitgeist. We will return to this story in discussing how 'patients appear when their category becomes defined' [2].

After defining the scope and limits of a retrospective epidemiology – with statistics from the period – the evolution of hysteria will be traced prior to Charcot, during his lifetime, and following his death in 1893. We will consider the emergence of certain phenomena or conditions related to the issue of hysteria in Charcot's time, then later on, during the TMI 'epidemics' appearing at the end of the 20th century.

Epidemiological Approach to Hysteria

According to its classical definition, epidemiology is 'the study of the distribution of diseases or disorders within human groups and of the various factors broadly related to this distribution'. For Lellouch [3], this relates poorly to psychiatry since knowledge of the mental health of a population, i.e. descriptive epidemiology, requires 'precise values of the prevalence or incidence of mental disorders within that population' and the essential problem is 'defining psychiatric disorders and ways of diagnosing them'. Nonetheless, within the framework of an 'explanatory epidemiology', he recommends finding extremely diverse factors associated with the appearance or evolution of the illness or disorder. This type of epidemiological study seems feasible, even retrospectively, in the case of hysteria in the late 19th century, given that it consists of studying the disorder as it was perceived at the time.

Epidemiology of Hysteria before Charcot

We have at our disposition – just before Charcot's time – a study which has been qualified as epidemiological [4]: the *Traité clinique et thérapeutique de l'hystérie* [5] published in 1859 by Pierre Briquet (1796–1881). However, in spite of the size of this work (430 observations collected over 10 years at La Charité), we learn very little in the way of real epidemiology of the illness from the mass of figures. It only serves to reveal the author's opinions.

Briquet visited all the women hospitalized in the various medical and surgical wards to monitor the frequency of the condition among women and concluded that a quarter of them were affected, and when including those who were considered highly impressionable (for him, a 'moral disposition peculiar to women') the figure grew to half of all female patients.

The principal interest of the work is its second part. Here he deals with symptomatology and one finds all the disorders qualified as hysteria by an eminent clinician of the period. Spectacular convulsive attacks did not subsume the condition since he noted that, of 421 patients, 116 had never been affected. For Briquet, the first manifestation was pain and one notes the frequency of myalgias (called '*myosalgies*') since out of these 430 patients he only found 20 who were not affected. These myalgias were spontaneous, but could be provoked by moderately pressing on the affected muscle.

What is noteworthy in this snapshot of hysteria in mid-19th-century Paris is that the author includes a group of functional somatic disorders under this diagnosis. This explains why DSM-III named a category of so-called somatoform disorders 'Briquet's syndrome', following the suppression of the term 'hysteria'.

Briquet indicated that the attacks should happen in a particular order – which remained to be discovered. Garrabé [6], in his analysis of the work, supposes that Charcot, who knew and admired the treatise (having himself commentated it), must have taken heed of this remark.

Hysteria 'à la Charcot'

Charcot, like Briquet, was an internist and it is only from 1867 onwards that most of his publications were dedicated to the nervous system [7].

His 1865 publication [8] is remarkable in being not only his first publication of a case of hysteria, but also the one which allowed him to discover the lateral spinal cord lesions in lateral amyotrophic sclerosis. This observation, though probably having nothing to do with hysteria, must have given him insight into the possibility of discovering an organic cause for the illness.

Even so, he needed to dispose of easily recognizable forms to bring the condition out from the shadow or 'chaos', as he put it. Hence, the importance of finding archetypes and his canonical description of hystero-epilepsy when he began devoting his works to the 'grande névrose'. His interest was growing and Swain [9] noted the steady increase in his lessons on the subject from 1870 to 1892.

A Defined Illness

The prototypical form is well-known even though not the most frequently occurring (see Medeiros De Bustos et al. [this vol., pp. 28–43]). Charcot accepted minor (or common) forms and even mixed forms combining hysteria and neurasthenia – an illness to which we will return. However, with his positivist and systematic approach, he required objective proof that the attacks belonged to the field of neurosis, and these were to become his stigmata. Among these he accorded much importance to the search for zones of anesthesia, an idea figuring in the thesis of Alfred-Géraud Alby (1854), which had a great influence on him.

Patients Appear

Though fin-de-siècle Paris is known for hysteria's 'heyday', it must be said that there are no figures showing that hysteria abounded during this period, and in 1883, when Henri Legrand du Saulle (1830–1886) claimed that there were 'in Paris around fifty thousand hysterics, of whom ten thousand experience attacks', he did not mention how he obtained these figures [10]. What little objective information we have is indirect.

Consultation or Hospitalization Rates: Ratio Men/Women

The few figures of the period were all obtained by Charcot's pupils, sometimes at his request, as in the statistics of Pierre Marie (1853–1940) obtained in May 1889 [11] by consulting the Central Admissions Office.

Bonduelle et al. [12] described how this worked. It was a triage center where young hospital doctors had to examine hundreds of patients in order to direct them to one of the Paris hospitals. Marie thus explains that since he was 'obliged to conduct rather rapid examinations', he chose anesthesia as a criterion: 'an easy phenomenon to look for' and 'presenting in all patients with symptoms of hysteria' (he does not cite these), and in those where hysteria was 'clearly obvious but not currently associated with cutaneous sensitivity disorders'. In all, he discovered 28 cases of hysteria in 525 men, and 6 cases in 172 women, or 5.4% in men against 3.5% in women. Marie admitted to being perplexed by this result. However, it did not persuade him to 'support that proposition too close to paradox, that hysteria be far more frequent in men than in women' and he explained the paradox in terms of the central bureau's particular recruitment: men of the lowest classes of society, i.e. those that he called 'irregulars' (see Edelman and Walusinski [this vol., pp 11–19]).

During the same period, Achille Souques (1860–1944) [13], an intern at Broussais Hospital under Chauffard, while gathering all the cases of hysteria observed in his department, noted a 'striking analogy' with the statistics of Pierre Marie since he obtained a percentage of 5.9% for men against 2.5% for women. Here too, the author is aware of biased recruitment: 'men who make up the hospital clientele are much more frequently exposed than women to those triggers of hysteria: traumatisms and intoxications'.

Admission statistics in Charcot's clinical department were provided by Georges Gilles de la

Tourette (1857–1904). From 1880 to 1889, he accounted [14] for 360 cases of hysteria in 1,232 women and 77 out of 872 men. Then, over 2 years, he noted the number of cases in the rooms he was supervising: he found 67 cases from 200 women and 37 cases from 123 men. He concluded that there was a ratio of one man for every two women affected. Finally, he provided figures for the recruitment of the 'policlinique', completed by Georges Guinon (1859–1932). For 9 months in 1891, out of 1,913 primary consultations, Guinon collected 806 for 'neuroses' including 177 for epilepsy, 214 for neurasthenia, and 244 for hysteria, which – extrapolated over 12 months – gives a 'round figure' of 325 new cases examined per year; however, he did not count the associated forms. These high figures confirmed their numerous cases of hysteria which, he says, are considered elsewhere as 'fables' [15].

Of course, these figures teach us nothing of the distribution of the illness in the population and they may simply interpret the interest given to the diagnosis – at that time and in these places – as well as to the new question of male hysteria, the frequency of which was given each time as a distinct statistic. The validity of diagnosis is not touched upon, so Pierre Marie does not discuss the value of his chosen criterion (in fact a sign), i.e. the presence of anesthesia (which can be very subjective), and he says nothing of his examination technique.

One could conclude, with Micale [4], that 'Past epidemiological data is notoriously unreliable [...] any number of factors may create the retrospective illusion of an epidemiological rise or decline.' This criticism, which is clearly addressed to Shorter [16], is perfectly justified from a logical point of view. It comforts Lellouch's [3] claim as to the difficulty (impossibility?) of establishing a descriptive epidemiology of mental illnesses. Nonetheless, large numbers of patients labelled as hysterics appeared during this period – notably men – and the number of these patients decreased rapidly thereafter.

Epidemiology of Hysteria after Charcot

The end of hysteria 'à la Charcot' is well known: the laws and psychophysiological interpretations were abandoned and replaced by purely psychological conceptions. Another indirect argument, which confirms the boom of the diagnosis, then its disappearance, is its use in registers where medical certificates were recorded upon committing mental patients without their consent. Effectively, if hysteria did not traditionally belong to the field of mental illness, the influence of Charcot and his school led alienists to accept the existence of hysterical madness and to adopt this diagnosis. Examination of the registers of the asylum section of La Salpêtrière [17] over 20 years – between 1870 and 1890 – thus reveals that nearly a third of the women committed without their consent were diagnosed as hysterical. The diagnosis disappeared gradually after 1900.

Other Patients Appear

At the same time as hysteria, or after its decline, other phenomena or conditions (and other patients) made their entrance on the clinical scene and eventually took front stage. Some of them undeniably belonged to the spectrum of hysteria, as was the case for ecmnesia, multiple personalities, and mad travelers, as well as – the most important – neurasthenia.

- It was Pitres, in his 52nd lesson [18], who described the first case of ecmnesia in Albertine: an 'interesting' hysterical woman. The phenomenon consisted of 'a partial retrograde amnesia in which the memory of events before a certain period of life is wholly conserved whilst the memory of events after this period is totally abolished'. Luauté [19] provides a good introduction to the current situation of ecmnesia.
- Multiple personality disorder dates back not from the end of the 19th century, but from

the end of the 20th century. Ellenberger [20], who had introduced a pertinent classification of its various forms, claimed that hysteria in Charcot's time had become the 'great synthesis' of magnetic illnesses (lethargy, catalepsy, ecstasy) and dual personality, and later with multiple personality.

- The history of 'mad travelers' is recounted by Philippe-Auguste Tissié (1852–1935) in his thesis and it constitutes Pitres' 56th lesson [18]. It has been retold by Hacking [1]. The 'cas princeps', 26-year-old Albert, was affected with 'ambulatory automatism'. From the age of 12 he ran away time and again, traversing the whole of Europe. He hardly had any memory of the places he had been, but under hypnosis was able to remember days, even years, that had been totally forgotten [1]. For Pitres, Albert – bearing 'sensitive-sensorial stigmata' – was hysterical. This hypothesis was contested by the Salpêtrière school, which considering other cases, raised that of epilepsy. Hacking considered that the description of the first cases had given rise to a small epidemic of compulsive mad travelers which spread throughout Europe for 22 years, though never reaching the USA.
- Neurasthenia, however, is the first mental illness to have been imported to Europe from the USA, and it also heralds a predominant, if not exclusive, sociogenesis: 'nervous' exhaustion due to the modern lifestyle. Following its description by George Miller Beard (1839–1883) in 1869 and a publication in 1880 in the USA, its success was overwhelming and the illness took on epidemic proportions in Europe. Charcot, at first reticent, eventually took it onboard [21]. We have seen in Guinon's statistics [15] that the rate of Tuesday consultations almost equaled that of hysteria. By the end of the century, it had dethroned hysteria as the 'illness of the century'.

'Explanatory Epidemiology'

The notion of a 'heyday' of hysteria at the end of the 19th century, rather than a veritable 'epidemic' of cases, corresponds more to the numerous literary and artistic influences contributing to the spread of a culture of the illness during this period in Paris. For our part, we are interested in what contributed to the medical knowledge of hysteria and how future patients were 'instructed'.

One can measure Charcot's academic influence and that of his school by the number of theses written on hysteria in France during his time. Swain [9], using Terrisse's statistics, notes that these multiplied from just 20 theses from 1800 to 1870, to 49 between 1871 and 1880, 65 from 1881 to 1890, and 111 from 1891 to 1900, before falling to 85 from 1901 to 1910 and then to less than 10 per year after World War I. Associated with an increased incidence of hysteria diagnoses in committed patients, these figures enable her to speak of 'a veritable climacteric moment of hysteria in France at the close of the century'.

It was Charcot's pupils who 'created an appropriate visual idea of the hysteric' [4], making its manifestations known through drawings [22] and photography [23]. Several treatises were published [14, 18, 22] with, first and foremost, the *Complete Works* gathering into volumes the lessons of Salpêtrière and the faculty. The pupils were responsible for transcribing the lessons and they began with a rapid publication in the press media created by Désiré-Magloire Bourneville (1840–1909): *Le Progrès médical, les Archives de neurologie.* The importance of this work of communication and diffusion of Charcot's ideas in the medical and scientific world must be emphasized. For Gelfand and colleagues [12], Bourneville's '*Iconographie Photographique* had on its agenda publicizing hysteria beyond a strictly medical context'.

Swain [9] claimed that it was the disciples who had systematized Charcot's thinking, while he himself remained 'as elusive as the hysterical Proteus that he sought to reduce'. His communication to the Academy of Sciences in 1882 [24], in which he presented his famous description of hystero-epilepsy, shows that it was indeed he who was calling the tune.

In fact, there existed between the master and his disciples a tacit sharing of roles which can only be understood in terms of the period and of Charcot's overwhelming personality [12]. Thereby, the relation of respect and usual hierarchical subordination was transformed into obedient and somewhat blind veneration.

Patients also found themselves at this time in a situation of dependence on doctors, which can be understood not only in terms of anxiety about their illness, but also of the prestige which these men of science enjoyed. The latter, full of the importance of their role, entrenched within their position as men of knowledge, were ready to swallow all the rantings and ravings of their patients, unaware that for the most part they themselves, through their expectations and suggestions, were the cause of them. Hacking [1] underlines the process that he calls 'accommodation', where a hypnotic relationship develops between clinician and patient, for example between Tissié and Albert in which 'the two (were) extremely accommodating of each other's needs and expectations'. Modern works have highlighted the active – even generative – role of the patient in the framework of an interactionist model of the doctor/patient relationship.

Hysteria 'à la Charcot' was, to all intents and purposes, just a fragile construction that became fissured, and then collapsed, after his death. The final blows were dealt, as we know, by Joseph Babinski (1857–1932) and Jules Dejerine (1849–1917). The image of hysteria was notably degraded after the pejorative descriptions of this 'mental state' by the alienists [17] and, later, by the psychiatrists' attempts to make an illness out of it, to be treated in their care [25].

On the other hand, neurasthenia remained (at the beginning) a somatic illness and its cause was, furthermore, blamed on society. Therein we can understand its success. This – sometimes massive – spread of certain nonorganic diseases in the population was rediscovered when TMIs appeared in the late 20th century. Some of them can be considered to be the current avatars of hysteria. In characteristic manner, they too are conditions whose causes are external to the subject.

Transient Mental Illnesses

Multiple personality disorder (now called dissociative identity disorders) has generally been attributed to sexual abuse suffered in childhood [26]. In the case of Gulf War syndrome, it was sufficient to have been exposed and to present compatible symptoms to benefit from the diagnosis and its related advantages.

Finally, though the search for an actual medical cause of chronic fatigue syndrome and fibromyalgia has been fruitless, those affected refuse to consider themselves as mental patients, as do the doctors who defend them. All of these conditions also have a strong 'epidemic' power in common. Multiple personality disorder is the most demonstrative; it affected 5% of the US population at the height of the epidemic, only to disappear almost entirely. The 'epidemic' lasted about 20 years and never affected France.

In introducing his concept of TMIs with the historical example of the mad travelers, Hacking [1] stated that in order to flourish, the illness required an 'ecological niche'. He listed the four principal vectors: a medical taxonomy providing choice of two diagnoses, rendering the condition interesting for doctors (as previously mentioned between hysteria and epilepsy); a cultural polarity between two social phenomena (valued romantic tourism and reprimanded criminal vagabondage); a surveillance system (compulsory travel documents, police checks), and a need for evasion. These vectors – unequally present depending on the country – explain for Hacking the propagation of the diagnosis of mad traveler in Europe but not in the USA.

We would add the need for an effective communication system to spread knowledge of these diagnoses to doctors and the public. For a long time, doctors acquired knowledge of new diseases through teaching, books, and specialized press articles. The times, however, have changed; now the media targets the public directly. The epidemic of multiple personality disorder has been attributed to the success of two 'popular' books: *The Three Faces of Eve* and *Sybil* [19, 26]. All the aforementioned TMIs have been popularized by magazine articles detailing the symptoms, often with checklists allowing self-diagnosis.

Some of these TMIs – the current avatars of hysteria – were already known in Charcot's day: Multiple Personality Disorder, neurasthenia – the ancestor of chronic fatigue syndrome [21] – and even fibromyalgia, whose symptoms were broadly described 'before his time' by Briquet. In all cases, medical diagnosis appears in response to a state of suffering, often perceived physically.

Was Hysteria a Transient Mental Illness?

Having wisely asked the question in his introduction whether hysteria belonged to the TMI framework, Hacking [1] answers later in the affirmative and identifies the four vectors: 'the notion of an ecological niche fits that protean disease surprisingly well'. However, he specifies that 'the ecological niche metaphor serves as a scheme' and refuses to adhere to theses which consider these illnesses to be socially constructed [2].

In all, this review of the epidemiology of hysteria in late 19th-century France has confirmed that this illness – hysteria 'à la Charcot' – which disappeared with its creator and with the cultural vectors that were the pillars of its conceptualization, corresponds effectively to a TMI. However, the true nature of hysteria remains an enigma and we cannot eliminate a fact of nature, a universal and transcultural illness, which could acquire different clinical aspects, depending on time and place. Attentive examination allowed the constants to be identified, as if patients were drawing from a pool of symptoms, as Shorter [25] puts it so well.

The official suppression of hysteria in the international nomenclatures was allegedly preceded by the disappearance of hysteria from the clinical scene, especially in its spectacular forms. Two well-known historians of hysteria, Veith [27] and Trillat [28] concluded their respective works with this claim. Nonetheless, hysteria has not disappeared: conversion phenomena are still observed, and sometimes even the more spectacular forms. The journalist Anna Politkovskaïa has reported the typical 'arching back' attitude of a young girl during an unrecognized hysteria epidemic in Chechnya [29].

But it is above all in neurology and rehabilitation departments [30] that these conversion phenomena are observed, and they are sometimes identical to those of Charcot's day, though without his systematization. These departments have reinitiated neurophysiological studies using advanced methods of functional exploration of the nervous system (brain imaging, electrophysiology, etc.). They have already enabled progress to be made in understanding hysterical conversion: the famous 'leap into the somatic'.

References

1 Hacking I: Mad Travelers. Reflections on the Reality of Transient Mental Illnesses. Cambridge, Harvard University Press, 1998.

2 Hacking I: La fabrication des maladies. La Recherche 2004;16(hors série):46–48.

3 Lellouch J: La représentativité en épidémiologie psychiatrique. Pour quoi?; in Lépine J-P (ed): Epidémiologie psychiatrique. Paris, Jean-Pierre Goureau, 1995, pp 49–57.

4 Micale MS: Approaching Hysteria. Disease and Its Interpretations. Princeton, Princeton University Press, 1995.

5 Briquet P: Traité clinique et thérapeutique de l'hystérie. Paris, JB Baillière, 1859.

6 Garrabé J: Le syndrome de Briquet. Perspectives Psy 2009;48:128–138.
7 Gasser J: Le rôle de Charcot dans la construction de la neurologie moderne; in Gauchet M, Swain G (eds): Le vrai Charcot. Les chemins imprévus de l'inconscient. Paris, Calmann-Lévy, 1997, pp 211–238.
8 Charcot J-M: Sclérose des cordons latéraux de la moelle épinière chez une femme hystérique atteinte de contracture permanente des quatre membres. L'Union Médicale 1865, pp 451–457, 467–472.
9 Swain G: L'appropriation neurologique de l'hystérie; in Gauchet M, Swain G (eds): Le vrai Charcot. Les chemins imprévus de l'inconscient. Paris, Calmann-Lévy, 1997, pp 15–95.
10 Legrand du Saulle H: Les Hystériques. Etat physique et état mental. Actes insolites, délictueux et criminels. Paris, JB Baillière, 1883.
11 Marie P: L'hystérie à la consultation du bureau central des hôpitaux de Paris, étude statistique. Le Progrès médical 27 July 1889, p 70.
12 Bonduelle M, Gelfand T, Goetz CG: Charcot un grand médecin dans son siècle. Paris, Michallon, 1996.
13 Souques A: De l'hystérie mâle dans un service hospitalier. Archives générales de médecine, 1890, pp 166–200.
14 Gilles de la Tourette G: Traité clinique et thérapeutique de l'hystérie d'après l'enseignement de la Salpêtrière. Paris, Plon, 1891.
15 Guinon G: La policlinique de M le Pr Charcot à la Salpêtrière; in: Clinique des maladies du système nerveux: professeur Charcot, Paris. Bureaux du Progrès médical, 1893, pp 430–444.
16 Shorter E: Paralysis: The rise and fall of a 'hysterical symptom'. J Soc Hist 1986; 19:549–582.
17 Edelman N: Les métamorphoses de l'hystérique. Paris, La Découverte, 2003.
18 Pitres A: Leçons cliniques sur l'hystérie et l'hypnotisme. Paris, Dion, 1891.
19 Luauté J-P: L'ecmnésie entre faits et fiction. Ann Med Psychol 2012;170:175–178.
20 Ellenberger HF: The Discovery of the Unconscious. The History and Evolution of Dynamic Psychiatry. New York, Basic Books, 1970.
21 Orsat M, Ernoul A, Canet J, Grandin-Goldstein E, Richard-Devantoy S: La neurasthénie du 19° au 21° siècle: figures de la première maladie psychosomatique. Ann Med Psychol 2013;171: 357–361.
22 Richer P: Etudes cliniques sur la grande hystérie ou hystéro-épilepsie. Paris, Delahaye et Lecrosnier, 1881.
23 Bourneville DM, Regnard P: Iconographie photographique de la Salpêtrière, service de M Charcot. Paris, Aux bureaux du Progrès médical, VA Delahaye, 1876–1880.
24 Charcot J-M: Physiologie pathologique. Sur les divers états nerveux déterminés par l'hypnotisation chez les hystériques. CR Acad Sci 1882;94:403–405.
25 Shorter E: From Paralysis to Fatigue. A History of Psychosomatic Illness in the Modern Era. New York, Free Press, 1992.
26 Hacking I: Rewriting the Soul. Multiple Personality and the Sciences of Memory. Princeton, Princeton University Press, 1995.
27 Veith I: Hysteria. The History of a Disease. Chicago, University of Chicago, 1965.
28 Trillat E: Histoire de l'hystérie. Paris, Seghers, 1986.
29 Luauté J-P, Saladini O: L'hystérie collective: un diagnostic politiquement incorrect? Formes juvéniles et dérivées. Ann Med Psychol 2007;165:263–268.
30 Stone J, Hewett R, Carson A, Warlow C, Sharpe M: The 'disappearance' of hysteria: historical mystery or illusion? J R Soc Med 2008;101:12–18.

Jean-Pierre Luauté, MD
Neuropsychiatrist
25 rue de la République
FR–26100 Romans (France)
E-Mail jean_pierre_luaute@hotmail.com

Bogousslavsky J (ed): Hysteria: The Rise of an Enigma. Front Neurol Neurosci. Basel, Karger, 2014, vol 35, pp 28–43
DOI: 10.1159/000360436

Clinical Manifestations of Hysteria: An Epistemological Perspective or How Historical Dynamics Illuminate Current Practice

Elisabeth Medeiros De Bustos[a, c] · Sylvio Galli[a] · Emmanuel Haffen[b, c] · Thierry Moulin[a, c]

Departments of [a]Neurology and [b]Psychiatry, Besançon University Hospital, and [c]CIC-IT 808, CHU Besançon – EA 481 'Laboratoire de Neurosciences', University of Franche-Comte, Besançon, France

Abstract

Hysteria has generated the most heated debates among physicians, from antiquity to the present day. It has been long confused with neuroses and neurological pathologies such as Parkinson's disease and epilepsy, principally associated with women and sexual disorders. The clinical manifestations must first be seen in their historical context, as interpretation varies according to the time period. Recently, the *Diagnostic and Statistical Manual of Mental Disorders* by the American Psychiatric Association marked a break in the consensus that previously seemed to apply to the concept of hysteria and approach to the clinical manifestations. The clinical manifestations of hysteria are numerous and multifaceted, comprising 3 main classifications: paroxysms, attacks, and acute manifestations; long-lasting functional syndromes, and visceral events. Each main classification can be subdivided into several subgroups. The first main group of paroxysms, attacks, and acute manifestations includes major hysterical attacks, such as prodrome, trance and epileptic states, minor hysterical attacks such as syncope and tetany, twilight states, paroxysmal amnesia, and cataleptic attacks. The second group includes focal hysterical symptoms, paralyses, contractures and spasms, anesthesia, and sensory disorders. Visceral manifestations can be subdivided into spasms, pain, and general and trophic disorders. The diversity of the symptoms of hysteria and its changing clinical presentation calls into question the same hysterical attacks and the same symptoms, which have had only a few differences for over 2,000 years. A new definition of hysteria should be proposed, in that it is a phenomenon that is not pathological, but physiological and expressional.

The principal signs of hysteria have been described since antiquity, covering a tradition of sine materia diseases that has generated the most heated discussions among physicians. The history of hysteria has long been confused with neuroses and disorders currently related to lesional neurological pathologies (Parkinson's disease, epilepsy, catatonia, etc.), so much that in 1682 Thomas Willis grouped half of chronic diseases under the name of hysteria. In order to understand the clinical manifestations of hysteria, one cannot ignore the historical context within which they developed. The following sections provide a brief historical overview.

History

Antiquity

During antiquity, hysteria was classified as a movement disorder, due to the frequency of seizures. Hysteria, as Hippocrates perceived its elusive nature, was a 'suffocation of the uterus'. It occurs in 'women who have not had sexual relations', emphasizing a possible element that would later develop into the sexual theory of neuroses. It was believed that when the uterus fastens itself to the liver and hypochondrium, it impedes the flow of breath, the whites of the eyes are reversed, the woman becomes cold, and even sometimes livid. She grits her teeth, saliva flows in her mouth, and she looks like an epileptic. If the uterus remains in the liver and hypochondrium for a long time, the woman suffocates [1].

This description foreshadows 'la grande hystérie' (the great hysteria). Hippocrates added that the uterus can fasten itself to other organs such as the heart, and that suffocation causes anxiety and bilious vomiting. Aretaeus of Cappadocia emphasized the acute and chronic nature of the disease, distinguishing hysteria from epilepsy. He spoke very briefly about the possibility of male hysteria, 'catoche', meaning 'possessed or inspired by a demon'. Soranus was the first at the end of the first century to oppose 'wandering womb' theories. Galen described three forms of hysteria: lethargic, suffocation, and motor. He was the first to establish the seminal theory of hysteria. His etiologic explanation raised the question of women with regard to unsatisfied sexuality and highlighted all areas of life relationships. The history of hysteria is closely linked to that of epilepsy, considered male, and hysteria, considered female [2].

Middle Ages

In the Middle Ages, hysteria left the medical field to become a deceiving evil. In the 15th century it was a means for identifying witches. At the end of the 17th century, the treatment for hysterics was often punishment. Sorcery was 'civilized', but the diabolical and deceptive nature of hysteria persisted. Hysteria resurfaced in medicine with Sydenham who placed it above all diseases, superimposed on a parallel plane, imitating all diseases. For Sydenham, the essential feature of the hysteric is to deceive the doctor and to simulate diseases. The symptom is an illusion, hiding what the patient does not know or want to know of their suffering, sexuality, or secrets. This popular conception still embodies contemporary thought. For the first time, and breaking with tradition, the cause of hysteria shifted from the uterus to the brain. Consequently, hysteria was desexualized and no longer the prerogative of women; men may also be hysterical. Sydenham insisted on the diversiform nature of hysteria [2]:

> This is a disease that takes a variety of different forms: it is a chameleon that endlessly changes its colours [...] its symptoms are not only numerous and varied, yet they have this peculiarity among all diseases, they follow no rules, and no uniform type and are just confused and irregular: hence it is difficult to give the history of hysterical affliction.

He saw hysteria as a chronic disease and not just acute attacks or fits, and amalgamated hysteria and hypochondria [2]:

> It imitates almost all diseases that come to humans, as in encountering any part of the body, it produces at once the symptoms that belong to this part, and if the doctor is not knowledgeable or experienced, he can be mistaken and easily assign a critical illness to this part, symptoms that depend solely on hysterical affliction.

Other authors also emphasize the role of imitation in hysteria, such as Paul Briquet (1859) who wrote that 'imitation is the privilege of women; it is above all a privilege of the hysterical. It is enough that a patient has seen a gesture just once, an act that strikes her, for her to unwittingly mimic it.' But imitation is not simulation, 'the hysteric is an actress on stage, a performer, but do not blame her, because she does not know what she plays, she sincerely believes in the reality of the situation' [2].

The 19th Century

The 19th century is quite clearly a turning point. It was necessary in this era to relocate hysteria in the context of more scientific and empirical medicine theorized by Claude Bernard, and to rely as much as possible on anatomopathological methods that had quickly demonstrated their relevance. At the time, clinicians aimed to provide a finer clinical picture of this protean disease, questioning its physiological and psychopathological basis, and empirically developing the first attempts at therapeutic evaluation. One must especially consider Paul Briquet, John Russell Reynolds, Jean-Martin Charcot and his 'students' (Bourneville, Richer, Babinski, Sollier, etc.), and Sigmund Freud, among many others [3].

According to Lasègue (1816–1883), hysteria cannot be included the field of general pathology and those of mental pathology [4]:

> The definition of hysteria has never been given and never will be. The symptoms are not sufficiently consistent, compliant, or equal in duration or intensity, so that a description can include all varieties… the laws that control pathological changes did not fit there, the exception does not prove the rule, but in fact becomes the rule and the characteristic.

In 1846 Landouzy suggested the term 'hystero-epilepsy', applied to two different clinical situations: epileptic patients with nonconvulsive and hysterical manifestations and epileptic patients who also had hysterical attacks [5]. It was reported that in hysteria, around 1 in 10 cases also had other attacks that could be 'intermediate' or 'mixed' forms of epilepsy, named by Briquet as 'epileptiform hysteria' [6]. These epileptiform hysteria attacks are characterized by a brief loss of consciousness followed by tonic seizures, interspersed with disordered movements. Briquet defined hysteria as:

> A neurosis of the brain of which the apparent phenomena are mainly in the disruption of vital acts which are the manifestation of affective sensations and passions… that is taken as a symptom of hysteria and the model still to be found in any of the acts that constitute the passionate demonstrations.

He first described patients who felt that they had been ill most of their lives and who complained of a multitude of symptoms pertaining to numerous different organic systems. These manifestations were coined as Briquet's syndrome by Guze [7]. By analyzing the symptoms of this disease, Briquet remarked that some of these were more or less permanent (sensory and motor disturbances), while others were presented as attacks. He classified the attacks into nine types (spasmic seizures with syncope, seizures with hysterical convulsions, epilepsy, catalepsy, ecstasy, sleepwalking, sleep, coma or lethargy, and delirium), clearly differentiating epileptic seizures presented by hysterics (group 4) from hysterical convulsions (group 3). At this time, although characterized by the lack of neuropsychiatric differentiation, the natural distinction between the two types of seizures was made, both in psychiatry and neurology, as well as the possibility of association [6, 8].

Charcot and his 'students' quickly occupied a medical no-man's land with regard to hysteria [9, 10]. To deal with the absence of morphological lesions in the brain, Charcot developed the concept of a 'dynamic lesion', which could not be seen under the microscope. In so doing, he was considering hysteria as an organic disease similar to any other organic disease of the nervous system, and the issue of psychological factors appeared in his work only shortly before his death in 1893. Although Charcot wrote that hysteria is 'largely a mental disease', this concept would crystallize only later, mainly with Pierre Janet [11] and Sigmund Freud [12]. In studying hypnotism and the mental state of hysterics, Charcot's followers implicitly recognized the importance and power of the 'unconscious', even though it was not immediately called as such. They emphasized the underground work of memory, which stores certain mental experiences in such a way that they are not accessible through conscious efforts of retrieval. Janet concluded that hysteria is characterized by a constant splitting of the personality, with each part ignoring the other, in a 'shrinkage of consciousness'. It is striking that the concept of the unconscious had its first developments in the medical field in neurology, and not within psychiatry. It is only after Babinski revised Charcot's concept of hysteria, and when Janet highlighted that it was no longer possible to consider hysteria as an organic brain disease, that the issue of a 'hysteric personality' really emerged and became a study topic for psychiatry.

In France, alienists rejected the great neurosis as being outside their field of investigation. Henceforth, hysteria became a matter for neurologists, with alienists only dealing with the most 'psychological or psychiatric aspects' of hysteria. This establishes a split between the neurological and psychological approaches. After Charcot, hysteria slowly took its place in a newly identified group of mental diseases, 'psychoneuroses', differentiating them from the 'vésanies' (psychoses) of the alienists, and amalgamating them in the neurasthenia of George Beard, psychoneuroses of defense of Freud, and psychasthenia of Janet [11].

In France, the evolution of ideas within Salpêtrière illustrates the diversity of the concept of hysteria [11–14]. While Charcot studied hysteria by the ordinary methods of medical observation, Babinski wished to define precisely the field and separate 'pithiatic' phenomena (that which can be reproduced by suggestion) from that of lesion neurology, Janet introduced it to the psychological field, and Freud further conceptualized it with the term 'conversion', based on his hypothesis that an intrapsychic conflict can convert into a physical symptom. As a result of the struggle between 'the Titans', the major contribution by Sollier unfortunately faded from thought (see Walusinski [this vol., pp. 126–138]) [15].

Finally, it is worth recalling sociological influences on the external manifestations of hysteria. No pathological form is more sensitive to the spirit of the time: the symptoms of hysteria vary across cultures, following the patterns and evolution of medicine.

Clinical Study of the Symptoms of Hysteria

Only an overall description will be made that will not take into account the discussions and quarrels of the different schools of thought. The multifaceted symptoms of hysteria can be classified into three groups: paroxysms, lasting clinical manifestations, and visceral disorders [16].

Paroxysms, Attacks, and Acute Manifestations

All these hysterical episodes are focused on hysterical attacks, which have become rare in their complete 'Charcot' form, and other paroxysmal manifestations are fragments or derivatives of it.

Major Hysterical Attacks

In the history of this neurosis, these attacks mark an epoch. The great 'Charcot' hysterical attack, first described by Richer in 1881 and 1885 [17, 18] consisted of 5 stages: (1) prodrome (hysterical aura), (2) epilepsy, (3) contortion (clownism), (4) trance or passion, and (5) terminal or verbal stage. The prodrome stage included ovarian pain, palpitations, globus hystericus, and visual disturbances, and resulted in a 'loss of consciousness with no sudden falls'. The next stage, epilepsy, was marked by tonic seizures with respiratory failure and immobilization of the whole body, and clonic seizures starting with small jerks and grimaces, de-

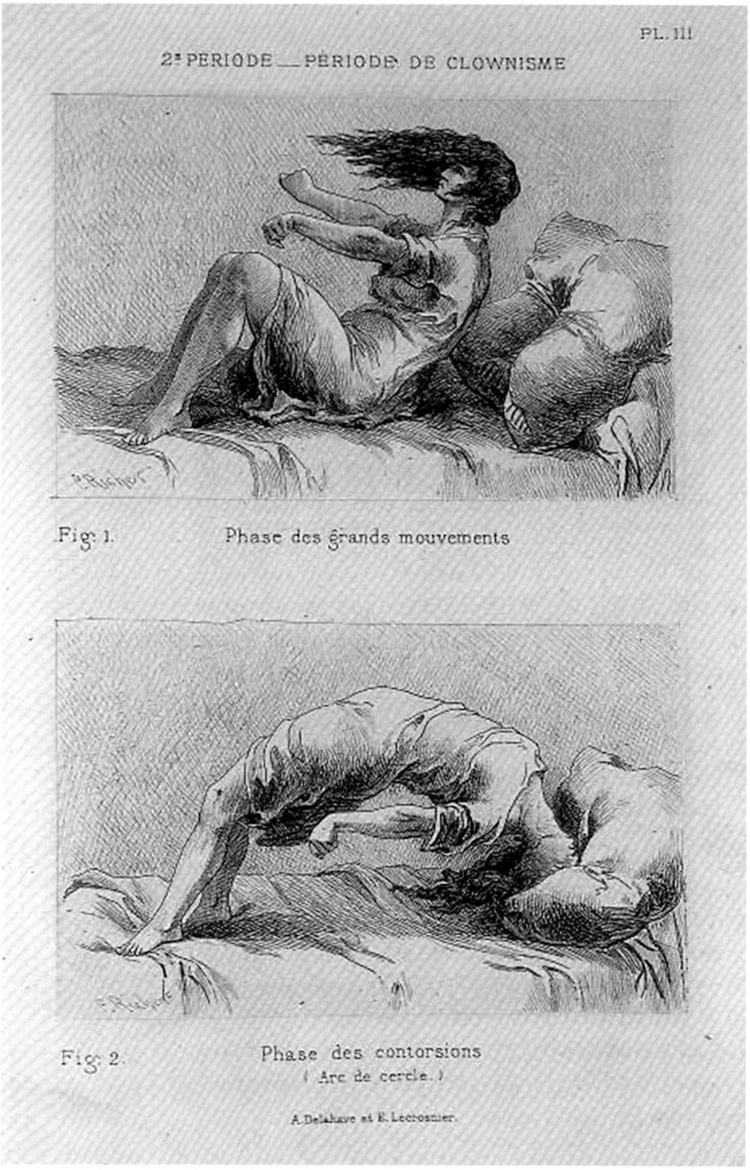

Fig. 1. Contortion phase. Richer, 1885 (BIU Santé, Paris).

veloping into large generalized tremors, and then resolution with stertor. Contortion (clownism) involved various movements accompanied by cries, similar to 'a struggle against an imaginary being' (fig. 1). In the trance or passion stage, the patient mimes violent, erotic, or demoniac scenes. This is a dream state, and usually the same theme is repeated in every attack (see Bogousslavsky [this vol., pp. 44–55; fig. 2]). Finally, in the terminal or verbal stage, the patient, rather rapidly, during the hallucinations, experiences residual contractures and a return to consciousness, but is still delusional. The stages can last anywhere from 15 min to several hours. In 1885, Richer [18] depicted the different stages in detail using brilliant drawings (fig. 2, 3) as well as photographs [19].

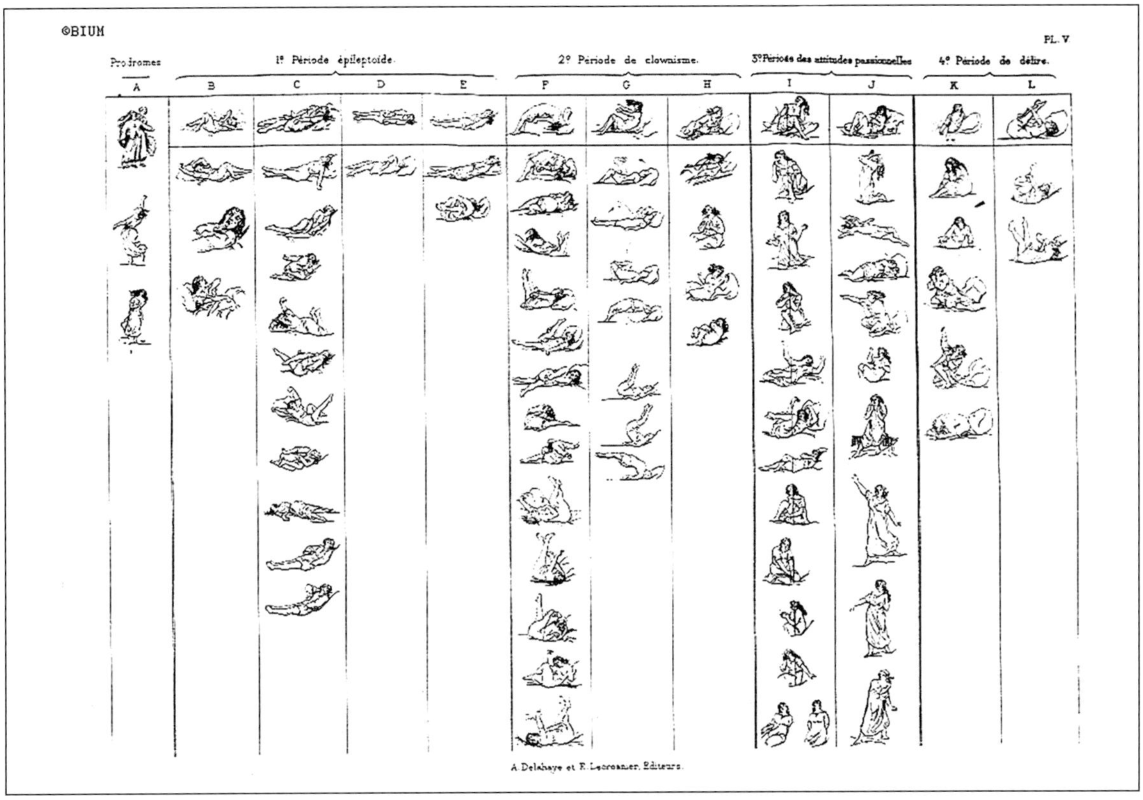

Fig. 2. Depictions of all phases of hysterical attacks. Richer, 1885 (BIU Santé, Paris).

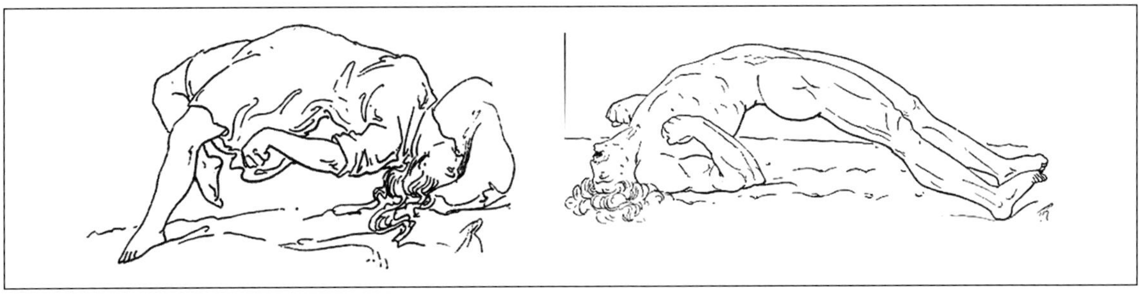

Fig. 3. Comparison of two drawings showing the 'Arc de cercle' described by Richer in 1881 (left) and opisthotonos by Bell in 1872 (right) (BIU Santé, Paris).

Minor Hysterical Forms

These are nervous attacks comprising agitation, grossly resembling epilepsy, expressive, emotional discharge, and the subsequent subsiding of these erotic or aggressive outbursts, retaining all the features of the classic attack. They are considered especially frequent in uncultivated persons or in certain ethnic or cultural groups [16, 20]. With a 'syncope' attack, the subject 'feels unwell,' pales, and collapses. There are signs of extreme vagotonia, i.e. a slow and weak pulse, and low blood pressure. Electrocardiogram reveals a normal heart rate. Fainting lasts a few minutes and is followed by a phase of fatigue without amnesia. Intermediary versions exist between simple fainting and true syncope. Patients may suffer from extrapyramidal symptoms, which include motor manifestations: fits of hiccups, yawning, sneezing, fits of laughter or uncontrollable crying, tremors, muscle twitching, tics, or large choreic movements. In hystero-epilepsy, some patients have 'emotional epilepsy' or neuropathic seizures and are confirmed epileptics. Some paroxysmal or intercritical aspects of epilepsy cannot be radically separated from hysterical manifestations. Finally there is hysteria and tetany. These two sets of disorders are linked and triggered by emotion as well as hyperpnoea, to the extent that it is no longer known if hyperpnoea occurs due to its emotional value or emotion due to humoral factors. These clinical forms of hysterical attacks demonstrate the borders of hysteria and certain syndromes.

Twilight States and Trance States

The twilight hysterical state consists of a change of consciousness that commences and finishes abruptly, ranging from simple confusion to stupor and semiconscious experiences of depersonalization. Ganser syndrome is a particular form of these states, characterized by nonsensical or wrong answers and acts associated with analgesia. It is a systematic nonrecognition of the surrounding reality [21, 22]. Patients do not take into account the environment, and their actions and words are addressed to an imagined situation. It is a hypnotic state of consciousness. The patient lives a 'twilight' experience, similar to some catatonic and cataleptic attacks [23]. For Sollier, it was even a new concept based on a notion of partial sleep and altered consciousness, limited to some brain regions: a state of 'vigilambulism' [24]:

Hysteria is a physical and functional disorder of the brain, involving localized or generalized, transitory or permanent numbness or drowsiness of cerebral areas, and resulting in (according to the affected areas) psychological, motor, sensorial, visceral, trophic, and vasomotor manifestations, and (depending on its variation, extent, and duration) in transitory attacks, permanent stigmata, or paroxysmal accidents.

Other twilight states, also known as trance states, are oneiroid syndromes with rich, visual imagery. These are trance states, isolated fragments that develop from the main attack. As for trance states in patients with 'multiple' personalities, this involves exceptional events in which real experience is replaced by dreamed experience, to the extent that the second personality (hysterical dream) alternates with the real personality (normal state). There are famous cases from Janet (Juliette), Morton Prince (Miss Beauchamp), and Azam (Félida). These twilight states are linked with hysterical somnambulism, which differs only by its occurrence during sleep. It is conventional to describe fugues in these semiconscious states, as the hysteric during these twilight or hypnotic states sometimes wanders as if fascinated by the suggestion of the images he or she perceives. These fugues have the same clinical value as amnesia [25].

Paroxysmal amnesia

The aforementioned states are generally deep or paradoxical memory problems, but amnesia can be presented as the only symptom. A hysterical amnesia attack is characterized by systematic, most often lacunar, amnesia consisting of forgetting a painful event or situation. Amnesia can be general and the hysteric is a 'traveler without luggage'. Reversibility, paradoxical evocation, relapse, and suggestion are characteristic of paroxysmal amnesia [11, 23, 25].

Cataleptic Attacks

This is 'hysterical sleep,' a term open to criticism since this state does not produce any clinical or electrical signs of sleep. The subject is

Table 1. Functional symptoms and syndromes in medical specialties

Disciplines	Symptoms or syndromes
Gastroenterology	Irritable bowel syndrome
Respiratory	Chronic cough, brittle asthma (some)
Rheumatology	Fibromyalgia, chronic back pain (some)
Gynecology	Chronic pelvic pain, dysmenorrhea (some)
Allergology	Multiple chemical sensitivity syndrome
Cardiology	Atypical/noncardiac chest pain, palpitations (some)
Infectious diseases (postviral)	Chronic fatigue syndrome, chronic Lyme disease (where the physician disagrees that there is ongoing infection)
Ears, nose, and throat	Globus, functional dysphonia

inert, eyes closed or open, but without the characteristic triad of sleep. Muscle tone is variable, especially as paralysis or contractures may be associated with catalepsy. Anesthesia or twitching can be observed. This patient is not completely unconscious or amnesic. It can last a few hours or days. If it persists, a slowing down of vegetative functions is observed with hypothermia, hypotension, cardiovascular or sphincter disorders, and sometimes an extreme decrease in metabolism [15, 16, 23]. Confusional states, delirium, hallucinations, and amnestic disorders can also be contained within this subgroup, and sometimes have been reported in particular psychoneurotic syndromes, such as 'bird syndrome' (see Tatu and Bogousslavsky [this vol., pp. 157–168]) [26].

Long-Lasting Functional Syndromes

Focal Hysterical Disorders: Clinical Presentation and Diagnosis

Hysteria is a difficult concern in medical practice. Several studies indicate an incidence of 5–10/100,000 in the general population, while it represents approximately 1% of consultations in a general hospital, and up to 10% of patients seen by neurologists or psychiatrists [27, 28]. These figures mirror those demonstrated in other specialties and table 1 lists functional symptoms and syndromes according to discipline. In practice and by principle, hysteria as a focal disorder should be diagnosed by exclusion. Thus, it is suspected clinically when the symptoms and physical signs are not consistent with basic anatomical or physiological principles, when symptoms change or evolve erratically over time, and when imaging or physiological tests show normal results [29, 30]. It is no longer a question of 'simple' diagnosis by exclusion. Positive clinical signs have greater specificity and these alone (clinical and paraclinical included) can make a quasi-certain diagnosis (table 2).

The diagnosis of functional neurologic disorder should be based on physical symptoms that are inconsistent or incongruent with neurologic disease (i.e. the Hoover sign), or 'positive' clinical signs, such as the Babinski sign. In addition, clinicians must be careful to consider the possibility of a comorbid neurologic disease and be aware of the unusual nature of some neurologic disorders, as well as the signs and evaluations that may be helpful in identifying functional weaknesses, none of which are flawless but can be used together to reach a clinical judgment [31]. Although these clinical signs are useful indices of preserved neurological functions, it is worth recalling that dissociations between conscious subjective experience and objective performance can also be observed in some patients with clearly organic brain disorders such as blindsight, neglect, or amnesia [32]. On the other hand, brain lesions may lead to obvious neurological deficits, such as anosogno-

Table 2. Functional neurological signs validated from study (adapted from Daum et al. [51])

Motor	Sensory	Gait
Hoover sign Abductor sign Abductor finger sign Spinal injury test Collapsing or give-away weakness Co-contraction Motor inconsistency	Midline splitting Splitting of vibration Nonanatomical sensory loss Inconsistency or changing pattern of sensory loss Systematic failure	Dragging monoplegic gait Chair test

sia, of which patients are unaware and even deny. This suggests that consciousness is associated with abilities which may be dissociated by brain lesions and psychological or emotional conditions [33]. While stressful situations or emotional factors frequently precede the onset of hysterical symptoms, the factors and their relation to the symptoms frequently interfere with the clinicians' subjective judgments (see Tatu and Bogousslavsky [this vol., pp. 157–168]). Moreover, the occurrence of psychological stress is rarely specific to be able to distinguish conversion from other disorders such as somatization, also known as Briquet's syndrome. It is worth recalling that in Briquet's syndrome, patients feel that they are always ill and have a multitude of symptoms pertaining to numerous different organ systems. This conviction of illness persists despite repeatedly negative consultations and diagnostic procedures, and patients continue to seek medical care, take treatments, and undergo needless diagnostic procedures. Nevertheless, the characteristics, as well as their impact on mental, emotional, or physiological processes are still poorly defined.

Detailed Description of Clinical Manifestations

The semiology of 'nervous' disorders can be described as follows, referring particularly to the proposed classification by Roussy and Lhermitte [34]. Paralyses are classified as systematic and localized. Functional deficit is paralysis of a movement or group coordinated by the same functional significance movements.

The major types and most common manifestations are gait disorders. Affected individuals demonstrate dissociation of the automatic reflex of walking (astasia-abasie) and emotional inhibition (staso-basophilia), with some clinical forms: the 'knock-kneed gait' (the knees flexed inwards with the trunk bowing on each side), the 'constrained gait' (hunched back, hands on hips), the 'swimmer's gait' (with the trunk thrown backwards as if the subject was struggling against the waves), the 'scrubber' (the lower limbs rub against one another), and the 'tightrope walker gait' (like a tightrope walker).

Localized paralysis can involve a limb or limb segment. In hysteria, paralyses do not follow the laws of anatomical organization, but instead an approximate pattern affecting a hand, arm, leg, etc. These functional paralyses are not associated with other signs indicating alteration of the pyramidal tract or other parts of the nervous system. They are, however, intermittent, paradoxical, and subject to intentionality, emotional inhibition, and suggestion [31].

Contractures and spasms are also a kind of active paralysis of which the systematization is paradoxical and variable under the influence of psychological factors. Limb and neck contractures (torticollis) can be observed, especially contractures of the trunk (camptocormia, see Tatu and

Bogousslavsky [this vol., pp. 157–168]). Camptocormia is characterized by hyperflexion of the trunk and pain in the lumbar region. Characteristically, the abnormal posture disappears entirely during sleep when the patient is lying down. Recognizing the syndrome enables easy diagnosis and treatment. Some other tonic or spasmodic manifestations are frequent (hiccups, vomiting, oculofacial spasms, etc.).

Psychogenic movement disorders are also a subtype of conversion disorder. Typical clinical characteristics of psychogenic movement disorders are acute onset, fast progression, movement patterns incongruent with organic movement disorders, distractibility, variability, suggestibility, and simultaneous occurrence of various abnormal movements and dysfunctions. Psychogenic movement disorders should not be diagnosed by exclusion. The cause is unknown and the underlying brain mechanisms remain uncertain. However, recent functional imaging studies have demonstrated altered blood flow in conversion disorders that may reflect changes in synaptic activity [35, 36].

Patients with hysteria can suffer from anesthesia, that is to say the loss of sensations of touch, pain, heat, etc., of body segments. These types of sensitivity disorders, their topography, and qualitative modalities of their alternations do not obey the laws of the innervation, conduction, and sensitivity, such as massive sensory loss of the entire hemibody. Sometimes all the skin, sensitive areas, and even sensory modalities (fakirs) can be affected by anesthesia. More rarely, the anesthesia can be present with inexplicable phenomena such as allochiria (sensitivity transferred from one side to the other of the body), synesthetic neuralgia (pain caused by the sight of an object, etc.), or more extensive cenesthesia of the different internal organs to the extent that the whole body is an illusion, such as inner internal autoscopia [37, 38].

Sensory disorders are sensory dysfunctions (blindness, deafness, anosmia, etc.), of which hysterical blindness is probably the most notable of these events, and is sometimes difficult to diagnose objectively. One can be certain of the hysteria when two other ocular symptoms have been described as part of the 'stigmata': concentric visual field constriction and monocular diplopia [11].

Visceral Manifestations

Visceral manifestations are vegetative in expression. Their existence in hysteria at the time of Charcot and Babinski was the subject of controversy with regard to both the reality of facts and their interpretation. These were simulated according to some, and functional consequences of attacks or inhibitions according to others. They are spasms, pains, and trophic disorders [15, 39].

Spasms

The most common are gastrointestinal, i.e. inability to swallow, nausea, and vomiting. The famous hysterical 'ball' felt in the neck or upper abdomen seems to be similar to an esophageal spasm. However, there are other spasms that are mainly urinary (retention) and genital (vaginismus, dyspareunia).

Pain

The frequency of pain symptoms in functional disorders of which patients complain is important. All locations and types of pain can be symptoms of hysteria. Quite often, the type of pain will be determined based on the presentation of the symptoms of the patient. Pain that cannot be explained must be hysteria. Pain is the only symptom that affects one or more anatomical sites, with psychological factors playing a dominant role in the onset and persistence of pain. Location, radiation, duration, intensity, and type are personal, unique, and incomparable, often located on the left side of the body as observed by Briquet [6]. In addition, Sollier determined a very precise and useful cartography of the main pain points (fig. 4) [15] and described a specific sign: 'hysterical cardialgia provoked by traction and

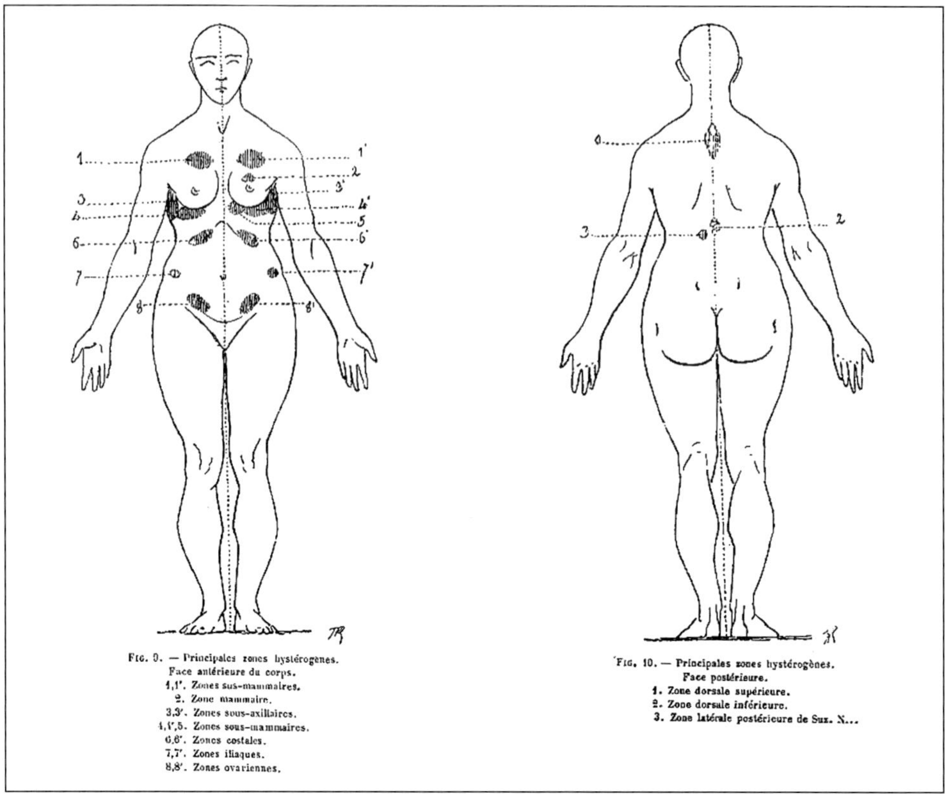

Fig. 4. Cartography of the different painful points of the body. Adapted from Sollier, 1897 [15].

forced recovery of the two last fingers of the left hand' [40].

General and Trophic Disorders

Some vegetative abnormalities have been shown mainly in catalepsy. When they persist, they can manifest as slow metabolism. Much more common are reductions in hunger bordering on anorexia, thirst, and excretions (oliguria and constipation). For Sollier, anorexia was the key symptom, always present in patients and its disappearance indicated the beginning of convalescence [41]. Other vegetative disorders have been reported such as respiratory disorders, cardiovascular phases of tachycardia or brachycardia, and sphincter disorders with urine incontinence or emotional diarrhea [15, 26].

Similar effects, but localized in the peripheral autonomic nervous system, can be observed. Under the name of physiopathic disorders, Babinski and Froment described vasomotor and trophic disorders that appear during certain hysterical paralyses. Paroxysmal disorders can be included in the same group, generally considered as belonging to the 'pathology of emotion', as well as some urticarial or angioedema attacks, and some vascular spasms. They appear as a pathological exaggeration of normal modes of expression. The reality of disorders such as localized hemorrhages or fever was not accepted by all authors, due to the lack of indisputable observations [42].

These aforementioned abnormalities are nonverbal expressions of emotion. The hysteric communicates via the 'language of the body', living metaphors instead of speaking them – the essence of the phenomenon of somatic conversion and stigmata [43].

Hysterical Characteristics: Personality and Collective Hysteria

Hysterical symptoms are produced by the pathological personality of the hysteric. Thus three basic aspects of hysterical 'characteristics' have been described: suggestibility, compulsive lying, and sexual dysfunction. Inconsistent personal identity and tendencies to repress real events and falsify experiences should also be included [43]. The hysteric, either sensitive to suggestion (especially hypnosis), or autosuggestion, is a 'malleable' individual. That is to say, the hysteric is suggestible and inconsistent because he or she fails to firmly establish an authentic personal identity. In addition, the hysteric continually gives 'theatrical performances', lies, and falsifies relationships with others (mythomania). They are always acting, for they perceive their life as a discontinuous series of scenes and imaginary adventures. Sexual dysfunction, however, is what gave its name to this neurosis. Indeed, in this dysfunction more than in others, emotional and passionate expressions are theatrical, excessive, and contrast with strong sexual inhibitions. The hysteric demonstrating this type of dysfunction hides impotence, frigidity, or perversions [16, 39, 43].

Mass psychogenic phenomena are better known as collective hysteria, which affect women and young people in particular. Mass hysteria is characterized by the rapid spread of functional disorder. In such episodes, psychological distress is converted into physical symptoms. There are two common types: anxiety hysteria and motor hysteria. Anxiety hysteria is usually short term in duration (a day), and is started by the sudden perception of threatening triggers. Symptoms could include headache, dizziness, nausea, breathlessness, and general weakness. Motor hysteria is mainly prevalent in intolerable social situations such as strict school and religious settings where discipline is excessive. From a neuropsychological point of view, the propagation of symptoms could be understood as imitation due to the involvement of the mirror neurons system. Symptoms include trance-like states and melodramatic acts of rebellion known as histrionics. Motor hysteria is long term in duration (weeks or months). The term 'mass hysteria' is often used inappropriately to describe collective delusions, as the overwhelming majority of participants do not exhibit hysteria, except in extremely rare cases. The main historical descriptions over the centuries were well summarized in 2000 by Bartholomew and Goode [44], and as also previously suggested by Bourneville and Teinturier [45].

Diagnosis

Analysis of functional, sensory-motor, and sensory disorders highlights their paradoxical nature or unconscious intentional expressiveness and enables a positive diagnosis. If one can discount the shortness of seizure and its fundamental symptoms (typical phases, terminal sleep, incontinence, tongue biting, unconsciousness, and total amnesia) and the theatrical nature of the hysterical attack (passions, emotional reactions and triggers, etc.), there are, as we have noted, cases of hysteroepilepsy that require careful observation. Hysteria is simulatory in all or almost all aspects of the disease. However, it should be noted that it is not sufficient that clinical and laboratory investigations are negative in order to prove hysteria and conversely find an organic cause to symptoms of which the semiological analysis may be hysteria [46].

The diagnosis of other neuroses is generally not difficult. However, phobia (rightly called 'anxiety hysteria') is very similar to hysterical neurosis. The extent of anxiety, systematization, and repetition of the same symptoms, always in the form of obsessive fear, usually enables diagnosis. This diagnosis is especially difficult to make in cases of schizophrenic psychoses. Due to its autistic organization, however, schizophrenia is quite different in its structure and evolution from hysteria. Mythomaniac tendencies, suggestibility, theatrical behavior, and superficial and variable symptoms favor the diagnosis of hysteria. In contrast, schizoid tendencies, the extent of delirium, introversion, development of autism, mental disorders, and progressive dissociation point to schizophrenia.

Contrary to pithiatism, Freud and Breuer consider seizures as a division of the contents of the conscience, attesting the return of an unconscious traumatic memory. This question, partly eclipsed by modern psychiatry, is resurfacing as a new clinical entity, psychogenic nonepileptic seizures. It can be defined as paroxysmal manifestations clinically resembling an epileptic seizure but relating to unconscious psychogenic processes. Clinical diagnosis is particularly difficult. Most patients with psychogenic nonepileptic seizures wrongly have anticonvulsant treatment, with no efficacy and adverse effects. In order to distinguish between psychogenic nonepileptic seizures and epilepsy, electroencephalography is the primary paraclinical examination, in conjunction with video recording. However, the psychotraumatic dimension of epileptoid phenomena, such as neuronal nonepileptic hyperexcitability, has been proven in recent studies. This might signify that recurrent dissociative disorders would be potentially the translation of a particular state of posttraumatic stress [47].

Classifications and Current Contribution of the *Diagnostic and Statistical Manual*

Insights Provided by the Classifications

The adoption of the *Diagnostic and Statistical Manual of Mental Disorders* (DSM) by the American Psychiatric Association marked a break in the consensus that seemed previously to apply the concept of neurosis. With DSM-IV in 1994, hysteria is found on two axes: axis I, a somatoform disorder, subdivided firstly into somatization, conversion and pain disorders, and secondly all dissociative syndromes (amnesia, fugue, identity disorder, and trance), and axis II, histrionic personality [48].

DSM-IV renamed paroxysmal somatic symptoms as excitomotor attacks, minor attacks, and atypical pseudoneurological aspects, with hiccups, yawning, trembling, trance, and choreiform or dyskinetic movement. These are the classic symptoms of somatoform disorders, corresponding to the three categories of DSM-IV. Somatization disorder corresponds to nonneurological, permanent, or paroxysmal symptoms, and is traditional in concept. Conversion disorder includes most permanent or paroxysmal pseudoneurologic symptoms (pseudoconvulsive attack). It is nevertheless more specifically related to hysteria than somatization disorder. Paralysis and hysterical anesthesia share some common points: lack of 'objectivity', pains, headaches, dizziness, and multiple and variable somatic complaints. Complaints of pain are the only symptoms that affect one or more anatomical sites, and psychological factors have a dominant role in the onset and persistence of symptoms. Dissociative disorders reflect an alteration in the organizational, integrative, structuring, and conscious expression of the self, particularly the affective and cognitive dimensions that characterize the sense of personal identity and memory of the self. They include intellectual inhibition, infantile amnesia, dissociative amnesia, dissociative fugue, dissociative identity disorder (formerly multiple personality), twilight and lethargic states, and the dissociative state of trance and possession.

Histrionic personality concerns axis II. The extent of frank emotional reactions defines the histrionic character. It is a general mode of excessive emotional responses and attention seeking, beginning in early adulthood, with at least five of the following for making a diagnosis: (1) dramatization, theatricality, and exaggeration of emotional expression, (2) suggestibility and easily influenced by others or by circumstances, (3) superficial and labile affectivity, (4) constant desire to distractions and activities in which the subject is the center of attention of others, (5) an aspect or behavior of inappropriate seduction, and (6) excessive preoccupation with the desire to please physically [48].

Histrionism is only one aspect of hysteria, of which its deep structure is especially characterized by simultaneous submission and rebellion. An obsessional personality also seems frequent and particularly concerns cognitive somatoform symptoms (which could be named 'cognitivoform' symptoms). The latter are not contained in the 'somatoform disorders' classification in the DSM-IV-TR. Consisting of so-called dissociative (mainly retrograde) amnesia, lacunar forgetfulness, attention or language disorders, they develop in the same way as somatoform somatic symptoms. As for somatoform somatic symptoms, semiological inconsistencies can be immediately striking, and networks of signifiers are recognizable. The role of language in the genesis of these disorders and the presence of focal cerebral hypometabolism require the application of inhibitory neuronal connections (directly or indirectly) between circuits of language and motor, sensory, or cognitive areas [30].

Limitations of the Classification and Perspective

The term 'somatoform disorders' appeared in DSM-III in 1980 to bring together, in a single chapter, disorders characterized by the presence of physical symptoms suggesting the existence of a somatic disease, without an organic lesion or pathophysiologic mechanism, defined on the basis of clinically significant suffering and/or social dysfunction, and for which there is strong evidence that the symptoms are related to psychological factors. It is conventional to propose four broad categories: (1) voluntary produced simulation with secondary benefits, (2) Munchausen syndrome, i.e. voluntary simulation without secondary benefit, (3) panic or somatization disorder, i.e. unintentional simulation without secondary benefits, and (4) conversion, i.e. unintentional simulation with secondary benefits. These different mechanisms do not have the same epidemiological weight. Simulation and Munchausen syndrome, which are factitious disorders during which the subject consciously develops deliberately misleading symptoms, are probably a minority of somatoform disorders. In contrast, panic and somatization disorders are particularly common in young adults and adolescents [49].

The definition of conversion, a somatoform disorder, has been revised in DSM-5, with reconsidered diagnostic criteria and designation [50]. For example, criterion B in DSM-IV-TR in which a psychological factor had to be associated with the initiation or exacerbation of symptoms is removed from DSM-5 because patients can be reluctant to discuss sexual abuse or other psychological trauma. Furthermore, it was a constraining condition to make a formal diagnosis of conversion disorder. The same applies to criterion C in which simulation had to be excluded; it seems to be extremely difficult in clinical practice to exclude feigners with certainty. Positive clinical signs are also methods of diagnosis [51].

If conversion disorders refer historically to psychoanalysis, this classic conception now competes with other approaches. For example, by showing a reduction in the activity of the contralateral thalamus in motor deficit, functional imaging suggests the existence of an unknown neurological dimension involving neuronal networks, and proves that the problem of conversion is not just psychology [35]. As opinions on the term 'conversion' itself are no longer unanimous, a more consensual designation is necessary to transcend the opposition to the original 'psychic' or 'neurological' origin of the disorders. Thus, the term 'functional neurological disorder' has been proposed to describe the symptoms as a 'functional weakness'. In a restrictive view of neurological psychogenic pathology, it is possible to maintain four major categories of disorders: psychogenic seizures, psychogenic movement disorders, psychogenic neurological deficits disorders, and neuropsychological psychogenic disorders, including amnesia [35].

Finally, the phylogenetic origin of psychopathological symptoms also has to be mentioned. The context of behavioral disturbances affecting humans in a natural environmental setting indicates the presence of phylogenetic components in their etiology. Claparède first established a phylogenetic parallel between hysteria and protective behavioral inhibition in response to a predator in the animal world [25]. Hysterical conversion disorders could provide a good illustration of this. The biological model to which they can be traced seems to be the 'distraction display', originally intended to deceive predators and lure them away from the offspring or threatened related individuals. Hysterical tendency to draw attention on oneself could thus paradoxically be seen as performing an altruistic function [52].

Conclusion

From a surrealist perspective, the clinical manifestations of hysteria are expressive and subliminal in nature [53]. Thus, André Breton (1896–1966) and Louis Aragon (1897–1982) invigorated the field of hysteria on the 50th anniversary of the invention of hysteria, considering hysteria as 'the greatest poetic discovery of the latter part of the century' [54]. They concluded by proposing a new definition of hysteria: 'hysteria is not a pathological phenomenon and may, in all respects, be considered a supreme means of expression'. It is true that Breton had studied the work of Charcot in his years as medical student and later was a student of Babinski!

The diversity of the symptoms of hysteria and its changing clinical presentation, once considered demonic and once predominantly female, calls into question the same hysterical attacks and the same symptoms, which have had only a few differences for over 2,000 years. Theories have thus succeeded in the following manner: Hippocrates and the wandering womb, Galen and the seeds, emblem of the devil in the Middle Ages, Sydenham and simulation, Babinski and pithiatism. All contributed to the contemporary ideas of hysteria, brilliantly emphasized by the functional, dynamic and physiological conceptions proposed by Charcot and affirmed by Sollier.

Acknowledgements

We would like to thank Holly Sandu for the translation and editing of this article.

References

1 Bogousslavsky J: Hysteria after Charcot: back to the future. Front Neurol Neurosci 2011;29:137–161.
2 Trillat E: L'histoire de l'hystérie. Paris, Editions Seghers, 1986.
3 Crommelinck M: Neurophysiology of conversion disorders: a historical perspective. Clin Neurophysiol 2013, in press.
4 Lasegue C: Etudes médicales. Paris, Asselin et Cie, 1884.
5 Landouzy H: Traité complet de l'hystérie. Paris, Baillière, 1846.
6 Briquet P: Traité clinique et thérapeutique de l'hystérie. Paris, Baillière, 1859.
7 Guze SB: The role of follow-up studies: their contribution to diagnostic classification as applied to hysteria. Semin Psychiatry 1970;2:392–402.
8 Reynolds JR: Epilepsy: Its symptoms, Treatment and Relation to Other Chronic Convulsive Diseases. London, Churchill, 1861.
9 Charcot JM: Leçons sur les maladies du système nerveux faites à la Salpêtrière. Paris, Delahaye, 1872–1873.
10 Charcot JM: Leçons sur les maladies du système nerveux faites à la Salpêtrière. Paris, Aux Bureaux du Progrès Médical, Delahaye et Lecrosnier, 1887, vol 3.
11 Janet P: Contribution à l'étude des accidents mentaux chez les hystériques. Thèse Paris n° 432. Paris, Rueff, 1893.
12 Freud S, Breuer J: (1895) Studies on Hysteria. New York, Basic Books/Hogarth Press, 1955.
13 Babinski J: Démembrement de l'hystérie traditionnelle, pithiatisme; in: Oeuvre scientifique, recueil des principaux travaux. Paris, Masson, 1909, pp 486–504.
14 Babinski J: Hystérie et pithiatisme, exposé des travaux scientifiques, in: Oeuvre scientifique, recueil des principaux travaux. Paris, Masson, 1913, pp 514–519.

15 Sollier P: Genèse et nature de l'hystérie. Recherches cliniques et expérimentales de psychophysiologie. Paris, Alcan, 1897.
16 Ey H: L'hystérie. Gaz Hôpit 1935;46: 797–836.
17 Richer P: Etudes Cliniques sur l'hystéro-épilepsie ou grande hystérie. Paris, Delahaye, 1881.
18 Richer P: Etudes cliniques sur l'hystéro-épilepsie ou grande hystérie, ed 2. Paris, Delahaye, 1885.
19 Regnard PML, Bourneville DM: Iconographie photographique de la Salpêtrière. Paris, Aux Bureaux du Progrès Médical, 1876–1880, vol 3.
20 De la Tourette G: Traité clinique et thérapeutique de l'hystérie. Seconde partie: hystérie paroxystique. Paris, Plon et Cie Editeurs, 1895.
21 Ganser SJ: Über einen eigenartigen hysterischen Dämmerzustand. Archiv für Pyschiatrie und Nervenkrankheiten 1898;30:633–640.
22 Ganser SJ: Zur Lehre vom hysterischen Dämmerzustande. Archiv für Pyschiatrie und Nervenkrankheiten 1904;38: 34–46.
23 Janet P: Etat mental des hystériques, les stigmates mentaux. Paris, Bibliothèque Charcot-Debove, Rueff, 1893.
24 Binet A, Sollier P: Genèse et nature de l'hystérie: L'année psychologique 1897; 4:669–678.
25 Claude H, Schnyder L: XVIIè congrès des médecins aliénistes et neurologistes de France et des pays de langue française. La Presse Médicale 1907;15:532–534.
26 Sollier P: Traité clinique de neurologie de guerre. Paris, Félix Alcan, 1918.
27 Carson AJ, Ringbauer B, Stone J, McKenzie L, Warlow C, Sharpe M: Do medically unexplained symptoms matter? A prospective cohort study of 300 new referrals to neurology outpatient clinics. J Neurol Neurosurg Psychiatry 2000;68: 207–210.
28 Dubas F, Thomas-Antérion C: Somatoform disorders in neurology visits: history and circumstances: Retrospective study of 124 cases (in French). Rev Neurol (Paris) 2012;168:887–900.
29 Stone J, Smyth R, Carson A, Lewis S, Prescott R, Warlow C, Sharpe M: Systematic review of misdiagnosis of conversion symptoms and 'hysteria'. BMJ 2005;331:989.
30 Dubas F, Thomas-Antérion C: Somatomorphic syndrome: proposed concepts and practices (in French). Rev Neurol (Paris) 2012;168:103–105.
31 Stone J, Carson A: Functional neurologic symptoms: assessment and management. Neurol Clin 2011;29:1–18.
32 Vuilleumier P: Anosognosia; in Bogousslavsky J, Cummings JL (eds): Disorders of Behavior and Mood in Focal Brain Lesions. Cambridge, Cambridge University Press, 2000, pp 465–519.
33 Vuilleumier P: Anosognosia: the neurology of beliefs and uncertainties. Cortex 2004;40:9–17.
34 Roussy G, Lhermitte J: Les Psychonévroses de guerre. Paris, Masson, 1917.
35 Vuilleumier P: The Neurophysiology of self-awareness disorders in conversion hysteria; in Laureys S, Tononi G (eds): The Neurology of Consciousness. San Diego, Academic Press, 2009, pp 282–302.
36 Magnin E, Thomas-Antèrion C, Sylvestre G, et al: Conversion, dissociative amnesia, and Ganser syndrome in a case of 'chameleon' syndrome: anatomo-functional findings. Neurocase 2014;20:27–36.
37 Janet P: L'anesthésie hystérique. Arch Neurol 1892;23:323–352.
38 Sollier P: L'autoscopie interne. Paris, Alcan, 1903.
39 Mace JC: Hysterical conversion. Br J Psychiatry 1992;161:369–377.
40 Sollier P: Signe particulier de cardialgie hystérique provoquée par la traction et le redressement force des 2 derniers doigts de la main gauche. Arch Générales de Médecine 1906;197:3123.
41 Sollier P: La définition et la nature de l'hystérie. Archives Générales de Médecine 1906;197:2585–2600.
42 Babinski J, Froment J: Hystérie-pithiatisme et troubles nerveux d'ordre réflexe. Paris, Masson, 1917.
43 Micale MS: Approaching Hysteria: Disease and Its Interpretations. Princeton, Princeton University Press, 1995.
44 Bartholomew RE, Goode E: Mass delusions and hysterias: highlights from the past millennium. Skeptical Inquirer 2000;24:20–28.
45 Bourneville DM, Teinturier E: Le sabbat des sorciers. ed 2. Paris, Lecrosnier et Babé, Paris, 1890.
46 Koehler PJ: Freud's comparative study of hysterical and organic paralyses: how Charcot's assignment turned out. Arch Neurol 2003;60:1646–1650.
47 Auxéméry Y: From hystero-epilepsy to psychogenic nonepileptic seizures: Continuity or discontinuity? Ann Med Psychol (Paris) 2012;170:609–614.
48 American Psychiatric Association. Diagnostic and Statistical Manual of Diseases, ed 4, text revision. Washington, American Psychiatric Association, 2000.
49 American Psychiatric Association. Diagnostic and Statistical Manual of Diseases, ed 3, text revision. Washington, American Psychiatric Association, 1980.
50 Stone JW, LaFrance C Jr, Brown R, Spiegel D, Levenson JL, Sharpe M: Conversion Disorder: current problems and potential solutions for DSM-5. J Psychosom Res 2011;71:369–376.
51 Daum C, Hubschmid M, Aybek S: The value of 'positive' clinical signs for weakness, sensory and gait disorders in conversion disorder: a systematic and narrative review. J Neurol Neurosurg Psychiatry 2014;85:180–190.
52 Demaret A: Origine phylogénétique des symptômes en psychopathologie. L'exemple de l'hystérie. Acta Psychiat Belg 1994;94:280–298.
53 Haan J, Koehler PJ, Bogousslavsky J: Neurology and Surrealism: André Breton and Joseph Babinski. Brain 2012;135: 3830–3838.
54 Aragon L, Breton A: Le Cinquantenaire de l'hystérie. Révolution Surréaliste 1928;4, 11, 15 Mars:20–22.

Dr. Elisabeth Medeiros De Bustos
Department of Neurology
CHU Besançon
FR–25000 Besançon (France)
E-Mail edebustosmedeiros@chu-besancon.fr

Bogousslavsky J (ed): Hysteria: The Rise of an Enigma. Front Neurol Neurosci. Basel, Karger, 2014, vol 35, pp 44–55
DOI: 10.1159/000359991

Jean-Martin Charcot and His Legacy

Julien Bogousslavsky

Center for Brain and Nervous System Diseases, GSMN Neurocenter, Clinique Valmont, Glion/Montreux, Switzerland

Abstract

Jean-Martin Charcot (1825–1893) rightly is considered the father of both modern neurology and psychiatry in France and much beyond. While he never was interested in mental disease and what was called 'alienism' at the time, his career at La Salpêtrière Hospital over 30 years was mainly marked by the development of a huge group of students which focused on the study and management of hysteria. When Charcot took office at the beginning of 1862, hysteria was a 'no-man's land', medically speaking, since neither the alienists nor the internists had much interest in this condition. At La Salpêtrière, these chronic patients were largely left to themselves before Désiré Bourneville, one of Charcot's first students, convinced his chief to care for them. Subsequently, the studies of Charcot with Paul Richer, Joseph Babinski, Georges Gilles de la Tourette, Paul Sollier, Pierre Janet, and many others allowed the condition to be addressed in detail. During his stay with Charcot in 1885–1866, Sigmund Freud, a young neuropathologist at the time, became fascinated by hysteria, an interest which probably was the main start of his interest in psychology. Charcot emphasized the concept of mental factors in hysteria, along with that of a 'dynamic' lesion, which accounted for the lack of neuropathological findings in the patients. While his ideas on hysteria and hypnotism were criticized after his death even by former pupils, such as Babinski, recent findings from functional studies using magnetic resonance imaging show how accurate and often visionary Charcot's thinking was in this field.

Between the 1860s and his death, Jean-Martin Charcot (1825–1893; fig. 1) developed the clinical and neuropathological bases of what would become modern neurology. Because he never moved to another position after his 1861 appointment as chief of the Cazalis service at La Salpêtrière until his death, he was able to build a remarkable and stable school with dedicated collaborators, among whom one would count several future 'stars' of neurology, including Désiré Bourneville, Pierre Marie, Joseph Babinski, Paul Sollier, and Georges Gilles de la Tourette. Among Charcot's many achievements, the study of hysteria has a particular place, as it had an impact largely beyond the medical world, which is still present today, as suggested by recent novels and films devoted to Charcot and hysteria [1, 2].

The term 'hystérique' (from 'uterus') dates back to 1568 to describe fits specific to women, while 'hystérie' appeared in 1731 [3]. While the relationship between hysteria and the brain

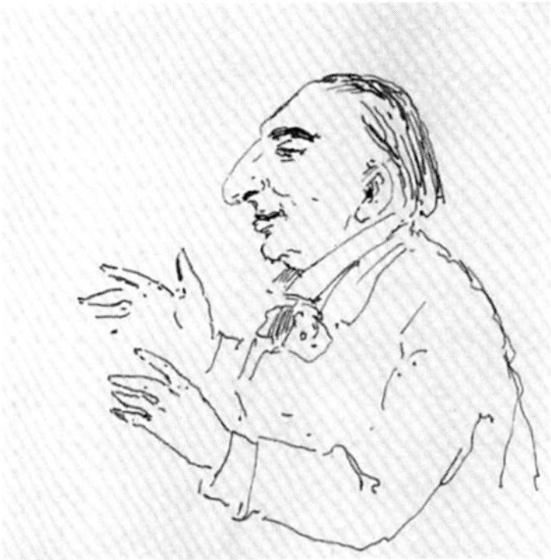

Fig. 1. Jean-Martin Charcot (1825–1893), self-portrait among other portraits, on his own stationary. Private collection.

(rather than the uterus) was already alluded to by Charles Lepois (1563–1633), Thomas Willis (1621–1675), Thomas Sydenham (1624–1689), and Pierre Pomme (1728–1814), it is only during the 19th century that this notion became accepted, and Charcot's work here was particularly critical. While hysteria today is considered as one of the 'great diseases' of the 19th century, when Charcot started his work at La Salpêtrière in the first days of 1862 along with his friend and colleague Félix Vulpian (1826–1887), hysteria was not a fashionable topic in medicine and alienism, and the patients were rather left to their fate in chronic wards. On the other hand, there was a general interest in the public in phenomena such as magnetism, 'mesmerization', somnambulism, and hypnotism. This general interest had already developed by the end of the 18th century, at the time of Franz Mesmer (1734–1815) and his pupil, artillery general Armand-Marie-Jacques de Chastenet, Marquis de Puységur (1751–1825), and of Abbé de Faria (1756–1819), who inspired Alexandre Dumas for the famous Abbé Faria figure in *Le comte de Monte-Christo* [4]. While Mesmer and Puységur developed the concept of a magnetic fluid leading to somnambulic states (mesmerization), Faria denied the existence of such a fluid and of animal magnetism, but emphasized a phenomenon, which he called 'awake sleep', with a particular state of mental concentration behind hypnotism [5]. Ecstatic crises and 'possession' with or without provoked changes in consciousness historically had always been associated with hysteria since Galen and Hippocrates, and this explained why these 'new' states were put into the perspective of hysteria, somnambulism, and hypnotism.

Charcot's Career

Charcot and Vulpian were 'internes' together at La Pitié, just beside La Salpêtrière, and they presented their doctorate thesis a few months apart in 1853: Charcot, on gout, on March 16, and Vulpian, on the origin of cranial nerves, on July 21 [6]. In 1857, one year after Charcot, Vulpian was appointed 'Médecin des Hôpitaux', allowing him to practice independently in the Parisian hospitals. The same year, Charcot failed at the 'agrégation' (professorship) contest, but in 1860, along with Carl Potain, both friends were successful (Vulpian at his first attempt), with close topics ('secondary pneumonias' for Vulpian and 'chronic pneumonia' for Charcot). In late 1861, both Charcot and Vulpian were appointed as Chief of Service at La Salpêtrière, where they started work at the beginning of 1862. For more than 5 years, the two young colleagues worked closely together, reorganizing their clinical services and classifying their patients into new diagnostic categories, while most of them had just been staying in hospital with a label of 'insanity'. This was the time when the scientific collaboration between Charcot and Vulpian was the most intense, the latter introducing the former to pathological anatomy in their shared laboratory, where their work was by far not limited to the nervous system. This collaboration increased their scientific and political weight in the local medical world, which was still recognized more than 10 years later when the correspondent of the *British Medical Journal* called the couple 'twin brothers' or the 'Castor and Pollux of experimental physiology and pathology' [6]. Charcot had taken up the Cazalis service, which he kept for over 32 years until his death, while Vulpian, who was in charge of the Jacquart service, first moved to La Pitié en 1868, and then to La Charité and to Hôtel-Dieu, thus interrupting their intimate scientific collaboration, but not their friendship.

Vulpian's move was triggered by his fulgurant academic rise, when in 1867 he was appointed the successor to Jean Cruvheilier, who had been the first holder of the Chair of Pathological Anatomy since 1835. It is striking that when Vulpian left this position in 1872 to be appointed the first holder of the newly created Chair of Experimental Pathology, his successor was Charcot, who still had not received a full professorship (he had failed in 1867 against Hardy and Axenfeld). Later, with the support of Vulpian, who now was Dean of Medicine in Paris, the celebrated Chair of Clinique des Maladies du Système Nerveux was created for Charcot in 1882. The more rapid ascension of Vulpian was not linked to political issues, but to his scientific excellence, as shown by the fact that in 1866 his enormous CV contained 169 publications, around twice Charcot's number, which made him the only credible candidate for the Chair of Pathological Anatomy, as recalled by Charcot himself after Vulpian's death [6].

During Charcot's time at the Cazalis service, Vulpian's successors at the Jacquart service included Jules Bernard Luys, Alix Joffroy, and Fulgence Raymond, who was followed by Jules Dejerine after Raymond was elected first successor to Charcot after a short interim by Édouard Brissaud in 1893–1894 [7]. While Vulpian succeeded so well in local medical affairs, Charcot spent his time building up a huge clinical service and teaching 'school' at La Salpêtrière, which he never left for over 31 years until his death. This 'school' progressively became synonymous with clinical neurology itself and perpetuated the master's memory for decades, while Vulpian never had such support, although Jules Dejerine was his pupil and Joseph Babinski was an 'interne' with him before becoming Charcot's 'Chef de Clinique' in 1885.

Charcot's Start with Hysteria

Charcot became interested in hysteria mainly after 1870, the year of his first lesson on that topic [8, p. 179], probably upon the influence of his collaborator Désiré Bourneville (1840–1909), who had been his 'interne' in 1868, after Victor Cornil and Charles Bouchard, and before Alix Joffroy, other famous pupils of Charcot. It is interesting that Bourneville was the only one among Charcot's 'internes' to have a background in alienism, while Charcot himself had absolutely no connection with it, having starting his clinical and scientific work in the field of 'clinique médicale', the predecessor of internal medicine. The first papers of Charcot on hysteria appeared in 1871–1872, dealing with ischuria, hemianesthesia, and contractures [9]. It is likely that the military events of the 'Commune' and of the 'Siège de Paris', with hysteria cases in fighters, stimulated his interest. Another trigger was the dismantling of the Delasiauve service at La Salpêtrière in 1870, eight years after Charcot's arrival to the hospital. Actually, because of building changes, the patients of that service who were not considered insane were transferred, along with Delasiauve's '*interne*' Bourneville, under the responsibility of Charcot in his service. They included mainly women with hysteria and epilepsy, conditions which at the time stimulated little interest with the alienists, who were mainly focusing on what we call today the psychoses. Just before the time when Charcot became interested in hysteria, alienists such as Wilhelm Griesinger (1845), Bénédict Morel (1860), Louis-Victor Marcé (1862), and Jacques-Joseph Moreau de Tours (1869) [10] were speaking of 'folie hystérique' or 'manie hystérique' ('hysterical insanity') [11]. Before them, Philippe

Pinel (1745–1826), who is considered the father of 19th-century psychiatry, had only scarcely mentioned hysteria [12], and during the first part of the 19th century, several great names (Louyer-Villermay and Foville in France, Romberg in Germany) still defended the Galenic-Hippocratic uterine theory. Étienne Jean Georget (1795–1828), who died at 33 years but was an extraordinary precursor in several fields of alienism, clearly highlighted the role of the brain in hysteria in his article of the *Dictionnaire de Médecine* (1824) [12], suggesting terms, such as 'attaques des nerfs' (nerve attacks) and 'encéphalite spasmodique' (spasmodic encephalitis), before Jean-Louis Brachet (1789–1858) in 1847 and Paul Briquet (1796–1881) in 1859 published their treatises on hysteria [13, 14]. They definitively discarded the uterine theory and reemphasized the role of the brain in such a masterly way that in the 20th century it was even suggested that hysteria now be called Briquet's disease [5]. It is interesting that at the time when Briquet's book was published, the poet Charles Baudelaire [15] wrote about Flaubert's *Madame Bovary*:

> Hysteria! Why would this physiological mystery not form the basis and the substance of a literary work, this mystery, which the *Académie de Médecine* has not solved yet, and which manifests itself in women through an asphyxiating ascending oppression (I mention only the main symptom), and in nervous men through all impotences, but also the ability to all excesses.

By the time Charcot became interested in hysteria, he had already studied several neurological diseases, such as multiple sclerosis, Parkinson's disease, and stroke, and what is now called internal medicine, but he claimed absolutely no interest in alienism (and would never) [16]. The only mentor quoted by Charcot with some connection with mental disease was a student of Étienne Esquirol, Jules Baillarger, who had been working as an alienist at La Salpêtrière for over a decade. Bourneville, who stimulated Charcot's interest in hysterical women, was only his third 'interne', and there was no 'school' around him. Indeed, this really was the study of hysteria which played this federating role within one decade. Because of the absence of detectable organic disease, the La Salpêtrière internists at the time were probably rather happy that the condition, for which the alienists also showed so little interest, was taken over by Charcot, who literally filled a 'no-man's land', where he was joined by numerous 'internes' and 'chefs de clinique' who would later become famous figures in neurology and psychiatry: Alix Joffroy, Fulgence Raymond, Albert Pitres, Paul Richer, and Édouard Brissaud in the 1870s, and Gilbert Ballet, Charles Féré, Pierre Marie, Georges Gilles de la Tourette, and Joseph Babinski in the 1880s [17].

It is interesting that Charcot played an instrumental role not only in the launch of neurology, but also in the development of modern psychiatry, which painfully emerged out of alienism during the last quarter of the 19th century [16]. Indeed, although Charcot himself always claimed his disinterest in mental medicine, he stimulated the development of an original scientific approach to nervous system conditions, along with a structured academic teaching, while alienism paradoxically remained stuck in organicism, after Antoine Bayle's report in 1822 of 'arachnitis' as the substratum of general paresis of the insane. Contrary to alienism, Charcot's young neurological school was capable of self-criticism, and already in the 1870s progressively underscored mental factors in hysteria. This led to the paradox that neurologists were active in a disease with a recognized lack of organic lesion, while alienists were postulating brain lesions in all mental disorders. The neurological activity thus indirectly and involuntarily led to the first developments of psychodynamic concepts in mental diseases. The academic evolution led to the launch of a faculty chair of mental and brain diseases in 1875, which was taken over for nearly half a century by students of Charcot: Benjamin Ball, Alix Joffroy, and Gilbert Ballet held the position until 1916, supporting the development of modern psychiatry in general hospitals, while alienism progressively disappeared at the turn of the century.

Hysteria in Charcot's Developing School

One is often surprised by the fact that Charcot's ideas on hysteria may commonly seem to be contradictory in his publications. This is mainly due to the fact that his concepts evolved significantly over the 20 years during which he was active in this field. After his first publications on the topic in the early 1870s, Charcot patronized the publication of Bourneville and Regnard's first volume of the monumental *Iconographie Photographique de la Salpêtrière* (1876–1877), which was devoted to hysteria [18]. Five spectacular cases of hysteria were reported in detail, together with comprehensive photographic illustrations (see Walusinski [this vol., pp. 65–77]). In this book and in other reports, Charcot and his collaborators described the main characteristics of 'hystero-epileptic' attacks (including its 'demoniacal' form) and other clinical manifestations, often underlining their sexual 'flavor', in now famous cases, including Geneviève, Rosalie, or Justine [19] (see Walusinski [this vol., pp. 65–77] and Goetz et al. [8, pp. 184–196] for a detailed account).The concepts elaborated by Charcot in his first studies on hysteria were mainly summarized by Paul Richer (1849–1933) in his *Études cliniques sur l'hystéro-épilepsie ou grande hystérie (Studies on Hystero-Epilepsy)* (1881; fig. 2) [20], while Georges Gilles de la Tourette (1857–1904), perhaps the most faithful student of Charcot, published his three-volume treatise on hysteria, *Traité clinique et thérapeutique de l'hystérie d'après l'enseignement de la Salpêtrière* (fig. 3) between 1891 and 1895 [21] (Charcot died in 1893). In short, Charcot emphasized two types of clinical manifestations: firstly, the stigmatas, which were chronic manifestations, including tunnel vision, hemianesthesia or paralysis, etc., and secondly, paroxysmal

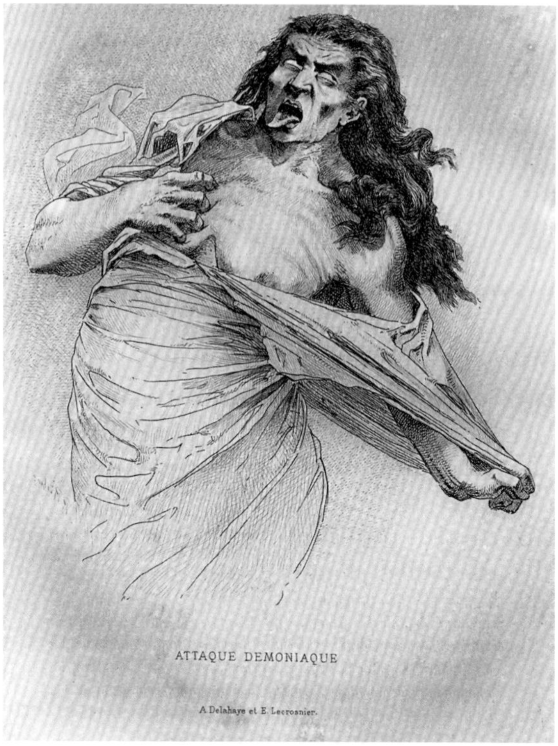

Fig. 2. Drawing by Richer of a hysterical attack. Private collection.

fits, among which the most spectacular event was the 'grande crise d'hystérie convulsive' ('the great hysteria crisis'), with its four successive phases (epileptoid period, clownism, passionate attitudes, which included the famous 'arc de cercle', and delirium). In his first theory on hysteria, Charcot put forward the necessity of the presence of stigmatas for the diagnosis, a claim which would subsequently be criticized after Charcot's death by two of his students, Freud and Babinski, while another of his students, Gilles de la Tourette, always defended his mentor's initial concept. Because of the absence of a detectable organic brain lesion, Charcot developed the concept of a 'dynamic lesion', in particular at the level of the motor cortex in the case of motor paralysis. In fact, this concept was not entirely new, as it had already been proposed by Briquet, on the

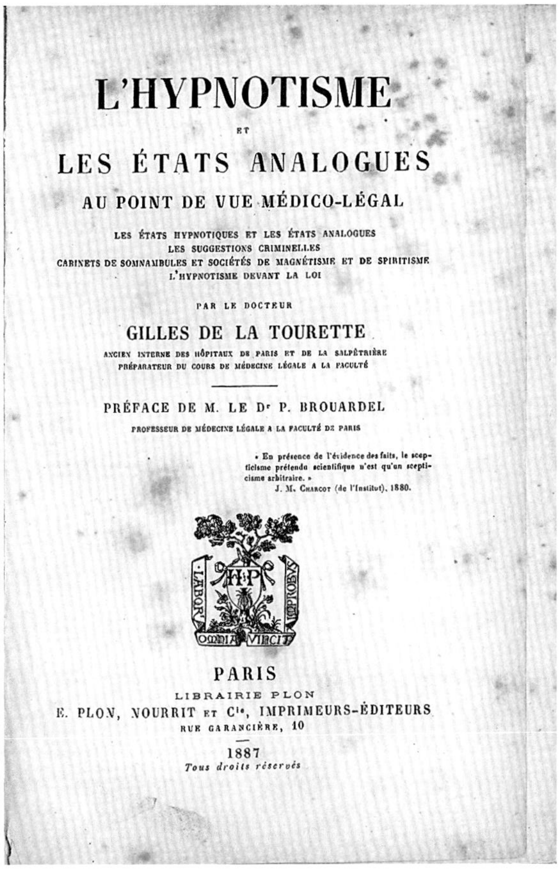
L'HYPNOTISME
ET
LES ÉTATS ANALOGUES
AU POINT DE VUE MÉDICO-LÉGAL
LES ÉTATS HYPNOTIQUES ET LES ÉTATS ANALOGUES
LES SUGGESTIONS CRIMINELLES
CABINETS DE SOMNAMBULES ET SOCIÉTÉS DE MAGNÉTISME ET DE SPIRITISME
L'HYPNOTISME DEVANT LA LOI
PAR LE DOCTEUR
GILLES DE LA TOURETTE
ANCIEN INTERNE DES HÔPITAUX DE PARIS ET DE LA SALPÊTRIÈRE
PRÉPARATEUR DU COURS DE MÉDECINE LÉGALE A LA FACULTÉ
PRÉFACE DE M. LE Dr P. BROUARDEL
PROFESSEUR DE MÉDECINE LÉGALE A LA FACULTÉ DE PARIS
« En présence de l'évidence des faits, le scepticisme prétendu scientifique n'est qu'un scepticisme arbitraire. »
J. M. CHARCOT (de l'Institut), 1880.
LABOR OMNIA VINCIT
PARIS
LIBRAIRIE PLON
E. PLON, NOURRIT ET Cie, IMPRIMEURS-ÉDITEURS
RUE GARANCIÈRE, 10
1887
Tous droits réservés

Fig. 3. Cover of the book of Gilles de la Tourette on hysteria and hypnotism.

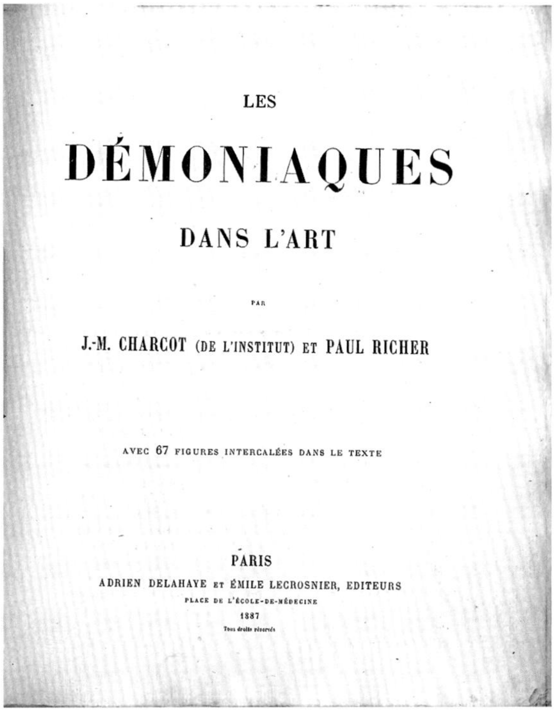
LES
DÉMONIAQUES
DANS L'ART
PAR
J.-M. CHARCOT (DE L'INSTITUT) ET PAUL RICHER
AVEC 67 FIGURES INTERCALÉES DANS LE TEXTE
PARIS
ADRIEN DELAHAYE ET ÉMILE LECROSNIER, EDITEURS
PLACE DE L'ÉCOLE-DE-MÉDECINE
1887
Tous droits réservés

Fig. 4. Cover of *Les démoniaques dans l'art* by Charcot and Richer.

basis of his 10-year experience with patients at La Charité (1859). Charcot and Richer also emphasized the cultural roots of hysteria, the representations of which could be found in religious and nonreligious art from the preceding centuries (fig. 4).

Around 1880, Charcot was defining hysteria as the ensemble of manifestations, which were taking the appearance of organic brain disease, but without a detectable lesion in the brain. In fact, he was mainly repeating Charles Lasègue's definition of 1864 [22]: 'One provisionallly calls hysteria an ensemble of nervous manifestations, which mainly develop in young women, exceptionally in young men, and which do not correspond to a known lesion of the nervous centers.' At this stage, the issue of psychological factors was not mentioned by Charcot, although the great alienist Bénédict Morel had claimed it several years before, and slightly older contemporaries of Charcot, such as Charles Lasègue and Jules Falret had reemphasized it around 1880. However, at about the same time, Charcot underlined 'traumatic factors' in the background of hysteria, especially with certain physical traumatisms (including sexual), where the subject had feared for his or her life. He also delineated two novel concepts, an 'incubation' phase, which was necessary for the symptoms to take place during an 'elaboration' process, explaining the commonly prolonged 'latency' between trauma and clinical manifestations. This was in studying the traumatic factors, which were often hidden behind hysteria, that

Charcot described cases of hysteria in men [9]. Shortly before, he had become fascinated by hypnosis, probably after having read Charles Richet's 1875 article on provoked somnambulism [23], and one of his innovative steps was to start the use of hypnosis in hysterics in 1878. In fact, Charcot and his closest followers (Richer, Gilles de la Tourette) considered that susceptibility to hypnosis was a characteristic, even a diagnostic feature, of hysteria, and that the stages of 'grande hystérie' corresponded to an identical mental state to that of hypnotism. There, Charcot and his school distinguished two major types of hysteria, i.e. 'grande' and 'petite hystérie', the former being typically associated with susceptibility of hypnotism (see Walusinski [this vol., pp. 78–89]).

For the La Salpêtrière school, susceptibility to hypnotism always meant a mental pathology, i.e. hysteria, a claim which was vigorously criticized by Hippolyte Bernheim (1840–1919) and other colleagues from Nancy (called by Charcot himself the 'Nancy school'), who denied hysteria was a specific entity and affirmed that virtually anyone could be hypnotized under favorable circumstances [24] (see Piechowski-Jozwiak and Bogousslavsky [this vol., pp. 56–64]). The controversy included the issue of possible simulation in La Salpêtrière patients [25], and it must be emphasized that while Charcot underscored the absence of an organic lesion in hysteria, he always considered that hysteria was totally distinct from simulation. Bernheim insisted that the issue of 'suggestion' was critical in hypnotism, a concept which would constitute the basis of Charcot's favorite student, Joseph Babinski, 10 years later, when he developed his revision of hysteria and introduced the term 'pithiatism' [26]. Along with public demonstrations of patients at La Salpêtrière, this dispute on suggestion, hypnosis, and hysteria went largely beyond medical circles, and sketches of Charcot and others appeared in the general press of the time.

The last years of Charcot were of major importance for his ideas on hysteria, and it must be emphasized that his sudden death in August 1893 certainly deprived us of fascinating developments in the concepts of hysteria, which in a way were made by his followers, including Sigmund Freud. Indeed, contrary to what he had initially claimed, and also at odds with all of his career, which had been made outside of the concepts and circles of alienism and mental pathology, Charcot became convinced of the critical importance of psychological factors in hysteria [16]. Firstly, he delineated the importance of old psychological traumas and of dreams in triggering hysterical manifestations, while he also observed that hysterical features could accompany organic symptoms of well-established organic diseases, such as multiple sclerosis. Charcot had the idea to reproduce under hypnosis hysterical paralyses using a minimal reproduction of an older physical trauma or its evocation to the patient. This provided the proof that this was the mental representation of the older trauma, and not the trauma itself, which was responsible for the clinical manifestation, a concept which subsequently gave birth to Freud and Breuer's first theories on hypnoid hysteria, i.e. the reactivation of the unconscious memory of a previous psychologically traumatic event [27, 28].

In several writings, including 'La foi qui guérit' (healing by faith), which appeared only 1 year prior to his death, Charcot developed the concept of a 'mental state' of hysterics favorable to suggestion, associated with either external factors or inner psychological processes [29]. In fact, 20 years earlier, Charcot had already supported the concept of a special individual background allowing hysteria to develop, which had been called 'hystericism' by Chambon in 1784, and which Armand Trousseau later had called 'nervous mobility' [30]. In his preface to the 1891 book of Gilles de la Tourette [21], Charcot clearly underlined the potential role of mental factors in hysteria, and in the words introducing Pierre Janet's doctorate thesis, 'The mental accidents of hysterics' [31] (presented to the faculty in July 1893, only a few days before Charcot's death), he highlighted the importance of psychological processes, also emphasizing the poorly delineated role of emotions in previous works on the topic. In fact, it is likely that the late evolution of Charcot towards important psychological factors in hysteria developed under the reciprocal interaction with Pierre Janet, who started work with him in 1889. According to Charcot's biographer and fourth successor at La Salpêtrière, Georges Guillain [32], Georges Guinon, who had been the last secretary to Charcot, said that shortly before his death his mentor had told him that certain concepts of his on hysteria had become obsolete, and that there was now the need for a thorough revision on the topic. Charcot was unable to pursue further, but this work was to be accomplished by his students and followers, mainly Pierre Janet, Joseph Babinski, and Sigmund Freud.

Developments on Hysteria Contemporary to Charcot

No other group than Charcot's really developed a specific interest in hysteria during the same period. The Nancy school (Babinski called it a 'village university') included only two or three senior people, and the controversy with La Salpêtrière mainly focused on hypnotism rather than the general concept on hysteria [33]. In fin-de-siècle alienism, there was no revival of interest in hysteria, which remained outside of the scope of studies and practices. In the same perspective, the statement of Jules Dejerine in the early 1900s that Charcot had taken hysteria out of the hands of the alienists is not really true since hysteria had stagnated into a no-man's land before Charcot, with neither the alienists nor the internists showing any enthusiasm for its scientific study and patient care. When what would become neurology became federated by Charcot around hysteria in the 1870s and 1880s, the alienists never challenged the issue. As we have shown previously [16], it is striking and paradoxical that while the developing neurologists were involved in a disease in which they emphasized more and more the psychological factors, the alienists remained stuck in primary organicism, where virtually all mental disorders could be explained by Morel's degenerescence or Bayle's general paresis inflammation.

The alienists did not study hysteria, but it is interesting that most of their descriptions of what is now called the psychoses included 'hysterical features'. For instance, in Karl Ludwig Kahlbaum's initial report on 'catatonia' (1874), clownishness, patheticism, or histrionic exaltation belong to the main manifestations, and this can also be found in Ewald Hecker's first description of 'hebephrenia' in 1871 [4]. Emil Kraepelin's introduced in his 1883 textbook the concept of 'dementia praecox', a term borrowed from Morel, and he stated that one fifth of the patients with that condition showed hysteriform attacks [34]. Later, when Eugen Bleuler introduced the group of schizophrenias in 1911, hysteria had become a mere adjective to qualify certain manifestations in specific conditions [35]. For the alienists, hysteria was now a 'free-floating symptomatological reaction that could develop with almost any physical or mental disorder', as a secondary psychological phenomenon [11]. The true renewal of interest in hysteria among mental disorders specialists developed in parallel with the work of Sigmund Freud, and with the launch of psychiatric private practices [5], while 19th-century alienism quickly disappeared from the scene during the first decades of the 20th century.

Other developments on hysteria remained isolated in the 19th century. In 1869, J. Russell Reynolds [36] (1828–1896) established a theory, according to which certain clinical manifestations were based on an 'idea, which should take possession of the mind and lead to its own fulfilment'. Over a century later, Hurwitz [37] would revive this theory of 'ideogenic neurologic deficits', with 'fixed beliefs of somatic dysfunction'.

Jules Bernard Luys was chief of a service at La Pitié, the adjoining hospital to La Salpêtrière, and he developed sessions with hysterics, which have often been compared to 'grand guignol' theatre [38], mainly because his 'Chef de Clinique' Gérard Encausse was also involved in secret occult ceremonies at night under the robes of 'Mage Papus'. The only contemporary of Charcot who developed a significantly original activity independently from his colleague (in fact prior to him) was Charles Lasègue (1816–1883), probably one of the brightest French physicians of the 19th century.

The name of Lasègue is of course associated with his 'sign' in lumbar root compression, although the written report was made by his assistant Forst in 1881 [39]. But Lasègue also developed an interesting activity in hysteria before and in parallel to that of Charcot: he was one of the first to emphasize the hysterical 'character' in 1881, and made the first description of hysterical anorexia in 8 cases in 1873 [40]. He also stated that 'hysteria borrows to the nervous system its pathological materials' [10]. Contrary to Charcot, he stated that hysteria could not be defined the same way as other diseases of the nervous system because it is associated with an infinity of manifestations, predicting that its future should be in mental medicine. His interest in hysteria preceded that of Charcot by 15 years, and between 1854 and 1864, he presented specific studies on hysterical cough, anesthesia, and ataxia [41, 42], which belonged to what Benjamin Brodie called 'local hysteria' in his 1837 lessons [8, p. 178]. Charcot and Lasègue officially cooperated at least once on hysteria when Fernand Espanet presented his doctorate thesis 'Hystericism and hysteria' on August 3, 1875, in front of Lasègue as chairman and Charcot as examiner [30]. Interestingly enough, when revising hysteria in the early 1900s, Joseph Babinski would quote Lasègue in parallel to a criticism of certain theories of his mentor Charcot. Contrary to his junior Charcot, Lasègue was a famous alienist, parallel to his neurological studies: he made the first report of 'persecution delirium' in 1851, and the first report of 'circular madness' with Jules Falret (the ancestor of bipolar disease) in 1854 and 'folie à deux' in 1877 [39]. In fact, Charles Lasègue certainly was one of the most brilliant physicians of the century. After philosophical studies and a teaching period at Louis-le-Grand College, where the poet Charles Baudelaire was one of his students, he switched to medicine and became a close friend of Claude Bernard, who introduced him to Falret, before he became 'Chef de Clinique' of Trousseau at Hôtel-Dieu. In 1853, the year when Charcot and Vulpian presented their doctorate thesis, he wrote his professorship thesis on general paresis [22]. In 1862 he was asked to deliver the first official series of faculty lectures on mental pathology, being appointed a full professor of general pathology in 1867, and Chairman of Clinical Medicine at La Pitié in 1869. He also became the first physician of the 'dépôt municipal des aliénés', which would become the celebrated unit of the 'infirmerie spéciale de la préfecture de police', where Ball, the future first holder of the chair for mental and brain diseases, worked for a time as his assistant.

Charcot's Hysteria after Charcot

Four main currents on hysteria came to light as a direct consequence of Charcot's work. The first one was just the continuation of his own studies, mainly with Gilles de la Tourette and Richer, who were often called the 'guardians of the temple'. By the way, it is likely that the devoted, often exaggerated, enthusiasm of these zealots contributed to the subsequent rejection of Charcot's ideas, as a counterreaction a few years after his death. The other developments were associated with three major figures in neuropsychiatry at the turn of the century, i.e. Pierre Janet (1859–1947), Sigmund Freud (1856–1939), and Joseph Babinski (1857–1932) – all of whom studied directly under Charcot. As their theories are specifically addressed in devoted chapters of this book, we will not discuss them here. We have also summarized them in a previous volume [42]. Another important follower of Charcot was Paul Sollier, who developed a neurophysiological approach to hysteria on the basis of the 'dynamic lesion' of Charcot [43], which put him into direct conflicts with his former colleague Babinski [44].

Charcot's concepts on hysteria are frequently presented as obsolete, usually on the basis of the 1908 sessions at the Société de Neurologie de Paris, which supposedly destroyed decades of Charcot's supremacy in a couple of days, with Charcot's former student Babinski leading the game [25]. This insistence is probably partly linked to Charcot's dominating personality, which would have explained why his 'erroneous ideas' would have been transformed for years into untouchable dogmas. However, in this perspective, only the early theories of Charcot are usually considered (ovary compression, the stigmatas), while the significant advances of the last part of his career, such as the emphasis on traumatic and mental factors, typically are not quoted. The detractors also borrow from Janet and Babinski the statement that Charcot's founding 'error' was to have started studying hysteria as if it were a condition similar to any organic disease [45]. However, this attitude in fact was the condition necessary for an unbiased scientific approach to a disorder, on which virtually nothing was known at the time (the uterine theory still had proponents). The criticisms also include the showy features of the hypnotism sessions at La Salpêtrière, and the easiness with which hysterical patients would have deceived the old man with staged fits and epidemics of 'grandes crises d'hystérie'.

With this perspective, Babinski typically is presented as the savior from obscure times, who swept away years of submission to the late dictator [42]. However, while Babinski indeed clarified the clinical criteria diagnosis, his own concepts on hysteria today seem rather retrograde and limited, with his reluctance to admit emotional factors, and his way to hide a lack of consideration of dynamic mental mechanisms behind fixed, rather primary, so-called 'psychological' factors (see Poirier and Derouesné [this vol., pp. 139–148]). In spite of the gross weaknesses of 'pithiatism', the longevity of Babinski's enterprise was clearly supported by the fact that neurologists saw here a very effective way to eliminate deeper psychological issues and to concentrate on overt clinical manifestations, on top of which the simplified Freudian concept of conversion of intrapsychic conflicts into somatic manifestations appeared as a sufficient psychological flavor. It is probable that Charcot's zealots, such as Gilles de la Tourette, indirectly also contributed to the need for destroying their mentor's image because of their intransigence to any step away from the 'doxa'. Charcot had well anticipated this risk at the time of the quarrel with the Nancy school: while Gilles de la Tourette proclaimed the supremacy of La Salpêtrière, Charcot was convinced that this 'victory' would harm advances on hysteria and hypnotism [33]. Actually, the dispute quickly became misinterpreted as Bernheim's defense of 'suggestion' against Charcot, while in fact Bernheim was negating the existence of hysteria itself. However, Charcot never contested 'suggestion', contrary to the common view that Bernheim, and Babinski 10 years later, had to contradict him on that issue in order to make their other points.

In this view, the survey of the evolving concepts of hysteria from the early years of the 19th century to the followers of Charcot and later demonstrate the astonishing modernity of many of Charcot's concepts, provided they are seen through the dynamic perspective of the evolution of emerging neurology and psychiatry. There are indeed several major examples of Charcot's precursory thinking in hysteria. Firstly, one should not forget that it was Charcot who launched a scientific interest in hysteria at a time when neurology did not exist, and when neither alienism nor medicine considered it as a field of study. Secondly, Charcot was the initiator of the traumatic theory lying behind hysteria, even emphasizing strong sexual factors 20 years before Freud. This issue also made him one of the earliest proponents of male hysteria. A recently discovered note by Charcot shows that he had a well-developed concept of the 'unconscious' in relation with past experiences and potential revivals of emotions [46]. Indeed, Charcot was the first to elaborate specifically on mental factors as critical determinants of hysteria and stimulated the early medical work of Janet on that topic by creating the first laboratory of experimental laboratory in a neurological service. Thirdly, several of the intuitive ideas of Charcot have in fact been confirmed by recent, modern imaging and neurophysiological studies [47, 48] (see LaFrance [this vol., pp. 198–204]). For instance, the concept of the 'dynamic lesion' is up to date with actual theories of brain functioning in normal and pathological situations. Interestingly enough, it is Paul Sollier, the brightest follower of Charcot on neurophysiological issues, who further elaborated on this issue, adding the concept of activation versus deactivation of different brain regions as the dynamic mechanism behind hysteria [49]. That concept has recently been validated by functional MRI studies [50], which have also shown that contrary to Babinski, Charcot was absolutely right to be firm in insisting that hysteria and simulation were two different conditions with different cerebral mechanisms [42]. Finally, one must underline that functional MRI studies have also confirmed one of Charcot's most cherished claims, i.e. the closeness of hypnotism with hysteria, the theory which had been the most vehemently criticized by Bernheim and his colleagues. Indeed, it was recently demonstrated that in hypnotic and hysterical palsy, the same preparatory activation takes place in the motor cortex, along with the same precuneus activation (a structure associated with self-related representations), while contrary to simulated palsy in instructed controls, there is no direct activation of the inhibitory frontal motor region [48]. Indeed, despite criticisms already made by direct followers, Charcot's work on hysteria certainly remains one of his major achievements.

Acknowledgement

Parts of this chapter have been adapted from [42].

References

1 Faulks S: Human Traces. London, Hutchinson, 2005.
2 Walusinski O, Poirier H, Déchy H: 'Augustine'. Eur Neurol 2013;69:226–228.
3 Rey A: Dictionnaire culturel en langue française. Paris, Dictionnaires Le Robert, 2005.
4 Ellenberger HF: À la découverte de l'inconscient. Histoire de la psychiatrie dynamique. Villeurbanne, Simep-Éditions, 1974.
5 Postel J, Quétel C: Nouvelle histoire de la psychiatrie. Paris, Privat, 1983.
6 Bogousslavsky J, Walusinski O, Moulin T: Alfred Vulpian and Jean-Martin Charcot in each other's shadow? From Castor and Pollux at La Salpêtrière to neurology forever. Eur Neurol 2011;65: 215–222.
7 Tatu L, Bogousslavsky J: The impossible succession of Charcot – the quest for a suitable heir. Eur Neurol 2011;65:193–197.
8 Goetz C, Bonduelle M, Gelfand T: Charcot. Constructing Neurology. New York, Oxford University Press, 1995.
9 Exposé des titres scientifiques du docteur J.-M. Charcot. Paris, Imprimerie Victor Goupy et Jourdan, 1883.
10 Cesbron H; Histoire critique de l'hystérie. Paris, Asselin et Houzeau, Libraires de la Faculté de Médecine, 1909.
11 Micale MS: On the 'disappearance' of hysteria. A study in the clinical deconstruction of a diagnosis. Isis 1993;84: 496–526.
12 Abricossof G: L'hystérie aux XVIIe et XVIIIe siècles. Étude historique et bibliographique. Paris, Steinheil, 1897.
13 Brachet JL : Traité de l'hystérie. Lyon, Savy Jeune, 1849.
14 Briquet P: Traité clinique et thérapeutique de l'hystérie. Paris, J.-B. Baillière & Fils, 1859.
15 Baudelaire C: Critique littéraire; in: Œuvres complètes. Paris, Bibliothèque de la Pléiade, NRF, Gallimard, 1976, vol 2, p 83.
16 Bogousslavsky J, Moulin T: From alienism to the birth of modern psychiatry: a neurological story? Eur Neurol 2009;62: 257–263.

17 Walusinski O: Jean-Martin Charcot's house officer at La Salpêtrière hospital; in Bogousslavsky J (ed): Following Charcot: A Forgotten History of Neurology and Psychiatry. Front Neurol Neurosci. Basel, Karger, 2011, vol 29, pp 9–35.
18 Iconographie photographique de la Salpêtrière, service de M. Charcot, par Bourneville et P. Regnard. Paris, Progrès Médical, V. Adrien Delahaye & Cie, 1877.
19 Hustvedt A: Medical Muses. Hysteria in Nineteenth Century in Paris. New York, WW Norton, 2011.
20 Richer P: Études clinique sur l'hystéro-épilepsie ou grande hystérie. Précédé d'une lettre-préface de M. le professeur J.-M. Charcot. Paris, Adrien Delahaye et Émile Lecrosnier, 1881.
21 Gilles de la Tourette G: Traité clinique et thérapeutique de l'hystérie d'après l'enseignement de la Salpêtrière. Paris, Librairie Plon, 1891 (vol 1), 1895 (vol 2, 3).
22 Lasègue C: Études médicales du professeur Ch. Lasègue. Paris, Asselin, 1884, vol 2.
23 Richet C: Le somnambulisme provoqué. Arch Physiol Norm Pathol 1875;11:348–378.
24 Bernheim H: Hypnotisme, suggestion, psychothérapie. Paris, Doin, 1891.
25 Laplane D, Bonduelle M: Le débat sur l'hystérie. Rev Neurol 1999;155:815–821.
26 Babinski J : Définition de l'hystérie. Rev Neurol 1901;9:1074–1080.
27 Breuer J, Freud S: Ueber den psychischen Mechanismus hysterischer Phänomene (vorläufige Mitteilung). Neurol Zentralbl 1893;12:4–10, 43–47.
28 Breuer J, Freud: Studien über Hysterie. Leipzig, Deuticke, 1895.
29 Charcot JM: La foi qui guérit. Revue Hebdomadaire 1892;5:112–132.
30 Espanet F: Hystéricisme et hystérie. Du sommeil hystérique en particulier. Paris, A. Parent imprimeur de la Faculté de Médecine, 1875.
31 Janet P: Les accidents mentaux des hystériques. Paris, Faculté de Médecine, 1893.
32 Guillain G: J.-M. Charcot, 1825–1893, sa vie, son œuvre. Paris, Masson & Cie, 1955.
33 Bogousslavsky J, Walusinski O, Veyrunes D: Crime, hysteria and Belle Époque hypnotism: the path traced by Jean-Martin Charcot and Georges Gilles de la Tourette. Eur Neurol 2009;62:193–199.
34 Kraepelin E: Compendium des Psychiatrie, zum Gebrauche zum Studierende und Aerzte. Leipzig, Abel, 1883.
35 Bleuler F: Dementia Praecox; oder, Gruppe der Schizophrenien. Leipzig, F. Deuticke, 1911.
36 Reynolds JR: Certain forms of paralysis depending on idea. Remarks on paralysis and other disorders of motion and sensation dependent on idea. BMJ, October 2, 1869, pp 378–379, November 6, 1869, 483–485.
37 Hurwitz T: Ideogenic neurological deficits, conscious mechanisms in conversion symptoms. Neuropsychiat Neuropsychol Behav Neurol 1988;1:301–308.
38 Parent A, Parent M, Leroux-Hugon V: Jules Bernard Luys: a singular figure of 19th century neurology. Can J Neurol Sci 2002;29:282–288.
39 Lasègue C: Écrits psychiatriques. Paris, Privat, 1971.
40 Lasègue C: Anorexie hystérique. Arch Gén Méd 1873;avril/Études Médicales, t.II: 45.
41 Lasègue C: De la toux hystérique. Arch Gén Méd, May 1854, pp 513.
42 Bogousslavsky J: Hysteria after Charcot: back to the future; in Bogousslavsky J (ed): Following Charcot: A Forgotten History of Neurology and Psychiatry. Front Neurol Neurosci, Basel, Karger, 2011, vol 29, pp 137–161.
43 Bogousslavsky J, Walusinski O: Paul Sollier: the first clinical neuropsychologist; in Bogousslavsky J (ed): Following Charcot: A Forgotten History of Neurology and Psychiatry. Front Neurol Neurosci. Basel, Karger, 2011, vol 29, pp 105–114.
44 Babinski J: Quelques remarques sur l'article de M. Sollier intitulé 'La définition et la nature de l'hystérie'. Extrait des Archives Générales de Médecine, mars 1907.
45 Derouesné C: Pithiatism versus Hysteria; in Philippon J, Poirier J (eds): Joseph Babinski, a Biography. Oxford, Oxford University Press, 2009, pp 297–319.
46 Bouchara C, Mazet P, Cohen D: Jean Martin Charcot, 1825–1893: did he anticipate Freud's first topology? Am J Psychiat 2010;167:387.
47 Cojan Y, Waber L, Carruzzo A, Vuilleumier P: Motor inhibition in hysterical conversion paralysis. Neuroimage 2009; 47:1026–1037.
48 Cojan Y, Waber L, Schwart S, Rossier L, Forster A, Vuilleumier P: The brain under self-control: modulation of inhibitory and monitoring cortical networks during hypnotic paralysis. Neuron 2009; 62:862–875.
49 Sollier P: L'hystérie et son traitement. Paris, Alcan, 1901.
50 Vuilleumier P: Hysterical conversion and brain function. Prog Brain Res 2005;150:309–329.

Julien Bogousslavsky, MD
Center for Brain and Nervous System Diseases
GSMN Neurocenter, Clinique Valmont
CH–1823 Glion/Montreux (Switzerland)
E-Mail jbogousslavsky@cliniquevalmont.ch

Bogousslavsky J (ed): Hysteria: The Rise of an Enigma. Front Neurol Neurosci. Basel, Karger, 2014, vol 35, pp 56–64
DOI: 10.1159/000359992

Hypnosis and the Nancy Quarrel

Bartlomiej Piechowski-Jozwiak[a, b] · Julien Bogousslavsky[c]

[a]Department of Neurology, King's College Hospital, London, UK; [b]Department of Neurology, The Medical University of Warsaw, Warsaw, Poland; [c]Center for Brain and Nervous Diseases, GSMN Neurocenter, Clinique Valmont, Glion/Montreux, Switzerland

Abstract

The theme of hysteria and hypnotism has been attracting the attention of medics, psychologists, writers, and the broad lay public. The role of hypnotism in the context of societal functioning, especially in crime, was a subject of research and significant debates between different neurology and psychology schools. One of these debates was between the Nancy and Salpêtrière schools of neurology at the end of the 19th century, and it was focused around a few cases of crime committed allegedly under hypnosis. In order to understand this particular quarrel, this chapter examines the history of mesmerism, hysteria, hypnosis, and fin-de-siècle neurology represented by both the Nancy and Salpêtrière schools.

The theme of hysteria and hypnotism has been attracting attention of medics, psychologists, writers, film makers, and the broad lay public. The role of hypnotism in the context of societal functioning especially in crime was a subject of research and significant debates between different neurology and psychology schools. One of these debates was between the Nancy and Salpêtrière schools of neurology at the end of 19th century [1]. In order to understand this particular quarrel, however, we may need to look at the history of mesmerism, hysteria, hypnosis, and fin-de-siècle neurology.

Before starting historical analysis of the link between mesmerism, hysteria, and hypnosis, it is important to acknowledge the current definition of the latter two. Hysteria and hypnosis have been defined differently by various authors. Contemporary dictionaries define both of these conditions as follows. Hysteria is a mental disorder characterized by emotional outbursts, susceptibility to autosuggestion, and, often, symptoms such as paralysis that mimic the effects of physical disorders. It can also be any frenzied emotional state, especially of laughter or crying [2]. Hypnosis is defined as an artificially induced state of relaxation and concentration in which deeper parts of the mind become more accessible; it is used clinically to reduce reaction to pain and encourage free association [2].

Mesmerism and Hypnosis

The influence of invisible forces like solar and lunar emanations on human behavior has been known since antiquity and the works of Aristotle, Ptolemy, and Galen [1]. The role of mechanical, chemical, and mathematical systems has been studied by the English physician Richard Mead (1673–1754) and James Gibbs (died 1724). These were the precursors of mesmerism. They regarded the body as a material mechanism ruled by the laws of matter alone. This was a concept of a human body functioning as a cartesian machine, in which physiological phenomena could be explained in terms of physics [3]. Mead's teacher, Archibald Pitcairne (1652–1713), developed a theory of 'hydraulic iatromechanism' in which the human body was conceptualized as a series of canals in which fluids circulated. In his work entitled *A Treatise Concerning the Influence of the Sun and Moon on Human Bodies and the Diseases Thereby Produced*, Mead applied Newton's gravitational theories to Pitcairne's hydraulic iatromechanism [4, 5]. He linked the influence of the gravitational effects of the sun and moon, such as the tides, on the pressure of vessels and fluids within the human body.

Franz Anton Mesmer (1734–1815), a German physician with an interest in astronomy, developed this idea further. He hypothesized the existence of a force or 'a universal fluid' present in animal and human bodies as well as filling the cosmos and all matter. He considered this fluid as a source of life and life force. This universal principle was a link between humans and the universe, which he named animal magnetism ('magnétisme animal') [6]. According to Mesmer, some people had the quality of using this principle as a base for therapeutic actions as they were able to direct their vital fluids in order to heal others [7]. These concepts were adopted into occult and medical practices. The subjects exposed had symptoms ranging from vomiting to convulsions, which was also known as 'crises'. The latter were to remove obstructions in the circulatory system that were causing sicknesses [8]. Mesmer propagated his theory in practice and moved to Paris and started treating the French aristocracy with his magnetic cures. He would have his patients surround an enclosed wooden tub with iron wands protruding from it. The patients would then hold the wands and bring them into contact with their afflicted parts. In this way, the animal magnetism would flow from the wooden tub through the wands to the patient. His patients were convinced that this healed them, and some even went into hysteric spasms or would pass out [9]. However, he was challenged by the French medical community. The French king called for a Board of Inquiry, which included, among others, Benjamin Franklin (US ambassador to France and an expert in electricity/magnetism), Jean Bailly (an astronomer), Antoine-Laurent de Jussieu (professor of botany), and Joseph Guillotin (the inventor of the guillotine). Mesmer decided not to be a part of this controlled experiment. Dr. Charles d'Eslon, Mesmer's collaborator, led the trials. The members of the commission underwent treatment themselves, but none of them felt any sensation. In one of the trials, d'Eslon magnetized a tree hoping that a susceptible and preselected patient would be affected by touching it. The patient was brought before four trees with the eyes covered, and was instructed to embrace them. Apparently each tree affected him and before he got to the fourth tree he fell into a crisis that resulted in fainting. During this time, d'Eslon was 'mesmerizing' a fifth tree. After a series of similar blindfolded trials, the Board concluded that mesmerism worked only by the action of the imagination [9]. During the French Revolution in the late 18th century, mesmerism was abandoned and forgotten.

A Goan Catholic monk, Abbé Faria (1756–1819), revived the notion of animal magnetism and started promoting a new doctrine of 'oriental' hypnosis in the early 19th century in Paris after leaving India. His approach was based on the practices of Sannyasa, Sadhus, Fakirs, and Yogis. This was based on self-hypnosis triggered by practicing rhythmic breathing exercises and meditation [10]. Faria's thinking went away from Mesmer's theory of magnetic fluid. He also dethroned the idea of the importance of the magnetizer, believing in the existence of autosuggestion instead. He postulated that everything came from the subject and took place in the subject's mind. The principle of hypnosis was based on the hypnotic subject's expectancy, cooperation, and ability to concentrate. Mesmeric magnetism was considered by Faria only as a form of sleep. According to Faria's theory, the operator was merely 'the concentrator' and somnambulism was viewed as lucid sleep [11].

Marquis de Puységur (Amand-Marie-Jacques de Chastenet, 1751–1825) was a French aristocrat and artillery officer with an interest in physics, and is considered to be one of the great forgotten contributors to the history of the psychological sciences and a founder of hypnotic induction [12]. He had his own 'cabinet de physique' in his majestic castle where he experimented with electricity. After being introduced to mesmerism by his brother Antoine-Hyacinthe, he started his own mesmeric practice. One of his most important patients was a young peasant, Victor Race, who was suffering from a mild respiratory disease. Race was easily magnetized and fell into a strange kind of trance in which he seemed to be more awake and aware than normal. He seemed to be far brighter than normal. Puységur tried the same on several other subjects, who once in that state were able to self-diagnose, foresee the course of disease evolution, and prescribe the treatments. Puységur observed the similarity between this sleeping trance and somnambulism, and he coined the term 'artificial somnambulism'. Puységur's practice blossomed and he started lecturing to the Masonic Society. During one of these lectures, he presented his view on the animal magnetism the following way [12]:

> I believe in the existence within myself of a power. From this belief derives my will to exert it. The entire doctrine of Animal Magnetism is contained in the two words: believe and want. I believe that I have the power to set into action the vital principle of my fellowmen; I want to make use of it; this is all my science and all my means. Believe and want, Sirs, and you will do as much as I.

He established an institute for training animal magnetism, Société Harmonique des Amis Réunis, which functioned until the French Revolution. The aim of it was to train magnetizers and to set up centers for magnetic treatment. After the revolution, Puységur was considered a patriarch of mesmerism and a founder of the method of inducing a sleeping trance, which differed from Mesmer's practices [12].

At the end of the 18th century, the young Mesmerist movement started slowly developing along new lines and spread in France and Germany. However, the spread of mesmerism outside these countries was slow. The brakethrough came in 1841 when the Scottish surgeon James Braid (1795–1860), after becoming impressed and convinced by demonstrations given by the French magnetizer Charles Lafontaine, gave a series of lectures in Manchester. However, instead of talking about 'magnetism', he used the more suitable term 'hypnotism', which made it more acceptable to certain medical circles. Braid opposed the theory of animal magnetism and the existence of paranormal powers such as telepathy. He also discarded the fluid theory, suggesting instead one based on brain physiology. As a result, he came to be considered the first true hypnotist as opposed to the Mesmerists. In his practice he adapted Faria's and Bertrand's old technique of fixating the hand by fixating a luminous object. Braid hypothesized that protracted ocular fixation fatigued certain parts of the brain and caused a trance compatible with a nervous sleep ('neurohypnosis'). Mesmerism later spread to Scotland and also became active in the USA, and eventually grew in intensity back in France in Nancy and Salpêtrière [12].

Nancy School

Ambroise-Auguste Liébeault (1823–1904), a French general physician, developed Faria's concepts further. This was a brave approach as in the second half of the 19th century hypnotism and magnetism were excluded from the accepted medical activities and he was conducting public hypnosis sessions. Liébeault's interest in hypnosis started during his undergraduate studies. As a medical student he found a book on magnetism and managed to magnetize a few patients [12]. Later on, Liébeault studied mental suggestion, clairvoyance, mediumship, and even poltergeists. He considered hypnosis as a normal phenomenon induced by suggestion, in contrast to others linking it to magnetism, hysteria, or psychophysiological phenomenon. He developed the concept of the overlap between hypnosis and potential of the mind and its subconscious activity [13]. Liébeault claimed that hypnotic sleep was identical to natural sleep. The hypnotic state significantly amplified the efficacy of the suggestions. He emphasized the importance of in-depth cooperation between the operator/hypnotizer and the subject (rapport). The proper rapport was facilitating the quality of suggestibility according to his hypothesis. Liébeault's methodology was based on delivering a sequence of suggestions using a monotonous but penetrating tone. The messages conveyed reassured the patient about the bodily functions [14]. Liébeault was an outcast in a rural area. His methods were criticized by the medical society, which considered him a fraudster since he was offering his services for free [12]. However, there was such a growing demand in society for magnetism that the number of patients treated by Liébeault grew very rapidly.

The rumors surrounding Liébeault's practices and spectacular results led to Hippolyte Bernheim (1840–1919), a renowned French physician, contacting him and later becoming his admirer and friend. Bernheim had an established reputation through his work on typhoid fever and heart and lung disease. He had left his position at the University of Strasbourg and was appointed a tenured professor of internal medicine in Nancy [12]. Bernheim was very skeptical of Liébeault's practices and questioned his clinical results. However, he joined Liébeault and they shared clinical and research activities. Together they treated more than 30,000 patients using suggestions under hypnosis.

Bernheim found higher rates of success in people from lower social classes such as factory workers and soldiers. Of note is the fact that these groups were accustomed to obeying orders and commands. He was not that successful with educated and wealthy subjects. He used hypnosis to treat patients with gastrointestinal, rheumatoid, and neurological disorders. In 1886, Bernheim published his book, which made him a leader of the Nancy school, in which he stated that hypnosis was not a pathological condition only found in hysterics, but an effect of suggestion. According to Bernheim, hypnosis was a stage of enforced suggestibility that was induced by suggestion. Bernheim defined the suggestibility as 'the aptitude to transform idea into an act'. He felt this was a natural property of every individual to some extent. Just before this publication, Charcot presented his paper on hypnotism at the Academy of Sciences. The two sides of interpretation of hypnosis met publically for the first time and was the starting point for an ongoing quarrel between the two schools [12].

Over time, however, Bernheim started using suggestion in a waking state – 'suggestion à l'état de veille' – and this later gave grounds for a new method of treatment called 'psychotherapeutics'. The other French collaborators from the Nancy school that require mentioning are physiologist and psychologist Henri-Étienne Beaunis (1830–1920) and legal expert Jules Liégeois. Beaunis and Liégeois were involved in the medicolegal aspects of suggestion and its implication in crime and legal responsibility. Due to his only general medical background, Bernheim was not able to create strong research and clinical foundations for the Nancy school to be more influential in the psychiatry and neurology societies. In this respect, the Nancy school should be viewed as a loose group of psychiatrists who adopted Bernheim's methods [12]. Two German physicians, sexologist Albert Moll and Albert von Schrenck-Notzing, were among Bernheim's followers. The latter devoted his MD thesis to the therapeutic application of hypnotism, in which he reported the cure of one of Jean-Martin Charcot's patients from chorea minor [15]. Richard Freiherr von Krafft-Ebing, an Austro-German neurologist psychologist and forensic specialist, was also among the Nancy school followers. He was the founder of the theory of 'masochism' based on Leopold von Sacher-Masoch's novel 'Venus im Pelz' [16].

Other prominent physicians of that time were also among the Nancy school followers. Auguste Forel (1848–1931), a Swiss psychiatrist, neurologist, and professor of psychiatry in Zurich, gained his experience in hypnosis from Bernheim. He was successful in using hypnosis in clinical practice to treat physical disorders. Of note is the fact that he used hypnosis in managing his hospital as he would hypnotize his personnel into a vigil state in order to improve their surveillance of agitated patients [12]. Last but not least is Sigmund Freud who visited Bernheim and Liébeault at Nancy many times. The main scope of their discussions was posthypnotic amnesia, which according to Bernheim could be overcome by skillful questioning and concentration [12].

Salpêtrière School

Victor Alphonse Amédée Dumontpallier (1826–1899) was a French physician. He started working at the Hôtel Dieu and later moved to the de la Pité Hospital. He was interested in hypnosis, mineral magnetism, and metalloscopy. He studied the effects of metal in hysteria. He was one of the founders of hypnosis of the Salpêtrière school and Charcot's teacher. He described the phenomenon of bilateral hallucinations and opposing expressions. He was able to demonstrate this on one of his patients under hypnosis, who showed expressions of joy on one side of her face and despair. This became an inspiration for his followers including Charcot [15].

Jean-Martin Charcot (1825–1923) and his followers are discussed extensively in other chapters of this book. Charcot was a precursor of modern neurology and psychiatry [1, 16]. Amongst his collaborators were Victor Cornil, Charles Bouchard, Charles Samson Féré, Paul Richer, Fulgence Raymond, Pierre Marie, Henri Mege, Joseph Babinski, Paul Sollier, and Georges Gilles de la Tourette. The latter was Charcot's student and later started working as an intern and advanced to the position of 'Chef de Clinique' and eventually to Charcot's personal secretary [1]. Charcot's interest in hysteria developed after he took over Delasiauve's service, which was a place for hysterics and epileptics. Charcot defined hysteria as a state of neurosis with an organic basis, but without demonstrable brain abnormality. He explained this as a 'dynamic lesion' of the brain causing, among the other permanent clinical symptoms, sensory dysfunction, hyperexcitability, and visual field defects. The other way hysteria manifested clinically was through paroxysmal fits ('grandes crises d'hystérie'). Charcot emphasized the importance of the 'dynamic lesion' as the organic etiology of hysteria with a lack of brain anatomical abnormalities [1]. Charcot was able to reproduce experimentally through hypnotism hysterical conditions including hysterical mutism, amnesia, coxalgia, etc. [12].

Charcot's approach evolved over time as he started recognizing trauma as a trigger and a mental representation, after a prolonged latency period, of hysteria [1]. Charcot had been using hypnosis in the management of hysterics since 1878. According to Charcot, the ability to be

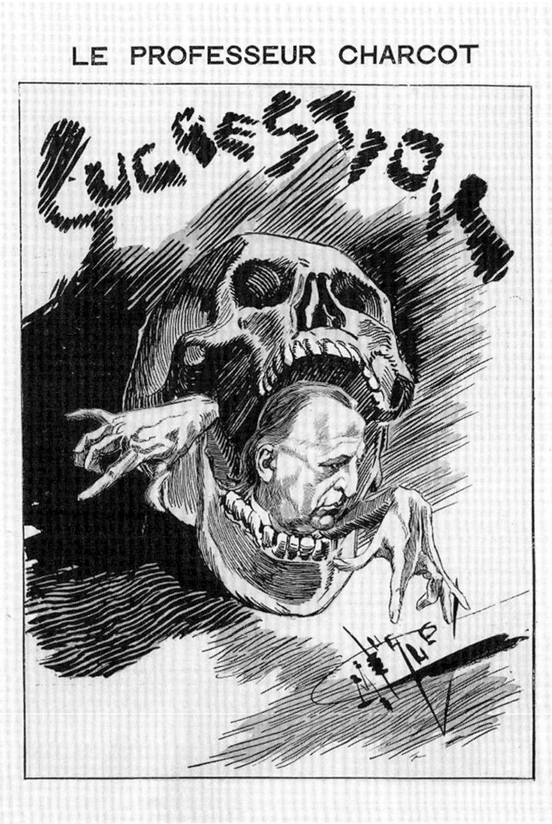

Fig. 1. Sketch of Jean-Martin Charcot at the time when hypnotic suggestion and 'mesmerization' were becoming highly popular in the public (with permission) [1].

hypnotized was a clinical feature of hysteria. He and his followers repeatedly used this phenomenon in front of the intellectual and lay public (fig. 1).

Susceptibility to hypnotism was considered synonymous with hysteria according to the Salpêtrière school. After confrontation with the Nancy school, however, this changed into dichotomized perception of hypnosis as a 'grand hypnotisme' in hysterics and a 'petit hypnotisme' in ordinary people [1]. The controversies between the Salpêtrière and Nancy schools started after a series of medicolegal cases in which the question of whether hypnosis could or could not influence people to commit crime was raised.

The Quarrel

It is important to highlight the role of Gilles de la Tourette (1857–1904) in the representation of the Salpêtrière school in these medicolegal aspects. Gilles de la Tourette's interest in this domain started after the training he had with Paul Camille Hippolyte Brouardel (1837–1906), a French pathologist, hygienist, and member of the Académie Nationale de Médecine. Brouardel became a professor of forensic medicine at the Faculté de Médecine de Paris and coauthored a book together with Charcot on the medicolegal aspects of hypnotism. Gilles de la Tourette had a strong view on the necessity of sentencing mentally disturbed criminals to asylums rather than sending them to prisons. This view was a very important part of the quarrel between the Nancy and Salpêtrière schools [1].

In 1887 Gilles de la Tourette published his book on the medicolegal aspects of hypnotism. He dedicated his work to Brouardel and Charcot [1, 17]. Gilles de la Tourette differentiated three states typical for 'grand hypnotisme': lethargy, catalepsy, and somnambulism. He also recognized initial states such as lucid lethargy, fascination, and charm states [1]. He stated that hypnotized individuals, he called them 'automatons', were in a conscious state and hence unable to perform acts that were against their inner beliefs. On the other hand, he postulated that hypnotized individuals, while in the lethargic state, could be submitted to rape. The latter would be possible due to muscle relaxation that would render the victim helpless against the perpetrator [1]. Gilles de la Tourette criticized Bernheim and Liégeois from the Nancy school for their assumptions that some crimes could have been committed by innocent individuals who were subjects to malevolent hypnosis. Gilles de la Tourette criticized the esoteric practices of hypnosis and he was a strong believer of reserving hypnosis for selected patients, especially hysterics [1].

In 1888 there was a major public debate on the case of Henri Chambige, a 22-year-old man arrested in Sidi-Mabrouk in Algeria for murdering a respected married woman, Madame Grille, in 1886 ('affaire Chambige'). During his trial, Chambige claimed that he and Madame Grille had a double-suicide pact. He was found injured beside the naked corpse of Madame Grille. He claimed he botched his suicide after killing Madame Grille [18]. The Nancy school approach represented by Bernheim argued that Madame Grille had been a subject of hypnosis and she had later been raped and killed by Chambige, who later tried to commit suicide. The controversy arose after Jean-Gabriel de Tarde, French sociologist and criminologist, claimed 'this is love, which is hypnosis'. Two years later Charcot published his article on hypnotism and crime in which he claimed that rape was the only crime that could be associated with hypnosis [1].

Gouffé's Trunk

The controversy between the Nancy and Salpêtrière schools flared up following a case of Toussaint-Augustin Gouffé's murder. Michel Eyraud and Gabrielle Bompard were accused of murder. The story is that Bompard lured Gouffé, who was a bailiff, to her place and she made him sit on a chaise longue. Behind it Eyraud was hidden with a hanging system he could operate remotely. During the foreplay, Bompard sat on the knees of Gouffé and pretended this was a part of the preliminaries as she put a belt of her peignoir around his neck and attached it to Eyraud's trap. The latter pulled the rope attached to it from behind the curtain, which in turn strangled Gouffé, who died soon after. The murder was a flop as no money could be found on the bailiff or at his office. Both Eyraud and Bompard left Paris and headed to Lyon with Gouffé's body hidden in a huge trunk. Both murderers abandoned the body and destroyed the trunk. A long investigation led to Bompard turning herself in to the police. Eyraud was subsequently arrested [1]. This crime was of great public interest and it made the news headlines in Europe and North America (fig. 2) [19].

After the arrest, the investigators observed childish, inappropriate, indifferent, and seductive behavior from Bompard. Her attorney alleged that she must have been hypnotized by Eyraud in the planning of the murder. This hypothesis was supported by the Nancy school. In addition to this, Bompard was successfully hypnotized several times in jail. Bernheim was unable to attend the trial and Liégeois replaced him. Liégeois was known for his own experiments of suggested murder with the use of fake weapons provoked by hypnotism. These arguments were counterattacked by the Salpêtrière team including Brouardel, Ballet, and Motet. They all claimed that no crime, particularly murder, could be committed under hypnosis. They considered Bompard being sane when committing this crime and that she lacked moral sense. The outcome of this trial was that Eyraud was sentenced to death and guillotined, while Bompard was sent to prison for 20 years. As a summary of this famous trial, Gilles de la Tourette published a famous epilogue in which he criticized Liégeois for his hypnotic experiments of murders committed with fake weapons and triggered by hypnosis [1].

The interesting point is that Gilles de la Tourette himself was conducting experiments with fake weapons and murder at Salpêtrière, which he documented in his book [17]. There was one case of a hysteric patient who was told under hypnosis to shoot a doctor after coming out of the hypnotic state. The reasoning for her to do so was that she was not treated well by him. She was given a ruler and she was led to believe it was a real gun. After she was awakened from her somnambulic state, she refused to give the ruler back and threatened to kill anyone who tried to take it away from her. When the 'targeted' doctor came, she waited until he was close enough and 'shot him' [1, 17].

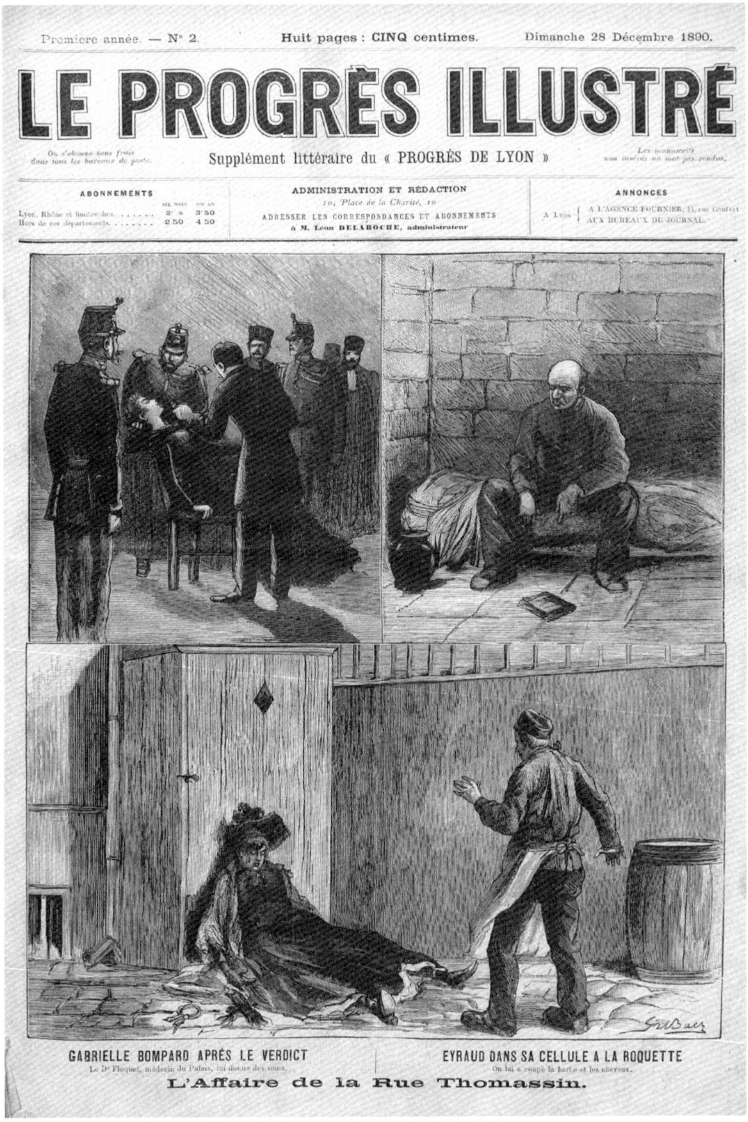
Première année. — N° 2. Huit pages : CINQ centimes. Dimanche 28 Décembre 1890.

LE PROGRÈS ILLUSTRÉ

On s'abonne sans frais dans tous les bureaux de poste.

Supplément littéraire du « PROGRÈS DE LYON »

Les manuscrits non insérés ne sont pas rendus.

ABONNEMENTS

	SIX MOIS	UN AN
Lyon, Rhône et limitrophes	2' »	3'50
Hors de ces départements	2 50	4 50

ADMINISTRATION ET RÉDACTION
10, Place de la Charité, 10
ADRESSER LES CORRESPONDANCES ET ABONNEMENTS
à M. Léon DELAROCHE, administrateur

ANNONCES
A Lyon { A L'AGENCE FOURNIER, 11, rue Confort
AUX BUREAUX DU JOURNAL.

GABRIELLE BOMPARD APRÈS LE VERDICT
Le Dr Floquet, médecin du Palais, lui donne des soins.

EYRAUD DANS SA CELLULE A LA ROQUETTE
On lui a coupé la barbe et les cheveux.

L'Affaire de la Rue Thomassin.

Fig. 2. Page of the newspaper *Le Progrès Illustré* showing Gabrielle Bompard and Michel Eyraud during 'Gouffé's trunk' case trial.

The atmosphere around hypnotism in the Belle Époque was so tense that it could have been cut with a knife. In light of this, Gilles de la Tourette became a victim of a crime related to hypnotism. His patient Rose Kamper-Lecoq came asking him for money and she claimed she was bankrupt because of hypnosis sessions which had altered her will. Gilles de la Tourette refused to give her any money and she shot him in the head. Luckily the shot was superficial and he survived it. Eventually, this patient was found to be paranoid as she claimed that Gilles de la Tourette was in love with her and that through hypnosis he transformed her by annihilating her will in a way that she would eventually kill him. She had delusions of communicating with the czar. She was eventually hospitalized in a mental unit and the association of hypnosis and the assault was finally discarded [1].

In summary, it is important to acknowledge the different opinions on hypnosis between the Nancy and Salpêtrière schools. Both originated from mesmerism and the works of Abbé Faria. The Nancy school claimed that hypnosis was the effect of suggestion. The Salpêtrière school claimed that hysteria and hypnosis were close conditions; however, subjects are unable to commit crime under hypnosis. The controversy between these two schools affected medical, legal, and public in the Belle Époque.

References

1 Bougousslavsky J, Walusinski O, Veyrunes D: Crime, hysteria and belle époque hypnotism: the path traced by Jean-Martin Charcot and Georges Gilles de la Tourette. Eur Neurol 2009;62:193–199.

2 Collins English Dictionary – Complete and Unabridged. London, HarperCollins Publishers, 2003.

3 Roos AM: Luminaries in medicine: Richard Mead, James Gibbs, and solar and lunar effects on the human body in early modern England. Bull Hist Med 2000;74:433–457.

4 Mead R: A Treatise Concerning the Influence of the Sun and Moon on Human Bodies and the Diseases Thereby Produced. London, Brindley, 1748.

5 Jones R: Richard Mead, Thomas Guy, the South Sea Bubble and the founding of Guy's Hospital. J R Soc Med 2010;103:87–92.

6 Mesmer FA: Dissertatio physico-medica de planetarum influxu, Vienna, Ghelen, 1766.

7 Wolfart C, Mesmer FA: Mesmerismus: Oder, System der Wechselwirkungen, Theorie und Anwendung des thierischen Magnetismus als die allgemeine Heilkunde zur Erhaltung des Menschen. Cambridge, Cambridge University Press, 2011.

8 Deleuze JPF: Practical Instruction in Animal Magnetism. London, Hippolyte Bailliere, 1850.

9 Best M, Neuhauser D, Slavin L: Evaluating Mesmerism, Paris, 1784: the controversy over the blinded placebo controlled trials has not stopped. Qual Saf Health Care 2003;12:232–233.

10 McGill O: Hypnotism and Mysticism of India. Glendale, Westwood Publishing Company, 1979.

11 Vas LSR: Abbé Faria: The Life of a Pioneer Indian Hypnotist and His Impact on Hypnotism. Panjim, Broadway Book Centre, 2007.

12 Ellenberger HF: The Discovery of the Unconscious: The History and Evolution of Dynamic Psychiatry. New York, Basic Books, 1970.

13 Alvarado CS: Ambroise August Liébeault and psychic phenomena. Am J Clin Hypn 2009;52:111–121.

14 Liebeault AA: Du sommeil et des états analogues considérés surtout au point de vue de l'action du moral sur le physique. Paris, Masson, 1866.

15 Sommer A: Policing epistemic deviance: Albert von Schrenck-Notzing and Albert Moll. Med Hist 2012;56:255–276.

16 Oosterhuis H: Sexual modernity in the works of Richard von Krafft-Ebing and Albert Moll. Med Hist 2012;56:133–155.

17 Harrington A: Metals and magnets in medicine: hysteria, hypnosis and medical culture in fin-de-siècle Paris. Psychol Med 1988;18:21–38.

18 Bogousslavsky J, Boller F: Jean-Martin Charcot and art: relationship of the 'founder of neurology' with various aspects of art. Prog Brain Res 2013;203:185–199.

19 Gilles de la Tourette G: L'hypnotisme et les états analogues au point de vue médico-légal. Paris, Librairie Plon, 1887.

Bartlomiej Piechowski-Jozwiak, MD
Consultant Stroke Neurologist
Department of Neurology, King's College Hospital
Denmark Hill, London SE5 9RS (UK)
E-Mail bartlomiejpj@gmail.com

Bogousslavsky J (ed): Hysteria: The Rise of an Enigma. Front Neurol Neurosci. Basel, Karger, 2014, vol 35, pp 65–77
DOI: 10.1159/000359993

The Girls of La Salpêtrière

Olivier Walusinski
Family Physician, Private Practice, Brou, France

Abstract

It was only by chance that French hospital authorities assigned Jean-Martin Charcot to the care of hysterics and epileptics, starting in 1870, at La Salpêtrière Hospital. The famous clinical work that resulted has been the subject of much discussion and, in many cases, misinterpretation. By referring to original sources, i.e. the medical observations written at the time by the department's staff, our aim is to bring the hospitalized patients to life. Many of these observations contain intimate details and reveal the painful experiences that led these young women to La Salpêtrière. To understand the gradual, 20-year evolution of Charcot's neurological thinking about hysteria, from organicity to psychology, in both clinical and therapeutic terms, it is more revealing to analyze all the physical and psychological miseries that make up this forgotten 'human material' than it is to examine the neurologist's famous lessons.

With the passage of time, Jean-Martin Charcot (1825–1893) and his work on hysteria have left only a distant, muffled echo in the minds of the general public. Medical historians in the 20th century focused on Charcot's concepts, often ridiculing them and taking greater interest in Freud. They rarely paid attention to his patients, who were mostly hospitalized women, since La Salpêtrière Hospital only treated women. To understand Charcot's conceptual changes and their gradual sedimentation in his thinking, we have retraced the lives of his patients to give some sense of the women Charcot examined in his department. This new perspective will help explain how Charcot developed the semiology of hysteria that made him famous, and also why he eventually evoked the role of emotions and trauma in the pathogenesis of the disease.

Imagine rows of several dozen beds, some closed off with curtains to hide the 'reposantes', prostrate patients who were often incurable. Heating during the winter was inadequate, provided by only a few stoves. Visitors were suffocated by pestilential odors. Charcot took particular care that the patients were correctly fed, meeting regularly with the cooks to discuss the menus. A few hospital gowns were provided, but detergent was at the expense of each patient. After an attack, if the patient had soiled herself, she was given a tub of lukewarm water, while the others knelt to scrub the floor. If they were lucky, the 'surveillante' might give them a piece of candy or a ribbon to decorate their beds. Some of the patients conspired with groundskeepers to plant vegetables between the bushes in the surrounding gardens. Ties were surreptitiously formed, and despite the close quarters, discreet relationships resulted in quasihouseholds [1]. But who were these women?

Abandonment, Violence, and Death

The women of La Salpêtrière were very young, ranging in age from 15 to 30 years when they entered the hospital. The typical patient was the eldest of a large number of children (5–12). In spite of herself and very early on, she became a substitute mother and had to witness little brothers and sisters dying from convulsions and fevers. She was thus familiar with death before adulthood. 'Of the seven children from the first marriage, only Marc... Célina survived. The others died as infants from convulsions. Of the eight children from the second marriage, two survived' [2]. Paternal violence, aggravated by alcoholism, destroyed family structure. Many of the patients were illegitimate children and bounced between religious institutions where spartan discipline, rather than affection, was the rule: 'Geneviève was born in Loudun on 2 January 1843 and immediately abandoned at the local hospice' [2]. Few of the patients had been to school or knew how to read and write. Their parents were unemployed or poor, and they themselves sought work as laundresses (the most scorned occupation at the time), linen maids, house servants, or florists (fig. 1, 2).

The Misery of Being a Woman

Accustomed only to the most extreme poverty, these women accepted miserable, cramped housing. Very often, their employers would come to harass them, demanding sexual favors. Eventually submitting in many cases, these women fled from shame into even greater misery. They carried the burden of guilt at a time when sexuality outside marriage was considered a sign of perversity and lewdness.

V.C., admitted on May 13, 1877 at the age of 24, recounted how 'a man supposedly made her drink an unknown liquid (or one she does not wish to name), then took advantage of her while she slept (fig. 1). This occurred on different occasions, more or less violently' [3]. Louise Augustine Gleizes, born on August 21, 1861 and admitted on October 21, 1875 to La Salpêtrière, 'is our patient whose plastic poses and passionate attitudes have the most regularity' says Paul Richer (1849–1933) [4, 5]. Due to her youth, fair skin, expressive face, and theatrical attacks, she was the hysteric who Paul Regnard (1850–1927) photographed the most ('the camera likes her'; fig. 3).

> 'L. was placed with C. supposedly to learn to sing, sew, etc., with his own children. She slept in a small, isolated closet. C., who was estranged from his wife, used her absences to try to take advantage of L., aged 13 and a half. His first attempt failed; he wanted to have her lie down under him. His second attempt ended with incomplete intercourse, due to her resistance. For his third attempt, C... tried to lure her with all sorts of promises, pretty dresses, etc. Seeing she did not want to give in, he threatened her with a razor, took advantage of her fear and made her drink alcohol. He then undressed her, threw her on the bed and had complete intercourse with her. The following day, L. was ill. She had lost a little blood, felt pain in her genitals and could not walk' [3].

Justine Etchevery suffered from a permanent hysterical contracture that set in after a hystero-epileptic attack in 1869. The attack took place as she was convalescing from severe burns. She had fallen in a fire after being raped. Once Charcot resumed his lessons after the 1870 Franco-Prussian War and the Commune, he devoted three of them to Justine in 1871: 'What is striking in this patient is the enormous contracture affecting her upper and lower left limbs. This contracture persists both during natural sleep and under chloroform.' Justine was color-blind and had hemianes-

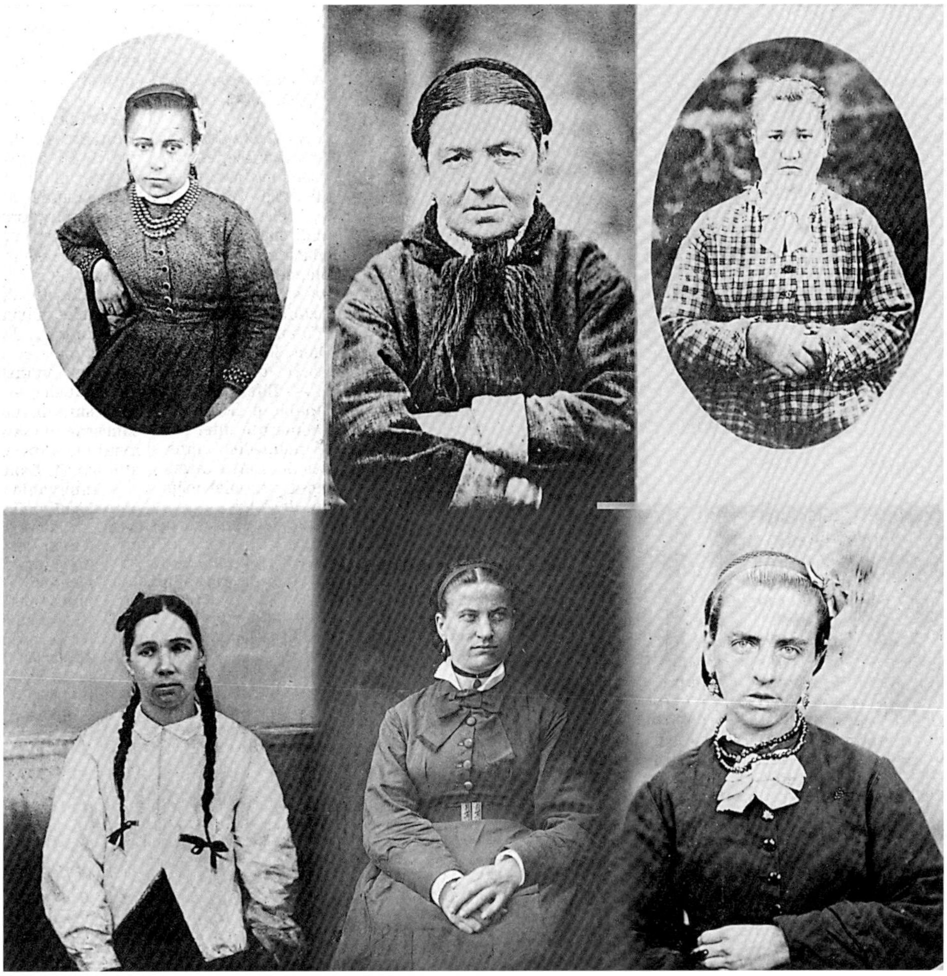

Fig. 1. Top row (left to right): L. Thérèse, L. Rosalie, and W. Madeleine. Bottom row (left to right): Geneviève de Loudun, V.C., M. Célina. Photos by Albert Londe, Iconographie photographique de La Salpêtrière 1877 and 1878. ©BIU Santé Paris, with kind permission.

thesia and ovarian hyperesthesia. She was the classic case for 'ischuria', which started for her in April 1871. 'Even before that, a woman who worked in the department and who felt the patient several times per day, noticed that sometimes the quantity of urine removed via catheter was very small; other times, there was no urine for two or three days, or longer, but the bedclothes were never wet'. Because she vomited daily, Charcot made her the classic case for a hysterical absence of urine [6, 7].

Accidents

The thesis of Paul Berbez (1859–?) showed that an accident following an emotional shock triggered 'traumatic hysteria', which could be resolved by persuasion. Clessienne A., an 18-year-old florist, had her first attack when she was 12 years old, in the street, just after the death of her mother from tuberculosis. She then had daily attacks, resulting in a hemianesthesia on the right side. One day, she fell from her bed and dislocated her left shoulder [8]:

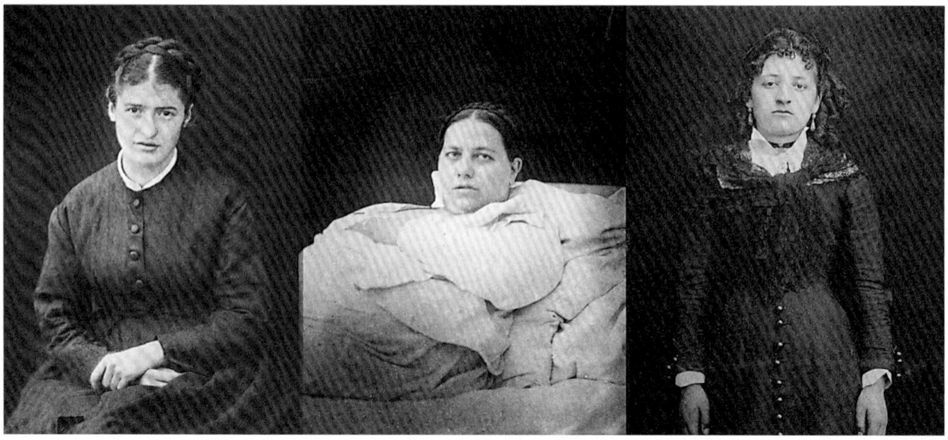

Fig. 2. From left to right: B… A, Hel… Eudoxie, Ma… dite N… Suzanne. Photos by Albert Londe, Iconographie photographique de La Salpêtrière 1878. ©BIU Santé Paris, with kind permission.

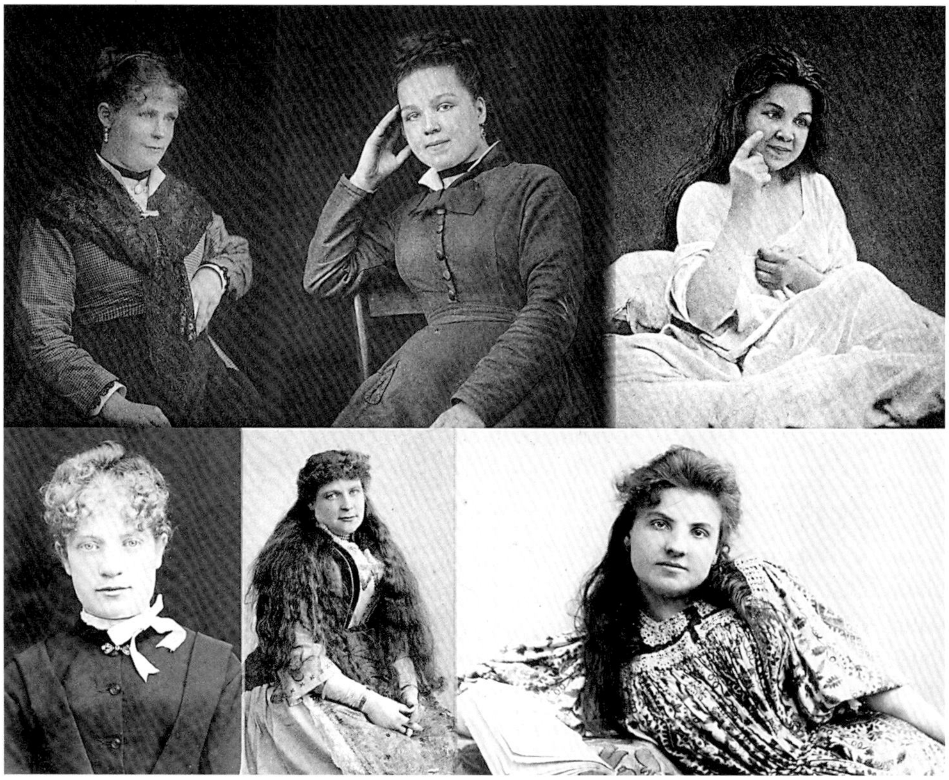

Fig. 3. Top row (left to right): Blanche Wittmann, Augustine Gleizes at rest and 'passionate attitudes'. Photos by Albert Londe, Iconographie photographique de La Salpêtrière 1878. ©BIU Santé Paris. With kind permission. Bottom row (left to right): Blanche Wittmann, Unknown hysterical. Original photos by Albert Londe, never published. Private collection of the author.

In her room, a few hours after the accident, the patient was found with monoplegia affecting her left arm, entirely the same as that which had hitherto been provoked by suggestion. While she had lost sensation in her left arm, the right arm had returned to normal; thus a transfer had occurred. A few days after reduction of the dislocated joint, everything returned as it had been. Her left arm recovered sensation while her right arm once again became insensitive.

Adolphe Dutil (1862–1899) related an observation of shaking which had developed following a dog attack on a blind patient [9]:

> Jeanne Kell... aged 23, admitted to La Salpêtrière on 7 July 1886 [...] is suddenly overcome by the sensation of a ball in the epigastric fossa, almost always in the evening. She has trouble breathing, she cries and the shaking immediately takes on considerable intensity. She can then no longer remain upright [...] The movements of her head and four limbs are perfectly rhythmical; the shaking is generalised [...] Her patellar reflexes are sharp; while percussion on the tendons activates the shaking, the sharp kick-out of her foot, rather than increasing it, causes a momentary cessation.

This patient was observed for more than 3 months with no change in her condition. Dutil did not indicate the effect of sleep, but all his treatments using electrification or hypnosis failed.

Still Women in the Masculine Medical Eye

Because he was depicting nature, Désiré-Magloire Bourneville (1840–1909) underscored the physical traits of his patients. He was also undoubtedly influenced by the academic art of the times, such as that of William Bouguereau (1825–1905), famous for his concupiscent nudes and their strikingly white skin. Marie 'Blanche' Wittmann (1859–1913) was known as the 'queen of the hysterics'. She is immortalized by Brouillet's painting (fig. 3). Bourneville described her as 'blond with a lymphatic complexion. Her skin is white with numerous freckles. She is very buxom' [5]. 'P. is tall, with white skin, light brown hair, regular features and an agreeable physiognomy' [10]. Augustine 'is tall and well developed (buxom, neck a bit thick, armpits and mons pubis covered with hair). Her tone and movements are decided, her mood is mobile and loud. She no longer has anything of a child's manner and seems almost like a grown woman, but she has never menstruated' (fig. 3). In contrast, 'Marc... is thin, short (1.43 m/4ft 8in) with a vulgar physiognomy' (fig. 1, 2) [2].

Illness and Hospitalization for Life?

While their arrival at La Salpêtrière is never clearly recounted, several of the patients apparently became 'filles de salle' (cleaning, simple care-giving), remaining at the hospital for years, or even until the end of their lives. After Charcot's death, Blanche W. became an aid in the photography laboratory, then one of the first victims of X-rays during the beginnings of radiology at La Salpêtrière. Conversely, B... A., who came to La Salpêtrière as a 'fille de service', was overcome a few days later with hysterical attacks. She was placed in the ward for epileptics and hysterics who were not considered lunatics. L. Rosalie, aged 56, stayed at La Salpêtrière for 33 years, reliving the terrors of her childhood in attacks lasting several hours [4]:

> 'Violent, rapid and large movements (fig. 1). Back arches. 'Ah! Ah!...' shouting. 'Monsters' – her agitation was extreme. Ler... would rise all the way up, then let herself fall back on her bed. She would throw herself from side to side, beating the bed with her feet. 'Help me... the thieves are here! [...] The murderer! [...] The monsters! [...] Death! Death! .

Many of the patients attempted to escape and were in some cases successful: 'On 31 August 1867, Geneviève returned to La Salpêtrière pregnant. She gave birth to a girl on 27 February 1868' [2]. 'M. ran away from La Salpêtrière on 7

September 1877 to be with "her Ernest" ' [2]. Augustine G. had a longer period of delirium than usual on March 14, 1878: 'She sat on her bed, head in her hands, and seemed to think. "No, I can't run away from La Salpêtrière to make you happy and follow you to England... I did give you a few days... . I don't like England... well, I'll try... . In what month? At the end of April? Too bad if I can't... no, I'm cured, I wasn't at La Salpêtrière... . They'll follow us everywhere; my father will spare nothing to find me" ' [4]. The hospitalizations were long and repeated: V.C. 'stayed 15 months in Lariboisière Hospital, and had frequent attacks over 11 months, almost every day' before coming to La Salpêtrière [4].

In light of all what they went through, it seems impossible not to understand 'their strong impressionability since childhood', their permanent anxiety which caused palpitations, throat tightness and abdominal pain, their passions, their signs of despondency and discouragement, and their jealousy – all states in which Charcot saw the cause 'of a higher suggestibility determined by symbolic representations'. A fact rarely noted, but one which Bourneville insisted upon, is that they all lived through the traumatic events of the Franco-Prussian War and the Commune [3, 10].

With their multiple daily attacks, these hysterics were not only manifesting their disturbance for Charcot; they were suffering significant psychological distress worsened by the close quarters (fig. 4–6). Charcot was aware of the possible contagiousness of hysterical attacks, and his thinking excluded the culture of hysteria he was unjustly accused of creating: 'Clearly, dispersion and dissemination of the group is the safest method to prevent the disease from propagating in such cases'. This could not be achieved at La Salpêtrière because the patients were crowded, living practically on top of each other [11]. However, the hospital remained a refuge from the misery outside, as noted by Jane Avril, the pseudonym of Jeanne Louise Beaudon (1868–1943),

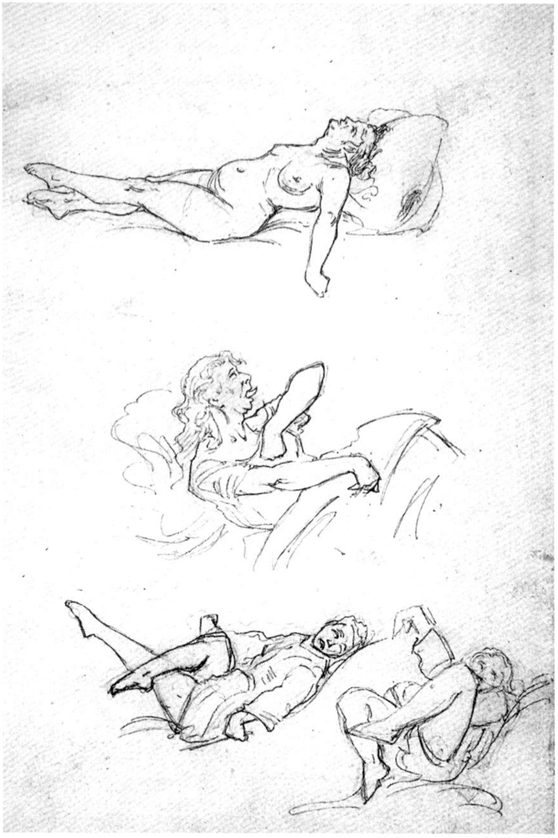

Fig. 4. Original graphite sketches by Paul Richer, drawn at patients' bedsides in La Salpêtrière Hospital. 1879. ©Paris, Ecole des Beaux-Arts, with kind permission.

one of the most famous dancers at the Parisian cabaret Le Moulin Rouge. Avril was treated in the department for hystero-epilepsy. In her 1933 memoir, she wrote: 'I stayed for two years in what for me was an Eden, everything down here on this earth being relative.' And about daily conditions, she added [12]:

It all came down to the one who could find some novelty to eclipse her peers, as a large group of students preceded by Charcot gathered around the patients' beds to watch their extravagant contortions, backarches, various acrobatics and other gymnastics. Several of the women had romantic adventures with the students, of which the living results became apparent after a few

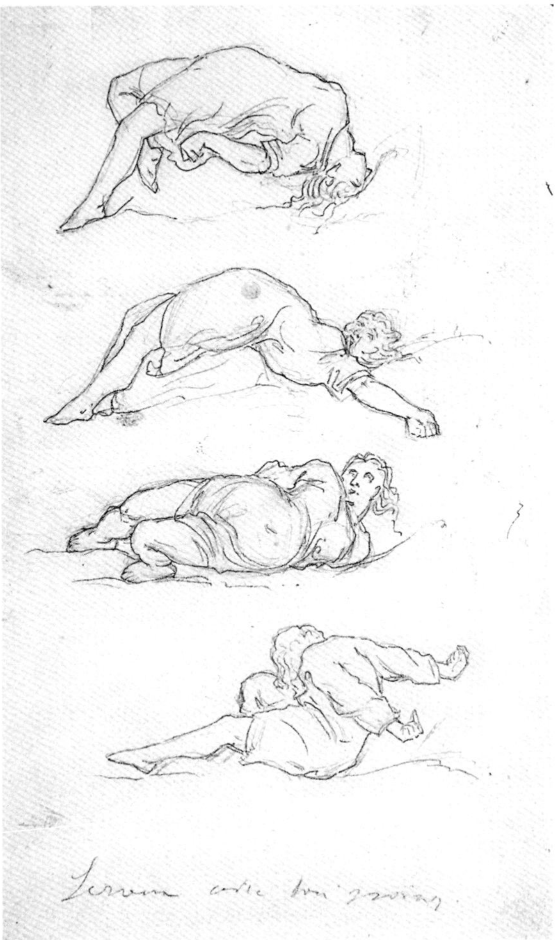

Fig. 5. Original graphite sketches by Paul Richer, drawn at patients' bedsides in La Salpêtrière Hospital. 1879. ©Paris, Ecole des Beaux-Arts. With kind permission.

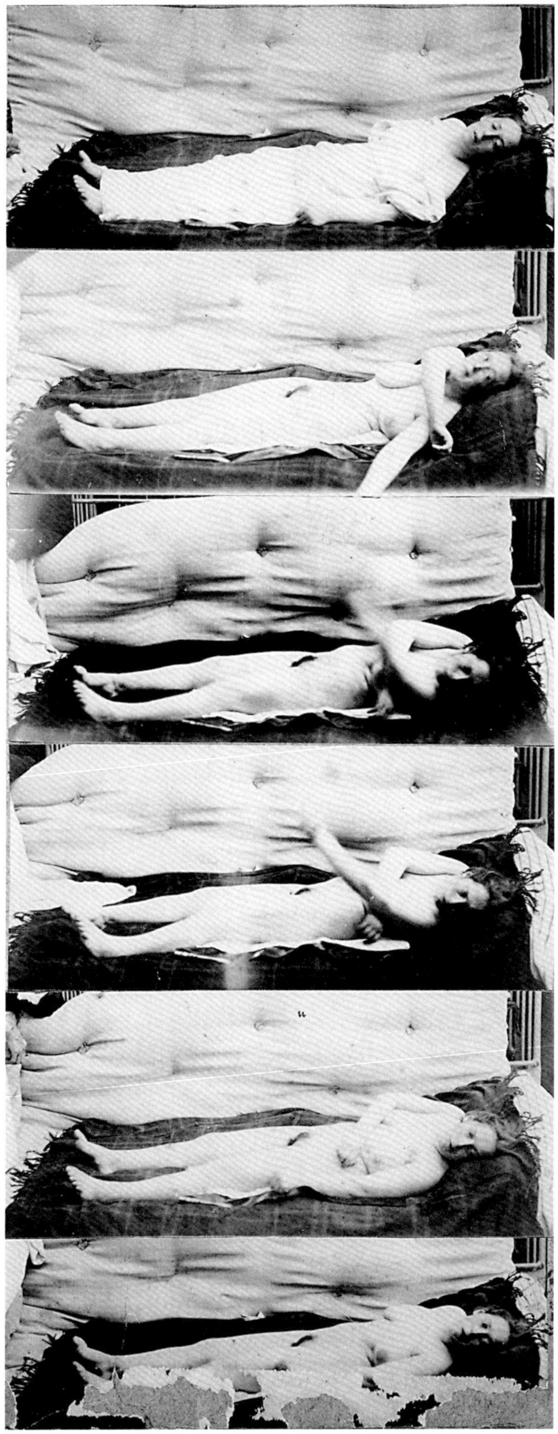

Fig. 6. Fall into hysterics, succesive phases by Albert Londe, October 29, 1882. A series of six photographs, albumen prints. ©Paris, Ecole des Beaux-Arts. With kind permission.

months. They were sent away during the time necessary for this sort of event. Then they'd come back like poor lost sheep, happy to return to the fold.

Treating the Attacks

Putting an end to the patients' violent and repeated attacks was a constant preoccupation. The consoling words of physicians and nurses, or isolation, could in some cases ease the emotional and physical shocks endured, but not permanently. Since both Bourneville and Charcot were convinced of the 'material' nature of the lesions 'in the sphere of ideas', they sought physical therapies. Charcot renewed the concept of ovarian hysteria, point of origin for the attack and a local sign of hyperesthesia: 'It may be concluded that the ovary, and the ovary alone, explains the fixed iliac pain of hysterics' [6]. It was not until 1882 that he defeminized hysteria by reporting cases in men. In 1879, Bourneville wrote: 'The ovarian region is the most well known of the hysterogenic regions. It has a dual property: using moderate pressure an attack may be triggered, then stopped by using more or less forceful compression. This fact has been highlighted by our great teacher Charcot' [5]. Bourneville's detailed accounts reveal many ambiguities as to the real effectiveness of this technique: 'Ovarian compression is difficult to put into practice. It is only after prolonged efforts that one overcomes the resistance of the abdominal muscles and penetrates the pelvis. Tetany then stops, but only for a short time' [3]. The ovary compressor was introduced in 1878 to increase the power and duration of the therapeutic effect. At his lesson on November 24, 1878, Charcot provoked an artificial contraction of Augustine G.'s tongue and larynx muscles. The patient remained aphonic. From November 25 to 30, Bourneville unsuccessfully applied a magnet, electricity, hypnotism, and ether. 'The ovary compressor was used for 36 hours without success' [3]. What terrible suffering was inflicted and endured!

Very surprisingly, Bourneville reported on a particularly cruel practice it is difficult to imagine him carrying out, a practice one would have thought abandoned long ago: '22 November 1873. Cauterisation of the cervix with a hot iron. Introducing the speculum was difficult and caused much suffering due severe vaginismus' [2]. The phenomenological ambiguity of a uterine etiology of hysteria can also be seen in the menstrual indications: 'Her periods are sometimes accompanied by attacks, but not in any absolute way. Often the attacks occur in the intervals between periods. Delays in menstruation do not appear to have any action. Finally, a very long amenorrhoea (19 months) did not prevent the attacks from returning for 10 months' [2].

Paul Blocq (1860–1896) reported: 'In Julie Antonine B., aged 32, both feet were affected by a strong equinus contracture. The patient could not stand up unassisted... . Only the toes of her feet and the anterior extremity of her metatarsals touched the ground; her heels were raised around 10 cm'. As manager of her father's failing clothing shop, she was present when he had a stroke. As he fell, he dragged her down with him. She then remained bedridden because the contracture of her feet made it impossible to walk. Although neither hydrotherapy, massage, orthopedic devices, nor chloroform corrected the deformity, Blocq [13] confirmed the patient's hysteria and had her Achilles tendons cut. She was then able to walk and leave the hospital!

The medications used at La Salpêtrière are now mostly considered narcotics. Amyl nitrite, which has been used since 1867 to treat angina, has become a component of aphrodisiac drugs known as 'poppers'. As Bourneville noted in *Iconographie de La Salpêtrière*, 'The inhalations stop the attacks'. Under the influence of amyl nitrite, L. Th. (an 18-year-old florist who had her first attack after being unjustly accused of theft) came to her senses after 20 s and said 'that she was suffocating, that she smelled a bad odour, that her throat hurt and she had a headache' [2]. She died shortly thereafter of tuberculosis. Bourneville reported on the disturbances experienced by V.C.: 'The effects of the medication are very marked: extreme cyanosis, discoloration of the fingers, purple fingernails; bluish tint to the tongue, the mucous membrane of the mouth and the eyelids. When the patient regained consciousness, she said, 'That's funny. Everything's green. Aren't my nails green?' [3]. While chloroform was used very frequently to put patients to sleep or loosen a contraction, ether was used even more often. Some women developed iatrogenic addictions. On March 3, 1878, Augustine G. inhaled '125 g of ether. From then until 8 March, she had fainting spells, strange ideas and nausea' [2]. As for Marie W., the following was noted on December 13, 1878: 'As the patient had experienced bothersome tremors for a few days, we gave her ether. This resulted in hilarity followed by delirium: "Give me more ether...". She laughed, twisting the compress against her nose and mouth. [...] She asked for ether...' [5]. Bourneville noted: 'Ether worked initially, but its action gradually decreased to the point that, to quell the attacks, an enormous dose was necessary, resulting in a long inhalation time. This led us to administer chloroform once the patient had inhaled ether for 10 to 15 min. This double anaesthetic was used on many occasions with W.' Static electricity was also used, 'causing sensitivity to return to the entire right side of the body' in Marie W., on January 10, 1879 (Ramsden equipment). On May 16, 1879 she underwent electrification: 'Her delirium continued nonetheless. Feeding by oesophageal tube' [5].

Charcot was certainly influenced by the demonstrations of Victor Burq (1823–1884) in 1851, which he had seen as an 'interne' under Pierre-Adolphe Piorry (1794–1879). This led him to continue experimenting with metals and magnets, which he applied to the hysterics' paralyzed limbs [6]. 'V. is sensitive to gold and zinc. A necklace of zinc plates, applied for five minutes, restores sensitivity of the bucco-pharyngeal mucous membrane. A single zinc plate, applied over the same time period to the left temple, momentarily restores the notion of colours on the left, but makes it disappear on the right' [3]. Geneviève, deemed a 'succubus' by Bourneville, was tortured by the nocturnal visits of her imaginary lover and fell victim to contractions: 'The magnet was applied to the right wrist; after about 10 min, the contraction disappeared on the left and overtook the right wrist' [3]. Referred to as 'transfer' by Charcot, this phenomenon led to experiments that steered his research from a neuropathological approach to a psychological one [6, 14]:

> Hysterical contraction can be artificially provoked in a woman who is subject to a hysterical diathesis. By itself, this surprising proposal reveals the cardinal importance of such a phenomenon and points to all the usefulness it will have for us in our future research to treat real hysterical contraction. Finally, the discovery of such laws will show us that hysteria is not one of these unknowns in which one sees all one wishes to see. Though it will not please sceptics and hysterophobes, hysteria has its laws and is no fiction.

Joseph Babinski (1857–1932) noted the case of a cook, aged 42. Following an event which frightened her at age 22, 'she had a series of convulsive hysterical attacks accompanied by delirium'. On April 4, 1892, she was struck by a car and taken unconscious to the hospital. When she regained consciousness, she had hematorrhea on the right side with facial paralysis and deafness. The exam also revealed hemianesthesia and a reduction of the visual field, both on the right side. Her reflexes were normal, which led Babinski to evoke post-traumatic hysteria [15]:

> On 20 April, around 4 pm, M. Jean Nageotte (1866–1948), an *interne* in the department, hypnotised the patient, who was then unable to open her eyes despite all her efforts. It was suggested to her that she

could walk normally. The immediate result was not satisfactory, but in the evening, the patient got up and found that she could walk much more easily. By the following morning, the locomotor impairment had completely disappeared. The patient's walking was no longer abnormal in any way, and has remained normal since then. Her facial paralysis, on the other hand, has not changed. On several occasions, we tried to improve this paralysis by suggestion, without obtaining any results.

Suggestion, Miracles, or Anticlerical Proselytism

Referring to Justine Etchevery and how her contracture disappeared by suggestion, Charcot noted in 1872: 'We must understand the possibility of these cures which, still today, make people speak of miracles, but which only charlatans boast of. Before our century, such facts were often evoked to convince the most gullible minds of the therapeutic influence of supernatural powers' [6]. As for Bourneville, after practically every clinical description, he added instructive historical accounts to decry how religious superstitions kept common people in ignorance. Without ever saying so clearly, Charcot shared Bourneville's anticlerical opinions, which were evident in *Iconographie de La Salpêtrière.* This medical publication also served as a cultural weapon: it compared clinical cases with women described as possessed, considered witches, exorcised, burnt at the stake, or otherwise stigmatized over the centuries. Geneviève was born on January 2, 1843, in Loudun, a city famous for its Ursuline nuns bewitched by Urbain Grandier in the 18th century and the subsequent witch trials. By a curious coincidence, Geneviève presented with 'nervous attacks, recurring daily. Her belly was very big as a result of them and also due to the irregularity of her menstruation. The nuns imagined that she was pregnant and persecuted her, claiming that she had tricked them.' Suffering from this hysterical pregnancy, Geneviève mutilated her breasts, was placed in a 'straitjacket', ran out on a roof to approach the workers there, had several attacks in which she removed her clothing, called for spectators, and said to one of them 'kiss me'. Treated with opium extracts, chloral, and strong doses of ether, she was the victim of hallucinations and a 'saltatory delirium' (fig. 1). Bourneville noted that 'her attitude is that attributed to visionaries such as Sainte-Thérèse, complete with ecstasies and prayer positions to conclude her erotic delirium', reminiscent of the Belgian stigmatic Louise Lateau [2]. It is likely that today, Geneviève would be treated for psychosis, perhaps schizophrenia, a clinical picture that had not yet been isolated in her day. In the case of M. Célina, there were 'demoniacal attacks' alternating with 'lewd positions'. Bourneville noted the crucifixion attacks of Léontine V., who 'would emit a long cry, spread her arms and fall slowly backwards... . Her arms were rigid, extended perpendicularly to her trunk in the shape of a cross' [2]. As for Richer, he also concluded his observations with historical notes: 'It is not surprising that religious excitation provoked, during certain periods of exaltation, these reactions of the nervous system which, in the final analysis, give rise to grande hystérie' [4]. Spectacular attacks were demythified, as Charcot wished them to be, according to a positivist and anticlerical ideology inspired by Auguste Comte (1798–1857) and Emile Littré (1801–1881). Charcot used this ideology to fit hysteria into the common clinical framework, which was subject to neurological and thus scientific reasoning.

Hypnotic Suggestion and Legal Repercussions

Based on the work of Charles Richet (1850–1935) concerning 'induced somnambulism', Charcot used hypnotism as a tool for pathophysiological exploration after conceding the failure of his anatomical-clinical method. An insidious conceptual shift led him to assimilate hysteria with hypnosis, which is described according to three stages: lethargy, catalepsy, and somnambulism. Then current events of the time took an unexpected turn, and La Salpêtrière patients were affected. Like Charcot, Georges Gilles de la Tourette (1857–1904) constantly sought to inform public opinion about the dangers of hypnosis, which was very much in fashion since Mesmer, and especially harmful hypnosis therapies. In the famous trial of the Gouffé affair, Gilles de la Tourette and Charcot opposed Hippolyte Bernheim (1840–1919) and Jules Liégeois (1833–1908) of the 'Nancy school' by maintaining that a crime could not be committed under hypnosis. Curiously, Gilles de la Tourette nonetheless recounted a crime suggested to a patient in a hypnotic state:

> 'We said to H.E., placed in the somnambulism stage, and who had had a few problems with our friend B. [Paul Berbez?], an *interne* within the department: 'You know Monsieur B.' 'Yes.' 'He's charming.' 'Oh, no! He won't give me my pills, he's not a good doctor.' 'Really! In that case, we're going to get rid of him, so that another *interne* will come and take better care of you.' 'I'd like nothing more.' 'You're going to be in charge of it: here's a pistol (and we placed a ruler in her hand); when you wake up, you'll fire at him once. He should come here; wait for him.' We blew on her eyes. After waking, H. E... continued to chat with us while toying with the revolver (or the ruler, which she took for a revolver). [...] Then our friend B. walked in. B. knew what awaited him. Once he had approached H., she coldly fired on him point blank. B. fell to the ground, crying: 'I'm dead!' 'What!' we said to H. 'You've killed Monsieur B.! What motives pushed you to commit such an act?' 'Monsieur B. was a bad doctor; I took my revenge.' 'That's no excuse.' 'Oh? Too bad. Besides, I had other reasons; he was supposed to be killed by me.' We put an end to the experiment, which had lasted long enough and was threatening to cause a state of nervous overexcitement in H. and potentially an attack of hysteria.'

Blanche W. also underwent an experiment involving a similar suggested crime. For Gilles de la Tourette, these were only experiments and 'the hypnotised patient always remains an individual who can manifest her will by resisting the suggestions... . A somnambulist, noted Monsieur Richer, can completely refuse to perform certain acts while offering no resistance to anything else' [16–18].

Redemption

All of these writings reveal the constant desire to improve the material and moral conditions of the women who ended up at the hospice. As Jules Clarétie reported: 'Originally, La Salpêtrière was, as Monsieur Gilles de la Tourette tells us, hellish. Charcot made of it what Pinel had once made of the holding place for poor, insane women: an asylum. Hope returned. There was consolation, relief from the horrible evils that gave rise to such cries and suffering' [19]. Jane Avril described herself as 'tossed about by life and for so long incapable of considering things normally; living in a perpetual dream without understanding the value of things or even seeking to find out!' She found solace at La Salpêtrière. Her account was published much later, in 1933: 'There were crazy girls, whose illness, called hysteria, was mostly a matter of faking.' It contrasts with that of Blanche W., recorded shortly before her death by Alphonse Baudouin (1876–1957): 'I'd like you to explain something about the attacks you used to have.' After hesitating a moment, she replied: 'Well! What do you want to know?' 'They claim that all these attacks were faked, that the patients pretended to be asleep and that the whole thing was a joke on the doctors (fig. 3). What's the truth in all that?' 'None of it's true. It's all lies; if we fell asleep, if we had attacks, it was because we were helpless to do otherwise. What's more, it was very unpleasant.' And she added: 'Fakery! Do you think it would have been easy to fool Monsieur Charcot? Yes, there were tricksters who tried; he simply gave them a look that said: Be still.' That was how this 'confession of a hysteric' ended, with a homage to the great deceased neurologist [12, 20, 21]. Indeed, Charcot was never fooled. As he wrote in 1872: 'We have met with simulation every step of the way in the history of hysteria, and we sometimes surprise ourselves by admiring the incredible cunning, sagacity and tenacity that these hysterics deploy to deceive... especially when the victim of the imposture is a physician' [6].

To Conclude

Several of these patients stayed in asylums directed by the alienists of La Salpêtrière, like Jules Falret (1824–1902), Louis Delasiauve, or Henri Legrand du Saulle. Comparing their various observations, as Nicole Edelman has done, highlights their different practices and concepts. Charcot developed a neurological semiology based on sensitivity, movement difficulties, and amaurosis. He described the manifestations, then classified and ordered what he had observed, but with little regard for the suffering experienced, going so far as to state during his Tuesday lesson on June 12, 1888: 'It is not always easy to question the patients. They offer up inaccurate facts or interpretations we have no use for' [22].

The alienists used psychiatric terms: hysterical psychosis, hallucinations, melancholy, erotic delirium, etc. They emphasized the mental state of the patients and attentively listened to their life stories. Trained under Delasiauve, Bourneville was very clearly the link between the two worlds, moving from one to the other with his empathy and his ability to listen. He took an interest in patients' pain, despair, imaginary guilt, and fears of abuse, which he was able to transcribe in his observations. Charcot's conceptual shift (1870–1893) from an organicist clinical approach to a social analysis taking poverty and its difficulties into account as causes of hysteria owes much to Bourneville, a pioneer in neuropsychology [23].

The opinion of Georges Guillain (1876–1961) is one we should share:

> The disdain expressed for the work of Charcot, who was an observer and clinician of the highest order, is not justified. Obviously Charcot, who studied neuroses at La Salpêtrière between 1862 and 1892, may have committed a few errors, but he described clinical types that have remained unchanged. He understood the role of suggestion in patients and was not unaware of the frequency of simulation. He indicated therapies to which we have nothing to add.

And in the same vein: 'Charcot's service to nosography is inestimable. He isolated types of psychoneurosis that continue to exist' [24]. Psychosis and anorexia are now treated by psychiatrists. But does hysteria not crop up periodically under new names, requiring concepts adapted to each age? Do the terms psychosomatic disorder, spasmophilia and fibromyalgia not mask entities described by the great neurologist of La Salpêtrière?

References

1 Bannour W: Jean-Martin Charcot et l'hystérie. Paris, Métaillé, 1992, p 256.
2 Bourneville DM, Regnard P: Iconographie photographique de la Salpêtrière, service de M. Charcot. Paris, Aux Bureaux du Progrès Médical, Delahaye, 1877, p 164.
3 Bourneville DM, Regnard P: Iconographie photographique de la Salpêtrière, service de M. Charcot. Paris, Aux Bureaux du Progrès Médical, Delahaye, 1878, p 232.
4 Richer P: Etudes cliniques sur l'hystéro-épilepsie ou grande hystérie. Paris, Delahaye et Lecrosnier, 1881, p 736.
5 Bourneville DM, Regnard P: Iconographie photographique de la Salpêtrière, service de M. Charcot. Paris, Aux Bureaux du Progrès Médical, Delahaye, 1879, p 259.
6 Charcot JM: Leçons sur les maladies du système nerveux recueillies et publiées par Bourneville. Paris, Delahaye, 1872, p 368.
7 Bourneville DM, de Montmeja A: De la contracture hystérique, leçon du Prof Charcot, juin 1870. Revue Photographique des Hôpitaux de Paris 1871; 3:192–203.
8 Berbez P: Hystérie et traumatisme. Paris, Aux Bureaux du Progrès Médical, Delahaye et Lecrosnier, 1887, p 127.
9 Dutil A: Contribution à l'étude clinique du tremblement hystérique. Paris, Lecrosnier et Babé, 1891, p 86.

10 Murat L: L'homme qui se prenait pour Napoléon. Pour une histoire politique de la folie. Paris, Gallimard, 2011, p 384.
11 Charcot JM: Toux et bruits laryngés chez les hystériques, les choréiques, les tiqueux et dans quelques autres maladies des centres nerveux. Clinique des maladies du système nerveux Mr Le Professeur Charcot. Paris, Le Progrès Médical et Félix Alcan, 1893, vol 2, pp 443–459.
12 Avril J, Morel JP, Brécourt-Villars C: Mes mémoires. Paris, Phébus, 2005, p 437.
13 Blocq P: Des contractures. Paris, Aux Bureaux du Progrès Médical, Delahaye et Lecrosnier, 1888, p 210.
14 Charcot JM: Oeuvres complètes. Paris, Delahaye et Lecrosnier, 1886–1894, vol 9.
15 Babinski J: Association de l'hystérie avec les maladies organiques du système nerveux, les névroses et diverses autres affections. Société Médicale des Hôpitaux de Paris, meeting of November 11, 1892. Bulletins et Mémoires de la Société Médicale des Hôpitaux de Paris 1892; 9:775–795.
16 Gilles de la Tourette G: L'hypnotisme et les états analogues au point de vue médico-légal. Paris, Plon et Nourrit, 1887, p 534.
17 Bogousslavsky J, Walusinski O: Gilles de la Tourette's criminal women: the many faces of fin de siècle hypnotism. Clin Neurol Neurosurg 2010;112:549–551.
18 Charcot JM: Accidents hystériques graves survenus chez une femme à la suite d'hypnotisations pratiquées par un magnétiseur dans une baraque de fête publique. Paris. Vigot. Revue de l'Hypnotisme et de la Psychologie Physiologique 1889;3:3–11.
19 Clarétie J. Charcot le consolateur. Les Annales Politiques et Littéraires 1903; 21:79–80.
20 Baudouin A: Quelques souvenirs de La Salpêtrière. La Presse Médicale 1925;21: 517–520.
21 Bonduelle M, Gelfand T: Hysteria behind the scenes: Jane Avril at the Salpêtrière. J Hist Neurosci 1999;8:35–42.
22 Charcot JM: Leçons de Mardi. Policliniques 1887–1888. Notes de cours de MM. Blin, Charcot et Colin. Paris, Delahaye et Lecrosnier, 1887, p 638.
23 Edelman N: Une hystérique ou des hystériques. Charcot et les aliénistes de la Salpêtrière (1870–1893); in Villa F, Fédida P (eds): Le cas en controverse, monographies de psychopathologie. Paris, Presses Universitaires de France, 1999, vol 1, pp 231–248.
24 Guillain G: Il est injustifié et erroné d'oublier l'oeuvre de J.-M. Charcot sur l'hystérie et les névroses. La Semaine des Hôpitaux 1949;25:147–160.

Olivier Walusinski, MD
20 rue de Chartres
FR–28160 Brou (France)
E-Mail walusinski@baillement.com

Bogousslavsky J (ed): Hysteria: The Rise of an Enigma. Front Neurol Neurosci. Basel, Karger, 2014, vol 35, pp 78–89
DOI: 10.1159/000360065

Public Medical Shows

Olivier Walusinski

Family Physician, Private Practice, Brou, France

Abstract

In the second half of the 19th century, Jean-Martin Charcot (1825–1893) became famous for the quality of his teaching and his innovative neurological discoveries, bringing many French and foreign students to Paris. A hunger for recognition, together with progressive and anticlerical ideals, led Charcot to invite writers, journalists, and politicians to his lessons, during which he presented the results of his work on hysteria. These events became public performances, for which physicians and patients were transformed into actors. Major newspapers ran accounts of these consultations, more like theatrical shows in some respects. The resultant enthusiasm prompted other physicians in Paris and throughout France to try and imitate them. We will compare the form and substance of Charcot's lessons with those given by Jules-Bernard Luys (1828–1897), Victor Dumontpallier (1826–1899), Ambroise-Auguste Liébault (1823–1904), Hippolyte Bernheim (1840–1919), Joseph Grasset (1849–1918), and Albert Pitres (1848–1928). We will also note their impact on contemporary cinema and theatre.

The history of hysteria is nothing if not dramatic.
Mark S. Micale, 1995

Four centuries ago, in his play *As You Like It*, William Shakespeare compared the world to a stage and its inhabitants to actors. In France, at the end of the 19th century, the microcosm of hysteria research seemed to place physicians and patients in the roles of actors playing to an audience of students, literary figures, and politicians.

Jean Martin Charcot at La Salpêtrière

Medical education in 19th-century France was 'dominated by the duality and the rivalry between medical schools and hospitals. Hospitals dominated as teaching centres, resulting in certain perverse effects' [1]. The teaching of Jean-Martin Charcot (1825–1893) perfectly illustrates this situation. Before the Chair of Nervous System Diseases was created for him in 1882 within the medical school, Charcot had been a professor of anatomical pathology since 1873. Already in the summer of 1866, however, he had begun giving lessons on all areas of medicine in an unused kitchen within his department at La Salpêtrière. These lessons were attended by hospital students as well as foreign visitors. Unhindered by any official program, Charcot was able to present his research and his multiple discoveries during the particularly fecund period between 1862 and 1882. In 1872, Désiré-Magloire Bourneville (1840–1909) published the first volume of his teacher's lessons [2]. Without abandoning the supervision of research he had assigned to his students, Charcot grew interested in hysteria, which from 1875 on he began to address more frequently in his teachings. On November 22, 1879, he explained [3]:

> This is the first time I have the honour of receiving you here, and I cannot hide my deep satisfaction to be inaugurating this hall with you. Work remains to be done, but we have here all the modern equipment for demonstrations. The construction of a room for teaching within this hospital has been a dream of mine ever since I took up my duties here in 1862. From that time, I've never ceased believing that this large, noble asylum of human miseries – where several Masters of French medicine, starting with Pinel, have carried out their illustrious work – would one day become a well-organised centre for instruction and research, or in other words, a Pathological Institute.

It was in this spacious room, with capacity for an audience of 100, that the famous Tuesday lessons would be held:

> We know that Charcot, independently of the value of his discoveries, was one of the most remarkable professors at the medical school. The clarity of his lessons and their pertinence have remained legendary. Not only were they rigorously constructed; they were as lively as performances. Charcot, who was passionate about teaching, prepared his classes with meticulous care [4].
>
> What did his teaching consist of? Lessons, mainly. They were the living representation of remarkable episodes of a disease in which the patients participated. They incorporated a branch of pathology where everything was to be revised or created: I'm speaking of the pathology of nervous centres. So what made this teaching attractive was its novelty [5].

Did Charcot grow bored of nervous system diseases, which were most often incurable? In 1870, he was put in charge of hysterics after a hospital reorganization, and he seemed taken with the spectacle of young women subject to eccentric attacks, their paralysis complete then instantaneously gone, their cabaret star poses often suggestive. For Charcot, hysteria was the sine qua non for hypnosis, which was to hysteria what anatomical pathology was to the study of organic pathology. Hypnosis made it possible to trigger or stop attacks, and to modify the symptoms. Charcot never considered hypnosis as a treatment, unlike others who imitated him. And he did not hypnotize his patients himself. As Alphonse Daudet described one lesson [6]:

> Lanky girl about 30 years old, with a small head, wavy pale hair; sunken.... She's at home at La Salpêtrière, in a straitjacket, with a scarf around her neck. 'Put her to sleep...', orders the professor. The house officer, standing behind the spindly creature, presses his hands over her eyes for a moment... . She sighs, and it's done. She's sleeping, rigidly straight. Her poor body takes on the imposed positions; one arm stretched out remains stretched out. As each muscle is lightly stroked, the fingers of the hand move one after the other, while the hand remains open and motionless. It's as if a mannequin could become even more docile and flexible. 'And there's no way she could trick us', declares Charcot. 'She'd have to know anatomy as well as we do.' [...] 'We mustn't tire her', says the Master. 'Go get Balmann.' But the house officer comes back alone. Balmann didn't want to come. She was furious that Daret had been called in before she was. The jealousy of celebrities, of stars linked these two cataleptics, the first subjects at La Salpêtrière. Sometimes disputes, heated words exchanged over the washing, some of them highly technical, turn the entire department into a madhouse.

Charcot's lessons took the form of lectures during which the professor described clinical cases. Although brief, the summaries were carefully constructed to have a long-term impact on the students. Since medicine is an art, Charcot selected the most presentable patients to definitively establish hysteria's clinical picture, proceeding as a painter might. This clinical picture, set up as a prototype that could easily be identified by all

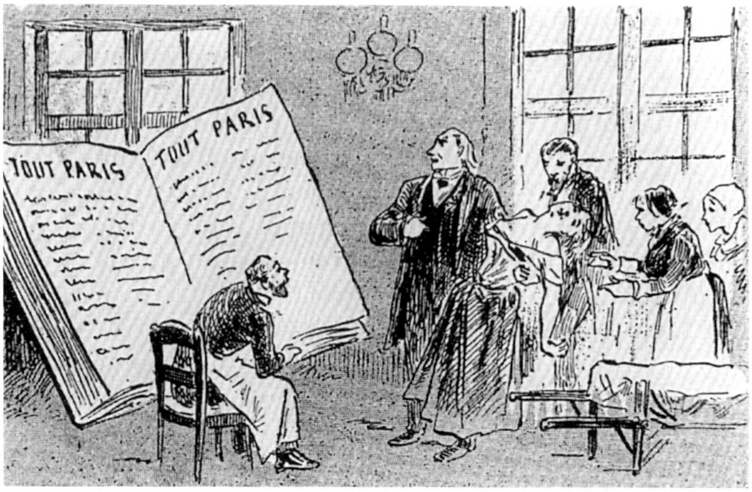

Fig. 1. Anonymous caricature of André Brouillet's painting *Une leçon clinique à La Salpêtrière.* Gilles de la Tourette on the left wearing an apron, Charcot, Babinski supporting Blanche Wittman in front of nurses Marguerite Bottard, and Mademoiselle Ecary. Private collection of the author.

physicians, gave rise to variants and complications underlying different clinical forms. Charcot's sole aim in putting forward this heuristic model was to leave a lasting impression by limiting the search for an exact etiology as much as possible and by focusing on symptomatic description. The presentation of hysteric patients followed these somewhat artificial rules. According to the Genevan neuropsychiatrist Georges de Morsier (1894–1982), only 24 hysterics were presented at the various lessons, compared to the more than 250 'hystero-epileptics' under the care of Charcot and his students [7].

Charcot presented himself to his audience as conducting experiments, aware of the attendant uncertainties [8]:

> This patient will help us show you what I have proposed. I will tell you, however, that while we are more or less certain of the expected result, the workings of an organism are not as exact as a mechanical device, and I won't be surprised if our operation does not succeed. It has been said that experiments on animals do not work as well in public as they do in the laboratory. The same logic applies, to an even greater degree, with the clinical experiments we perform here. If we don't succeed as we hope to, you will still be able to learn something from the experiment.

At the end of the 19th century, medicine was turning the rapid advances in science and technology to its advantage. Scientific ideology, colored by anticlericalism to which Charcot adhered, transformed Claude Bernard (1813–1878), Louis Pasteur (1822–1895), and Charcot himself into high priests who officiated not in cathedrals but in their lecture halls: 'The ambience was unique, resembling a whirlwind of knowledge and high aspirations, endangered by a whirlwind of errors' [6]. Initially, Charcot's lessons were no different than those of other famous physicians, whose students left us lively accounts by compiling their lessons in books, notably for Armand Trousseau (1801–1867), Ernest-Charles Lasègue (1816–1883), or Sigismond Jaccoud (1830–1913). What eventually differentiated Charcot was how he brought physicians and artists together around his lessons (fig. 1). Charcot was an artist himself, and with the help of his brilliant house officer and illustrator Paul Richer (1849–1933), he compared his patients during their attacks with old pictorial representations. He also became a source of inspiration for his friends who were writers and philosophers, including Jules Clarétie (1840–1913), Octave Mirbeau (1848–1917), Joris-Karl Huysmans (1848–1907), Jules Lermina (1839–1915), and Henri Bergson (1859–1941): 'We have simply set out to demonstrate the role that exterior accidents of hysterical neurosis have played in Art, when they were considered not as a disease, but as a perversion of the soul caused by the devil' [9].

Charcot's fame grew rapidly and well beyond scientific circles with the success of his demonstrations. He thus obtained the recognition he had sought and was seen as demystifying hysteria [10]:

> Sunday morning, Gambetta accompanied the deputies Paul Bert and Henri Liouville on a visit of the hysterics division of La Salpêtrière Hospital, which is directed by Professor Charcot. It is a well-known fact that Professor Charcot conducts scientific magnotherapy at La Salpêtrière that involves no trickery. Mr. Gambetta witnessed several experiments which he found fascinating. Before leaving, he congratulated Professor Charcot on his work.

The physician Maximin Legrand, in one of his chronicles, painted a lively picture that captures the ambiance of the lesson/show and what went on behind the scenes [11]:

> A beautiful young woman is brought into the room adjoining the lecture hall on a stretcher. She has a fine figure and a mass of blond hair. She is struggling against the constraints of her straitjacket. 'There you are!' says the professor. 'But, my girl, it's not time to leave us yet.' The stretcher is placed on the ground. Mr. Charcot presses his hand into the right ovary of the patient, who grimaces and immediately calms down. 'Let's put the compressor on her.' [...] On another stretcher, a second patient is brought in. She's thin with brown hair and twisting in every direction, markedly different than the first patient, more typical of the demonically possessed seen in church paintings. 'And M...', says the professor. 'Is she ready? Does she have her leggings on?' 'Yes, sir!' [...] Charcot: 'The demonstration is difficult because my personnel is always on the edge of revolt. But today, I've prepared these patients with their consent; we've given them ether.' [...] In a lesson that is very substantial and marvellously clear, Mr. Charcot presents the characteristics of Hysteria Major, and explains the differential diagnosis that distinguishes the attacks of this condition from epileptic attacks... . Mr. Charcot's house officer Mr. Richer has used his remarkable talent to draw a diagram on a black canvas showing all the aspects of a hysterical attack. Mr. Charcot uses it to explain that the attacks are divided into four periods... . These periods, with their various phases, occur in succession over two or three minutes, or longer, and sometimes it all ends there. Other times, a series of up to 150 successive attacks takes place without interruption. The lesson lasts around three quarters of an hour, during which time the young blond woman lies on her stretcher. In her straitjacket and fitted with the compressor, she appears to follow the professor's demonstration with intelligence and interest... . The straitjacket and compressor are then removed from the patient; the stretcher is set down so that she can be seen by everyone in the hall... . An attack of grande hystérie begins. The four periods, divided into successive phases, occur in the expected order, and all the details on the diagram are reproduced with surprising exactitude... . I only wish to relate what I saw and attempt to explain why everyone who witnessed this lesson was convinced, as I was, that, despite the nature of hysteria, nothing had been left to chance... . This was Professor Charcot's aim. Once again, he has achieved it marvellously.

Lessons in Paris outside La Salpêtrière: Jules Luys and Victor Dumontpallier

The success of the lessons at La Salpêtrière encouraged others to imitate them, notably Jules-Bernard Luys (1828–1897) and Victor Dumontpallier (1826–1899). Charcot, Luys, and Dumontpallier were members of a commission appointed by Claude Bernard (1813–1878), president of the French Biological Society. The commission's task was to verify the results of the metalloscopy and metallotherapy research conducted by Victor Burq (1823–1884). Two highly favorable reports submitted in 1877 and 1878 were met with great enthusiasm by the scientific world and well-informed outsiders, which very likely encouraged these three researchers to pursue their studies of hysteria and hypnotism.

Luys is famous for his innovative work on anatomy and his physiological hypotheses concerning the basal ganglia. However, 'suddenly

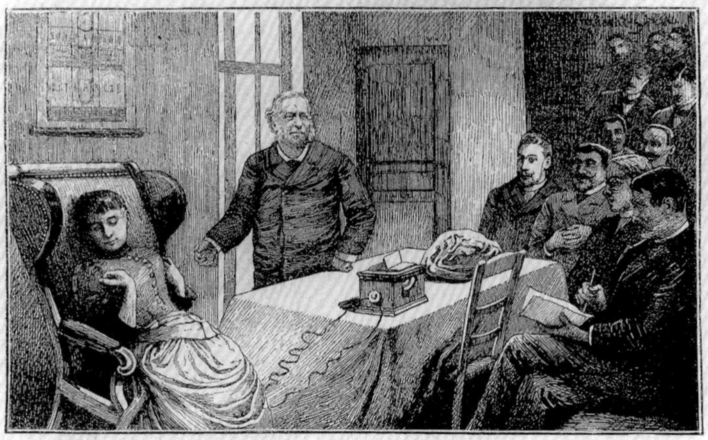

Leçon du docteur Luys à la Charité.

Fig. 2. Etching by Alexandre Laurent Gsell published in *Hypnotisme*. Dr Foveau Courmelles. 1890. Private collection of the author.

abandoning the clearly mapped route he had taken up until then, Luys stepped onto the mysterious path of hypnotism and suggestion, riddled with pitfalls. He fell into these subtle traps, but in good faith, and all of his adversaries paid homage to his honest sincerity' [12]. With the passion of a neophyte, Luys began studying hysteria in 1884 [13]. His unscrupulous entourage took advantage of his gullibility, and was able to deceive him in experiments like those designed to show the remote action of medications [14] (fig. 2).

Luys wrote: 'I had the good fortune to have hypnotisable female subjects whom I'd known for several years and whose normal traits and pathological manifestations were familiar to me' [15]. On August 30, 1887, Luys distributed photos of Esther and Gabrielle, 'his hysterics', to his fellow academicians. The photos showed the women in their normal state, and also after Luys had applied a tube containing essences of fennel, thyme, pepper, etc., to an eye, the neck, or a cheek. In this way, he triggered fear, dread, or cheerfulness. In one subject, he provoked a 'split' response; the same substance produced suffering on one side and joy when applied to the other (fig. 3). Following the information communicated by Luys, and on behalf of the Academy, Paul Brouardel (1837–1906) declared: 'These problems are the most considerable of their type that have ever been presented to the Academy, and as they engage its moral responsibility in an unprecedented way, each of us must be capable of verifying these and similar experiments, in order to provide a well-informed opinion'. The conclusion rendered on September 6, 1887 by the appointed commission of experts, was definitive [16]:

> Mindful of the task assigned to it, the Commission deems that its mission is hereby complete. While it recognises without question the good faith of Mr. Luys, the Commission has sufficiently demonstrated that the effects of tubes placed at a distance from hypnotisable subjects appears to depend more on the fancy, imagination and memory of the subject than on the medicinal substances in these tubes... .

But Luys' experiments had considerable impact, despite the rejection of his results by the French Academy of Medicine. Luys, who remained convinced his discoveries were real, conducted sessions at his home. These events were covered extensively in mainstream newspapers, which showed little indulgence for a learned man who had strayed into irrationality.

Having already ridiculed Charcot and Luys by means of the composite character of Dr. Foutange

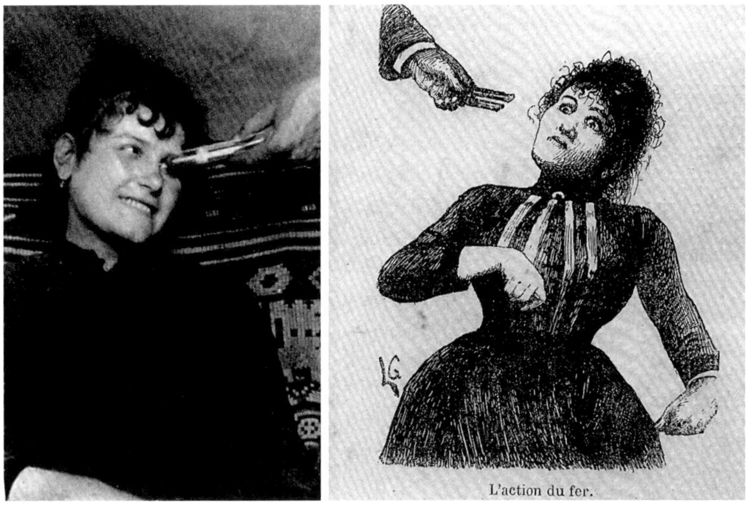

Fig. 3. Left: photo of Esther by Jules Luys. Right: Esther engraving by Alexandre Laurent Gsell. Luys: 'A tube, containing fennel oil to the left eye, determines the hilarity, presented to the right eye triggers a heightened repulsion.' Private collection of the author.

in his satirical 1894 novel *'Les Morticoles'*, Léon Daudet (1867–1942) offered a most ruthless description in his memoir, published in 1915 [16]:

> One hardly ever speaks of the work of Doctor Luys, who made the mistake of tackling hysteria and hypnotism at the same time as the great Charcot. At La Charité Hospital, he housed all the neurotic impostors in Paris, scheming women who were corrupt to the bone and quite pretty in some cases. They knew their way around hospitals and were practised in false attacks, dream states and suggestion. Confident and resembling a fat white parakeet, Luys used colourful visual aids to describe the extraordinary 'somnambulic well' of Sarah, Suzanne and Lucie, along with the phases of their customary hallucinations, while Sarah, Suzanne and Lucie, sitting obediently in their chairs, shook and pinched each other to keep from laughing.

Dumontpallier, who studied under Armand Trousseau (1801–1867) and Charles Lasègue (1816–1883), was most interested in gynecology (his name is associated with a certain type of pessary used for uterine prolapse). He showed no particular interest in neurology until he came across the studies of Burq. With his two students, Paul Magnin (1854–1913) and Edgar Bérillon (1859–1948), Dumontpallier founded *La Revue de l'Hypnotisme expérimental et thérapeutique* in 1886, and from then on, he devoted himself exclusively to hypnosis experiments at La Pitié Hospital in Paris. He eulogized Charcot in 1893 before the French Hypnology Society, claiming that shortly before his death, Charcot accepted the theories of Hippolyte Bernheim (1840–1919) and the Nancy school, which he had always opposed [17]. With his exceptional corpulence and immense beard, Dumontpallier was famous for serving as the sculptor's model for the statue of Charlemagne in front of Notre-Dame Cathedral in Paris [18] (fig. 4). The work of Dumontpallier, who considered himself head of the La Pitié school, was primarily focused on metallotherapy, hypnosis, and hysteria, and remained very faithful to the ideas of Burq.

Like Charcot, Dumontpallier invited journalists to attend his experiments. Henri de Parville, the pen name of François-Henri Peudefer (1838–1909) was an editor at *La Nature*, *La Revue scientifique,* and *Le Journal des débats*, in which he had written an article on January 10, 1879 concerning Charcot's 'impressive' experiments at La Salpêtrière. On February 1, 1882, he wrote a long piece for *Le Journal des débats* on the 'singular action of the application of metals on the bodies of patients' [19]:

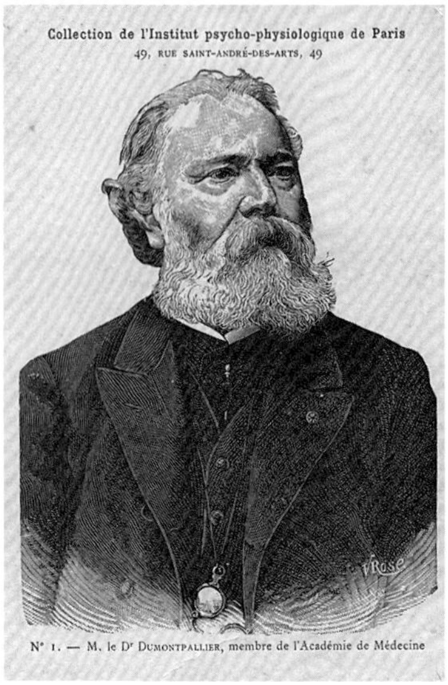
Collection de l'Institut psycho-physiologique de Paris
49, rue Saint-André-des-Arts, 49
N° 1. — M. le Dr Dumontpallier, membre de l'Académie de Médecine

Fig. 4. Victor Dumontpallier (1826–1899). Private collection of the author.

> Suffice it to say that the application of certain metals specific to each patient temporarily restores sensitivity to anaesthetic subjects.... With plates applied to various regions of the body, the subject becomes a sort of puppet controlled by multiple springs. Press her forehead, and an arm lifts on one side, a leg on the other... . Use a bellows on her anterior leg muscles, and she develops a club foot; with another burst of air from the bellows, everything returns to normal. The bellows of Mr. Dumontpallier is sure to become the stuff of legends.

In 1884, Bérillon defended his thesis on 'experimental hypnotism, cerebral duality and functional independence of the two hemispheres of the brain'. The experiments were always conducted with the same patients, who had in fact grown conditioned. Amongst the surprising conclusions: The activity on one side of the brain can be transferred to the other side by application of metal plates on one side, demonstrating the crosswise action of peripheral excitation', or 'In hysterics with unilateral morbid manifestations, the peripheral functional disturbances are located in only one of the brain hemispheres.' Some of the conclusions are even more improbable: 'While one experimenter tells the patient the weather is fine in her left ear, the other tells her it's raining in her right ear; it is then clearly observed that the patient's face expresses the distinct characteristics of laughter on the left side, while the right side reveals a sullen expression.' Bérillon concluded his thesis with this peremptory statement: 'Given that each hemisphere is complete in itself and carries out a particular activity within the limits of its attributions, man is in fact binary from a psychic, sensory and motor point of view; in a word, he possesses two organs of ideation, two brains' (fig. 5). The implausibility of these conclusions, which were nonetheless presented as the pathophysiological basis for split personality in hysterics, reveals that Bérillon and Dumontpallier ultimately lacked critical insight into their work, as did Luys [20].

Outside Paris: Nancy, Bordeaux, and Montpellier

It was by chance that Ambroise-Auguste Liébault (1823–1904), a rural physician in the Lorraine region of France, discovered the therapeutic effectiveness of suggestion, which he called attention. After 10 years of practice, he opened an office in a shed outside Nancy, where he treated a steady stream of poor patients at no cost. Having no interest in research, he only became famous after a meeting with Hippolyte Bernheim (1840–1919) (fig. 6), who had sought out this locally renowned physician, considered by many to be a healer, to learn more about his practices (fig. 7). Joseph Delboeuf (1831–1896), a Belgian mathematician and philosopher who became a psychologist, left us this account [21]:

> Only the most desperate patients go to see Dr. Liébault, those who have been to all the doctors, taken all the drugs including antipyrine, undergone all the tortures from vesicatories and hot cauters, to showers and inductive currents.... Although Mr. Liébault's approach is somewhat naïve and simple, what sets it apart

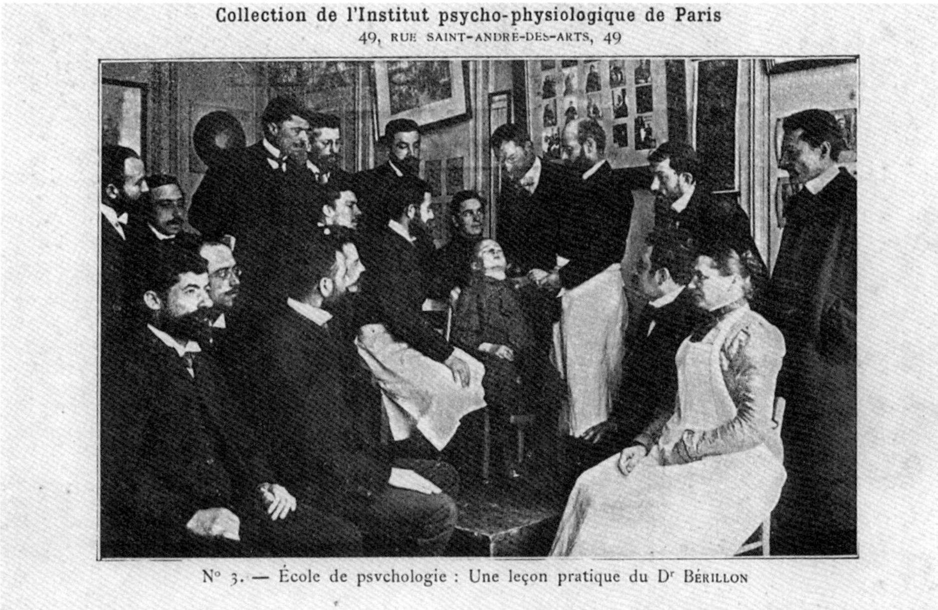
Collection de l'Institut psycho-physiologique de Paris
49, rue Saint-André-des-Arts, 49
N° 3. — École de psychologie : Une leçon pratique du Dr Bérillon

Fig. 5. A public lesson by Edgar Bérillon (1859–1948). Private collection of the author.

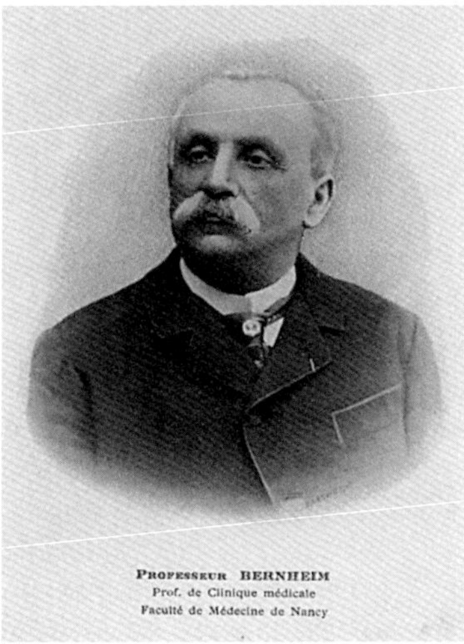
Professeur Bernheim
Prof. de Clinique médicale
Faculté de Médecine de Nancy

Fig. 6. Hippolyte Bernheim (1840–1919). Private collection of the author.

is his air and tone of profound conviction. His words have such communicative warmth that both he and his clients are enchanted. After asking what's wrong, if this is indeed necessary, and without any sort of examination, he has the patient sit down, places a hand on his forehead, and without even looking at him, says: 'You will now sleep'; then, which is to say immediately, he closes the patient's eyelids, ensuring that he is asleep [...] and he speaks, he speaks unceasingly in a strong, vibrant voice. Then the suggestions begin: 'You will heal; your digestion will be good; your sleep will be good; you will no longer cough; your circulation will be free and regular; you will feel great strength in your limbs; you will walk easily'; etc. He hardly varies this refrain. Every disease is mentioned; the client must recognise his particular condition. Undoubtedly, he makes a few special recommendations, related to the patient's disease, but the general recommendations are the principle component.

Despite his scientific skepticism, Bernheim began using hypnosis and suggestion after visiting Liébault. He found these techniques could both bring relief and do harm. Bernheim, who had been a professor of clinical medicine since 1868, was a general practitioner, without any specific training in either neurology or psychology. In the preface to the thesis of his student Gaston Amselle (1881–?), defended 14 years after Char-

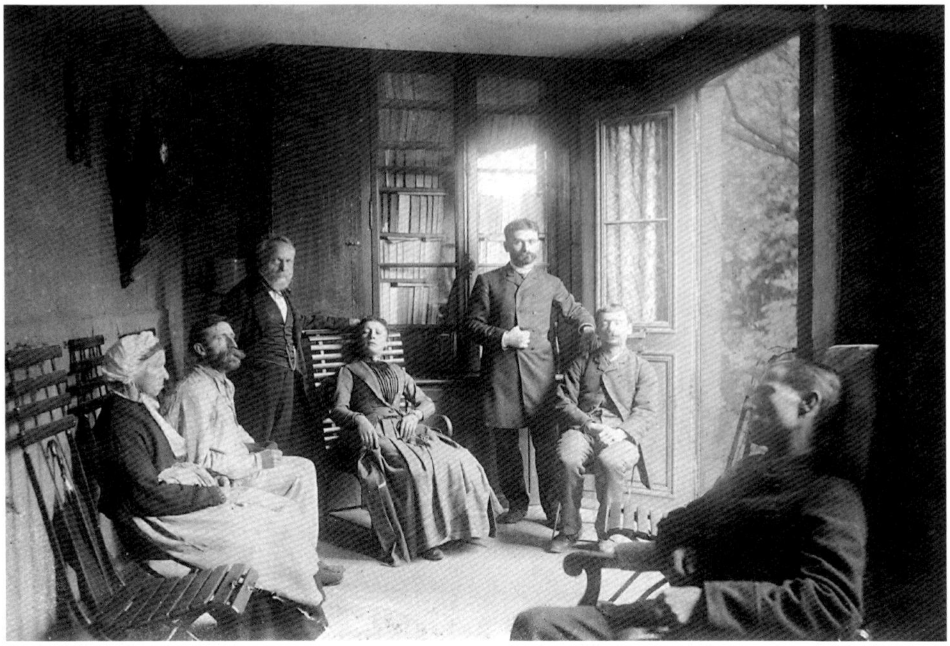

Fig. 7. Ambroise-Auguste Liébault, on the left, at his clinic in Nancy in 1873. He stands surrounded by patients, in the presence of Dr. Levinsson of St. Petersburg. With permission from Collection D. Morque, Centre Image Lorraine©.

cot died, Bernheim declared he was convinced this study would help 'destroy the classical doctrine, universally accepted before my time'. Amselle noted [22]:

> I had seen him use various treatments for convulsive attacks. It was quite surprising to see Mr. Bernheim put an end to highly violent attacks in a few seconds. I attended his clinical lessons, which he gave at the patients' bedsides. With his habitual simplicity, but also with remarkable clarity, he developed his conception of hysteria, and I couldn't help but think that much of what I'd read on the question had been false, as the clinical lessons revealed the inaccuracy of the authors' descriptions'.

As Amselle noted, Bernheim taught while treating his patients; there was no lecture hall or stage in Nancy. He treated a variety of diseases: infectious, tumorous, and psychiatric pathologies. Bernheim, accompanied by his learned assembly, went from bed to bed, dissertating with his patients as well as his students. He used suggestion on both. Delboeuf relates this anecdote [21]:

> We return to the men's room. The previous evening, a 19-year-old cobbler was admitted. Mr. Bernheim carries out a brief examination, observing a coryza with flu. The patient develops a violent headache. He's heard about magnotherapy: 'Is that a joke?' 'You're going to fall asleep and be rid of your headache. You're already starting to feel sleepy.' The patient laughs. 'Go on and laugh. No more pain! You fall deeper and deeper into sleep!' Turning towards us: 'He doesn't hear anything but me now. He's hypnotised!' The subject laughs once again, incredulous. 'Come, my friend, you're going to sleep now. I'm not here to make you laugh, and I don't have any time to lose. Sleep! This time, you fall asleep. I lift your hand; try to lower it. It's impossible for you. I turn your arms; if you try to stop them, they'll turn faster and faster.' And they do. The cobbler's face grows serious; his arms turn rapidly. 'You've lost sensation; I give you an injection, you don't feel anything!' And the

patient doesn't. 'Take this, it's a glass of beer. Drink it.' He makes a drinking gesture. 'You no longer have a headache.' The patient nods. 'While you sleep, I draw your portrait. But, to make you laugh, I give you a red nose. You'll see it when you wake up.' The patient is awakened. He is given his hospital admission file, which is intended for him but still has no writing on it. He looks at it for a few moments, then begins to laugh. He recognises himself and imagines a red nose. 'A farce! I'll keep it, though. It looks a lot like me.' He no longer has a headache and has no memory of what happened.

As Bernheim explained: 'Suggestion is the act by which an idea is introduced in the brain and accepted by it' [23].

Joseph Grasset (1849–1918) spent his entire career in Montpellier, a city in southern France with the world's oldest medical school. From 1885 to 1890, he dedicated his research to hysteria. Amédée Dechambre (1812–1886) asked Grasset rather than Charcot to write the article on hysteria for his monumental dictionary. Grasset began with an etiological theory based on degeneration, close to that of Charcot, but through the various editions, he shifted to a psychological origin and later, after Charcot's death, to a theory of 'deux psyches' that may have been linked to the ideas of Pierre Janet (1859–1947) on 'upper' conscious brain activity and 'lower' unconscious activity. Grasset argued that hysteria resulted from impaired articulation between these two psyches. The value of his lessons lies more in the numerous cases reported than in any original content; Grasset's ideas seem to have evolved with the times, rather than through his own thinking [24].

Albert Pitres (1848–1928) returned to Bordeaux after his training at La Salpêtrière with Charcot. He gave clinical lessons on hysteria, remaining aligned with the teachings in Paris. Charcot used the preface he wrote for *Leçons cliniques sur l'hystérie* published by Pitres in 1891, to justify his positions [25]:

> It is with great satisfaction that I see your studies confirm the research results obtained at La Salpêtrière on the same subjects, not only the essential points, but in most cases even down to the smallest details. The legitimacy of our descriptions has been questioned on several occasions by objections that the patients who served as our models, as they were confined to a special ward, must have been subject to a sort of learning through mutual contamination, thus acquiring a strange and excessively complicated symptomatology, which does not correspond to normal cases. This is why a unique type of hysteria at La Salpêtrière has been alluded to, albeit never with any proof, an artificial, cultivated hysteria, improved so to speak by education, which would not be observed in other environments. For many years, we have been responding to this criticism, solely based on speculative views, by presenting numerous clinical facts, for example showing that relative to an attack of grand hystérie, 'imitation' and 'suggestion' – considered to modify morbid appearance, and while very interesting to study – are relatively restricted and strongly limited in their role, contrary to what has been gratuitously suggested… . I am happy to observe that your lessons also lend strong support to the thesis I am defending. They categorically prove that hysteria is absolutely no different in the Provinces than it is here in Paris, provided that the available neuropathological means are sufficient to cover all its forms, and to reveal its major aspects.

Hysteria, Theater, and Cinema

In addition to inspiring numerous novels by the authors mentioned above, the consultations on hysteria provided rich material for theater and cinema directors. While we cannot give a complete list here, a few examples include *Freud: The Secret Passion*, a 1962 John Houston film in which Sigmund Freud attends one of Charcot's consultations in Paris; *Augustine*, a well-documented film by Jacques Monod and Jean-Christophe Valat that captures the atmosphere of La Salpêtrière and Charcot's lessons; *Augustine*, a 2012 film by Alice Winocour that uses the consultations to weave a metaphorical romance drawing more on feminism than historical fact [26]; *Le Mystère des roches de Kador* (1912), a film directed by Léonce Perret with Suzanne Grandais and Emile Keppens playing Professor Williams (a pseudonym of Charcot) which was presented only 2 years after the Babinski's seminal publication in which he coined the term 'pithiatism', and *Half a Man,* a 1925 American silent comedy film starring Stan Laurel. *Half a Man* combines an iconographic borrowing of passionate attitudes and a scenario of romantic fantasies directly inspired by 'l'Ecole de La Salpêtrière'. Another comedy, *Good Night, Nurse!* is a 1918 short film written and directed by Fatty Arbuckle and starring Buster Keaton, which takes place in a sanitarium where a young patient simulates lethargy, and several figures are inspired by the 'Iconographie de La Salpêtrière'; There is also *The Mask of Dijon* (1946) directed by Lew Landers with Jeanne Bates and Erich von Stroheim who is cast as Dijon, a stage magician specializing in a gruesome guillotine act. Long retired, when he runs out of money, Dijon is forced to make a comeback as a nightclub hypnotist and utilizes his hypnotic powers to cause a crime [27].

Inspired by Mady Schutzman's 1990 article *Dr. Charcot's Hysteria Shows*, Dianne Hunter, a professor at Trinity College in Hartford, Connecticut, wrote and produced a theatre/dance piece, directed by Lenora Champagne. The production's feminism and its historical qualities were not enough to ensure its long-term success, but it is described in Hunter's book [28, 29].

In 2001, Rae Beth Gordon wrote an extensive artistic review entitled *From Charcot to Charlot: Unconscious Imitation and Spectatorship in French Cabaret and Early Cinema*, which was recently translated into French [30, 31].

Hysteria: From Disease to Spectacle

While the primary goal of the physicians mentioned above was study and teaching, the transformation of lessons into spectacles clearly provided inspiration for music halls, circuses, and carnivals until after World War I. The convulsive movements and cataleptic postures became acrobatic contortions and grimaces aimed at provoking anxiety and hilarity. Transformed into an automaton, the body illustrated the dissociation between voluntary gestures and involuntary or unconscious ones. This provided a visual representation of the concept of degeneration, which was the etiology proposed for hysteria before Janet and Paul Sollier (1861–1933). Such burlesque performances caused spectators to feel discomfort, for which laughter was the natural remedy. A regular at Charcot's lessons, Bergson drew inspiration from them for his book *Laughter* (originally published in 1900): 'The attitudes, gestures and movements of the human body are laughable in exact proportion as that body reminds us of a mere machine' [32]. 'We no longer know whether art imitates the clinical, or vice versa' [33].

References

1 Poirier J: L'externat des hôpitaux de Paris (1802–1968). Paris, Hermann, 2012.
2 Goetz CG, Bonduelle M, Gelfand T: Charcot: Constructing Neurology. New York, Oxford University Press, 1995.
3 Charcot JM: La clinique médicale de l'Hospice de La Salpêtrière. Le Progrès Médical 1879;7:913.
4 Janet P: J-M Charcot et son œuvres psychologique. Revue Philosophique de la France et de l'Etranger 1895;39:569–604.
5 Raymond F: Leçons sur les maladies du système nerveux. Première Série recueillies et publiées par MM. E. Ricklin & A. Souques. Paris, Doin, 1896.
6 Daudet A: La Salpêtrière. La Chronique médicale: revue bi-mensuelle de médecine historique, littéraire & anecdotique 1898;4:16–20.
7 Morsier de G: Jean-Martin Charcot (1825–1893); in Kolle K (ed): Grosse Nervenärtze: Lebensbilder in Gemeinschaft. Stuttgart, Thieme, 1956–1963, vol 3.
8 Charcot JM: Leçons de Mardi. Policliniques 1887–1888. Notes de cours de MM. Blin, Charcot et Colin. Paris, Delahaye et Lecrosnier, 1887.
9 Charcot JM, Richer P: Les démoniaques dans l'art. Paris, Delahaye et Lecrosnier, 1887.
10 Anonyme: Magnétisme scientifique à La Salpêtrière. L'Union Médicale 1878; 3s:828.

11 Legrand M: Un dimanche à La Salpêtrière. L'Union Médicale 1878; 3s:893–894.
12 Cadet de Gassicourt E: Eloge de Jules Luys. Bulletin de l'Académie Nationale de Médecine 1897;38:624–627.
13 Parent M, Parent A: Jules Luys in Charcot's penumbra. Front Neurol Neurosci 2011;29:125–136.
14 Luys J: Les émotions chez le sujet en état d'hypnotisme: études de psychologie expérimentale faites à l'aide de substances médicamenteuses ou toxiques impressionnant à distance les réseaux nerveux périphériques. Paris, Baillière, 1887.
15 Brouardel P: Nomination de la commission d'enquête MM Hérard, Charcot, Marey, Gariel et Brouardel. Bulletin de l'Académie nationale de Médecine 1887; 51:336.
16 Daudet L: Devant la douleur. Souvenirs des milieux littéraires, politiques, artistiques et médicaux de 1880 à 1905. Paris, Nouvelle Librairie Nationale, 1915.
17 Dumontpallier V: Eloge de J.-M. Charcot. Revue de l'hypnotisme et de la psychologie physiologique 1894;8:170–171.
18 Miloche P: Un méconnu de l'hystérie, Victor Dumontpallier 1826–1899; thèse, Caen, 1982.
19 de Parville H: Hypnotisme and magnétisme. Journal des Débats politiques et littéraires 1882;68:1–3.
20 Bérillon E: Hypnotisme expérimental: la dualité cérébrale et l'indépendance fonctionnelle des deux hémisphères cérébraux. Paris, Delahaye, 1884.
21 Delboeuf J: Le magnétisme animal: à propos d'une visite à l'Ecole de Nancy. Revue de Belgique 1888;60:241–260, 386–408.
22 Amselle G: Conception de l'hystérie, étude historique et clinique. Paris, Doin, 1907.
23 Bernheim H: Hypnotisme, suggestion psychothérapie. Paris, Doin, 1891.
24 Grasset J: Leçons de clinique médicales faites à l'hôpital Saint-Eloi de Montpellier. Montpellier, Coulet & fils, 1895–1898, vol 3.
25 Pitres A: Leçons cliniques sur l'hystérie et l'hypnotisme faites à l'Hôpital Saint-André de Bordeaux. Paris, Doin, 1891, vol 2.
26 Walusinski O, Poirier J, Déchy H: 'Augustine'. Eur Neurol 2013;69:226–228.
27 André E: Le choc du sujet, de l'hystérie au cinéma (XIXè–XXIè siècle). Rennes, Presses universitaires de Rennes, 2011.
28 Schutzman M: Performance review of Dr Charcot's hysteria shows. Women Performance 1990;5:183–189.
29 Hunter D: The Makings of Dr Charcot's Hysteria Shows. Lewiston, Edwin Mellen Press, 1998.
30 Gordon RB: From Charcot to Charlot: Unconscious Imitation and Spectatorship in French Cabaret and Early Cinema. Critical Inquiry. Chicago, University of Chicago Press, 2001, vol 27, pp 515–549.
31 Gordon RB: De Charcot à Charlot, mises en scène du corps pathologique. Rennes, Presses universitaires de Rennes, 2013.
32 Bergson H: Le rire: essai sur la signification du comique. Paris, Alcan, 1900.
33 Carroy-Thirard J: Possession, extase, hystérie au XIXè siècle. Psychanalyse à l'Université 1980;5:498–515.

Dr. Olivier Walusinski
20 rue de Chartres
FR–28160 Brou (France)
E-Mail walusinski@baillement.com

Bogousslavsky J (ed): Hysteria: The Rise of an Enigma. Front Neurol Neurosci. Basel, Karger, 2014, vol 35, pp 90–98
DOI: 10.1159/000360052

Emma Bovary, Hedda Gabler, and Harold Brodkey Would Not Have Lived without Charcot: Hysteria in Novels

A.A. Kaptein

Medical Psychology, Leiden University Medical Centre, Leiden, The Netherlands

Abstract

Medical humanities is the interdisciplinary field of humanities (literature, philosophy, ethics, history, and religion), social science (anthropology, cultural studies, psychology, and sociology), and the arts (literature, theater, film, and visual arts), and their application to medical education and practice. In this chapter, the concept of 'hysteria' is put into a medical humanities perspective. We review the concept of hysteria concisely. Two novels and one autobiographical story are used as material in order to study how 'hysteria' is represented in literary work. *Madame Bovary* (Gustave Flaubert), *Hedda Gabler* (Henrik Ibsen), and *A Story in an Almost Classical Mode* (Harold Brodkey) were searched for elements that are characteristic of hysteria. Excessive emotion, dramatics, attention-seeking behavior, physical symptoms of unknown and unidentifiable organic causes, self-centered behavior, and flirtatious behavior are the six elements used to operationalize hysteria. It was found that these elements were present in both a quantitative and qualitative manner in the literary works examined. Acknowledging some limitations and suggesting some research areas and clinical implications, we conclude that literary works are useful in analyzing concepts in medicine. Also, more generally, using literary works seems to have a positive impact on readers, healthcare providers, and researchers in the healthcare domain. Studying novels and related literary work contributes to the body of knowledge of medical humanities.

'No results matching your search were found' – this is the outcome of entering 'hysteria' as a search term in the electronic version of DSM-5 [1]. The word 'enigma' in the title of the book with the current chapter seems well chosen. Only time will tell whether the DSM-VI will see a rebirth of the concept 'hysteria'.

Hysteria: Hydrotherapy, Clitoridectomy, Leeches on Wombs, and Addressing Illness Perceptions

Andrew Scull's biography *Hysteria* represents a wonderful analysis of the history of 'a diagnostic waste bin', pertaining to 'a chameleon-like disease that can mimic the symptoms of any other, and one that somehow seems to mold itself to the culture in which it happens' [2, pp. 6–7]. A quite bizarre list of approaches has been applied to 'hysterics', people who display a set of behaviors, emotions and thoughts, which has varied over time, place, and culture, but seems to encompass: excessive emotion, dramatics, attention-seeking behavior, physical symptoms with unknown and unidentifiable organic causes, self-centered behavior, and flirtatious behavior [2].

Over the past centuries, diagnostic and 'therapeutic' approaches to persons displaying all or part of this set of symptoms and behaviors make for fascinating reading. In Hippocratic and Galenic medicine, the uterus and its malfunctions are the seat of hysterical behavior. In 17th-century England, purges, vomits, and bleeding were applied to remedy what was seen as a deep-seated disturbance of the body's equilibrium. Observing that human beings without a uterus also suffered from 'hysteria' necessitated a new model to explain the affliction. A disorder of the nerves served this observation well. Electricity and steel magnets found their place in treating the oversensitive nerves. With 'the birth of the clinic', psychiatric patients, including patients who received the diagnosis 'hysteria', were managed in psychiatric institutions. Bleeding, cupping, applying leeches, and water therapies ('hydrotherapy') were some of the therapeutic methods of choice. However, 'a course of injections of ice water into the rectum, introduction of ice into the vagina, and leeching of the labia and cervix' were also part of the therapeutic arsenal [2, p. 66]. Clitoridectomy was the pinnacle of the arsenal – an approach that (luckily) was viewed too unscientific and harsh by almost all gynecologists and other MDs.

Other harsh and highly invasive methods, such as electrotherapy and ovariotomy (or oophorectomy) followed, soon to be replaced by therapeutic methods that followed from conceptualizing 'hysteria' as a neurological disorder. The 'rest cure' replaced more aggressive and invasive 'therapeutic' approaches. American psychiatrist Weir Mitchell and a female patient in *The Yellow Wallpaper* (1890) exemplify this approach [3]. In hindsight, the doctor's order 'never touch pen, brush or pencil as long as you live' [p. 46] to a patient who desperately wanted to express her despair over her unbearable position in life and love is a tragic side effect of this 'cure' (see Smyth et al. [4, 5] with their work that demonstrates the effectiveness of expressive writing in patients and healthy respondents).

Charcot conceptualized 'hysteria' as a disorder of the nervous system, 'as real and as somatic a disease as any of the other neurological catastrophes' [2, p. 105]. His demonstrations of patients with hysterical behavior became famous in medical and psychiatric circles, and developed into 'Charcot's circus'. Increasingly, his medical colleagues, from France and abroad, viewed 'hysterics' as theatrical learned behavior, thereby dismissing Charcot's views.

It was Freud who argued in his psychoanalytic writings how 'hysteria' should be viewed as a psychiatric – not neurological – affliction. Unconscious conflicts, repressed sexual impulses, and fantasies about incest all contributed to the initiation and maintenance of 'hysteria'. Psychoanalytic therapy was, therefore, the answer.

Learning theory gave rise to behavior therapy. Hysterical behavior was conceptualized as learned behavior – which, therefore, can be unlearned. Cognitive behavioral therapy became vogue in 20th century psychotherapy. Patients with medically unexplained diseases encountered psychotherapists who challenged their cognitions and associated emotions, transforming maladaptive cognitions and emotions into more constructive and helpful thoughts and feelings [6, 7].

The Common Sense Model is currently the most successful theoretically based approach to patients' coping with somatic and psychiatric disorders [8]. In this model, illness representations (cognitions and emotions in response to the disorder) determine coping and self-management of a patient with an illness. Adequate (i.e. adaptive, conducive to reducing stress and to constructive coping) illness perceptions are associated with adaptive outcomes. Inadequate illness perceptions (i.e. maintaining stress, impeding coping) are associated with inadequate self-management skills, and therefore, poor outcome. This implies that therapeutic approaches aimed at transforming inadequate illness perceptions into more adaptive ones, lead to improved outcomes. Meta-analyses support this statement [9].

In patients with somatoform disorders (sometimes labeled as 'conversion disorders'), interventions aiming at changing inadequate illness perceptions appear to lead to positive outcomes, expressed as reductions in symptoms, increased participation in societal activities (work), and quality of life [10, 11]. Encouraging 'hysterical' patients to become a more active participant in his/her problem and its potential solution seems the current psychotherapeutic approach of patients in this category.

After having given this concise but broad-brushed view on hysteria, we now will see whether novels and other literary work can help clarify hysterical behavior.

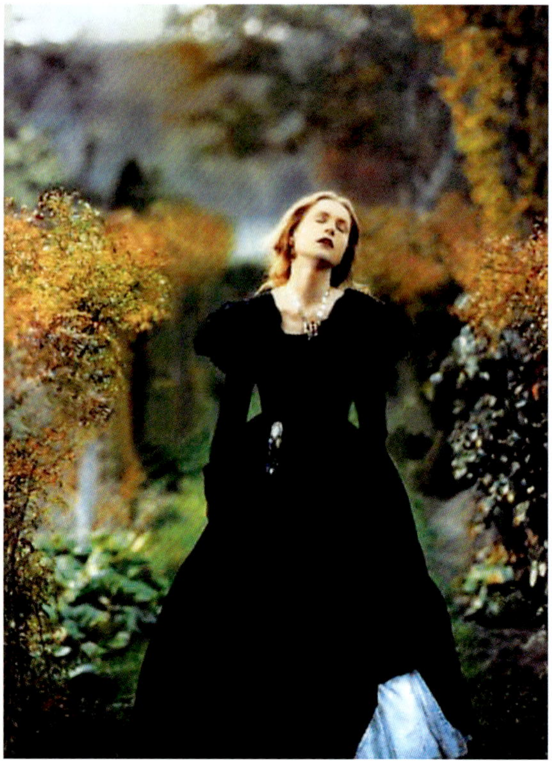

Fig. 1. Isabelle Huppert as Emma Bovary in Claude Chabrol's film (Collection Christophel).

Methods

Literary works were selected via a search using the Columbia University of New York website (www.litmed.med.nyu.edu) under the heading 'hysteria'. Three works were selected, based on literary quality, and with the wish to have the views of a 'hysteric' her/himself, and those of someone who must cope with the hysterical behavior of a close relative. *Madame Bovary* (Gustave Flaubert), *Hedda Gabler* (Henrik Ibsen), and *A Story in an Almost Classical Mode* (Harold Brodkey) were the selected works [12–14].

The six criteria for 'hysterical behavior' mentioned earlier were studied in those works: excessive emotion, dramatics, attention-seeking behavior, physical symptoms of unknown and unidentifiable organic causes, self-centered behavior, and flirtatious behavior. Similar to comparable studies [15], 'chunks' of text containing these criteria in the three works were identified and listed.

Our essay is a descriptive, exploratory study, given the virtual absence of a body of knowledge on how to analyze in a theoretically based and empirically founded manner [16]. We follow a method that we described and applied earlier when analyzing a novel on patient-physician relations [17] and on illness perceptions [18], rendering acceptable and meaningful results.

Madame Bovary

She is false, she is deceitful by nature: she deceives Charles from the very start before actually committing adultery. She lives among philistines, and she is a philistine herself. [...] In Emma the vulgarity, the philistinism, is veiled by her grace, her cunning, her beauty, her meandering intelligence, her power of idealization, her moments of tenderness and understanding, and by the fact that her brief bird life ends in human tragedy [19, p. 142] (fig. 1).

Madame Bovary was published in 1857. It brought the author, Gustave Flaubert (1821–1880), both a trial for writing a scandalous and blasphemous novel, and fame – almost immediately after the book was published, literary critics and the public loved the book, continuing into this day. The novel describes the rise and fall of a middle-aged woman in rural France in the middle of the 19th century. The story line itself is not that remarkable – it is the detailed and precise depiction of the major characters that draws the reader toward the dramatic finish of the book. The protagonist marries, has affairs with two lovers, swallows a handful of arsenic from an apothecary bottle, and dies. If anything, Madame Bovary is a classic example of a hysteric woman.

Excessive Emotion

Accustomed to calm aspects of life, she turned, on the contrary, to those of excitement. She loved the sea only for the sake of its storms, and the green fields only when broken up by ruins. She wanted to get some personal profit out of things, and she rejected as useless all that did not contribute to the immediate desires of her heart, being of a temperament more sentimental than artistic, looking for emotions, not landscapes' (p. 75). [...] So at last she was to know those joys of love, that fever of happiness of which she had despaired! She was entering upon marvels where all would be passion, ecstasy, delirium (p. 273).

Dramatics

Madame Bovary's death could hardly be less dramatic. Dying after ingesting a huge amount of arsenic is a dramatic affair – the author studied the details of the phenomenon in medical books. Less dramatic but nevertheless impressive is Madame Bovary's shopping behavior: spending a lot more money than available, with disastrous consequences. Drama surrounds her life: 'Love, she thought, must come suddenly, with great outbursts and lightings – a hurricane of the skies, which falls upon life, revolutionizes it, roots up the will like a leaf, and sweeps the whole heart into the abyss' (p. 175).

Attention-Seeking Behavior

She envied lives of stir; longed for masked balls, for violent pleasures, with all the wildness that she did not know, but that these must surely yield (p. 123). [...] Her looks grew bolder, her speech more free; she even committed the impropriety of walking out with Monsieur Rodolphe, a cigarette in her mouth, 'as if to defy the people' (p. 319).

Physical Symptoms

Madame Bovary is a collector of a very impressive list of symptoms. Psychiatrists specializing in medically unexplained symptoms would have a field day if they were to use the novel as a source of symptoms:

From that moment she drank vinegar, contracted a sharp little cough, and completely lost her appetite (p. 123). [...] She was seized with giddiness, and from that evening her illness recommenced, with a more uncertain character, it is true, and more complex symptoms. Now she suffered in her heart, then in the chest, the head, the limbs; she had vomitings, in which Charles thought he saw the first signs of cancer (p. 349).

Self-Centered Behavior

Emma Bovary seems to be in love with herself, mainly: 'She could have wished this name of Bovary, which was hers, had been illustrious, to see it displayed at the booksellers, repeated in the newspapers, known to all France (p. 115). [...] Emma was growing difficult, capricious' (p. 121).

Flirtatious Behavior

The novel is about flirting, about seeking the attention of men, about passion, including sexual passion. Emma has relations with at least two lovers in the novel. Giving samples of text on this criterion would do injustice to the literary work itself, in our view. May the reader of Madame Bovary find out for himself/herself!

Hedda Gabler

Henrik Ibsen (1828–1906) wrote *Hedda Gabler* in 1890. The work is considered to be one of the classic plays where 'hysteria' plays a crucial role. It is a relatively short piece, with the action taking place in a couple of hours. The number of players is limited, but their interactions are many – and very emotional, complex, and deadly. At the end of the play, two players end up fatally wounded – by their own hand (fig. 2).

Applying the criteria for hysterical behavior as outlined earlier, the following observations can be made.

Excessive Emotion
Hedda spends months on their honeymoon. She tells a relative: 'I've been bored to death. [...] Try passing six months without meeting a single person you can talk to' (p. 32). Concerning the house the newlyweds have just moved into, Hedda remarks: 'There is something of the mortuary about it. It smells of rot' (p. 37).

Dramatics
'I'm going to die! I'm going to die of all of this!' (p. 71). And, after her husband's colleague/competitor committed suicide, Hedda starts playing dance music on the piano. One minute later, Hedda commits suicide.

Attention-Seeking Behavior
The maid predicts Hedda's behavior already on the second page of the play: 'I have a feeling she'll be very demanding' (p. 6). The protagonist herself wonders: 'Well, what in God's name am I supposed to do with myself?' (p. 31).

Physical Symptoms
Hedda Gabler does not seem to exhibit any.

Self-Centered Behavior
When her husband is relieved that his rival will not compete for a professorship, he exclaims: 'He will not stand in our way!' Hedda retorts: 'Our' way. Please leave me out of it' (p. 42). And when a relative's friend is dying, she comments: 'I don't care to look at sickness, or death, it's ugly. I want nothing to do with it' (p. 58).

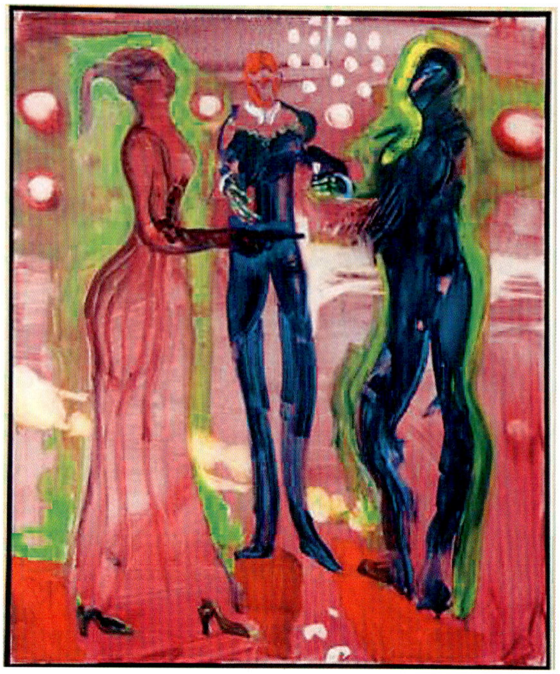

Fig. 2. Haakon Bleken: *Overrekelse av pistolen (The Handing-Over of the Pistol).* ©ProLitteris, Zurich.

Flirtatious Behavior
Hedda: 'Doesn't it seem, Judge, like an absolute eternity since we last spoke? Some small talk last night and this morning, but I don't count that.' Judge: 'You mean, a talk like this, just the two of us?' Hedda: 'I guess that's roughly what I mean.' Judge: 'Every day I've wandered around wishing you were back home.' Hedda: 'The same goes for me' (p. 31).

A Story in an Almost Classical Mode

This story begins ominously: 'My protagonists are my mother's voice and the mind I had when I was thirteen' (p. 221). How 'hysterical behaviour' is perceived by persons in the immediate psychological and social environment of 'the hysterical patient' is described in painful detail by Harold Brodkey (1930–1996). Harold is adopted by his

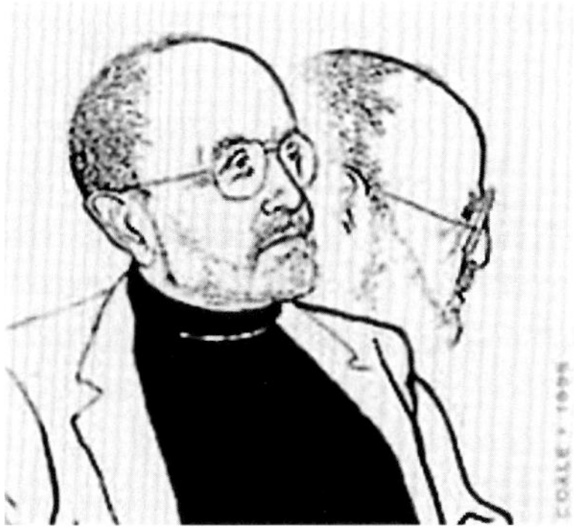

Fig. 3. H. Brodkey, by Howard Coale for The New Yorker, 1995 [32].

stepmother when he is 2 years old, after his mother and father died. In the 45-page short autobiographical story, the author describes the struggle he battles out with his stepmother during her illness (she suffers from breast cancer, among other diseases). At the end of the story, she dies. We will analyze the story with the six characteristics of hysteric behavior as in the previous two novels, this time as perceived by the son (albeit stepson) of the 'patient' (fig. 3).

Excessive Emotion
That is, if I came in and said, 'Hello, Momma,' she would demand, 'Is that all you can say? I'm in *pain.* Don't you care? My God, my God, what kind of selfish person are you? I can't stand it.' If I said, 'Hello, Momma, how is your pain?' she would shriek, 'You fool, I don't want to think about it! It was all right for a moment! Look what you've done – you've brought it back. [...] *I don't want to be reminded of my pain all the time!*' (p. 233). [...] She said that I came from filthy people and what I was was more filth, that I came from the scum of the earth and was more scum. [...] She threw an ashtray at me. She ordered me out of the house (p. 255).

Dramatics
Doris [the stepmother] yelled, 'What do you think it does to me to see you exercising in your room – when I have to die?' I said, 'I don't know. Does it bother you a lot?' 'You're a fool!' she screamed. 'Don't make me wish you'd get cancer so you'd know what I'm going through!' (pp. 229–230). [...] God, how she screamed (p. 255).

Attention-Seeking Behavior
Doris insisted I give her what money I earned. And usually I did, so that I would not have to listen to her self-righteous begging and angry persuasiveness (p. 229). [...] If I ignored her or argued with her, she became violent, and then temper and fright – even the breath she drew – spoiled the balance of pain and morphine in her; sometimes then she would howl (p. 230).

Physical Symptoms
Sometimes she would apologize; she would say, 'It's not me who says those things; it's the pain. It's not fair for me to have this pain: You don't know what it's like' (p. 230). [...] She said, 'Look at what they've done to me. My God, look what they've done to me.' She lowered her nightgown to her waist. The eerie colors of her carapace and the jumble of scars moved into my consciousness... . That gargoylish torso. [...] She said, 'I scratched myself while I slept – look, there's blood' (p. 231).

Self-Centered Behavior
She wanted those women to telephone and come and be present at her tragedy (p. 225). [...] She would yell, 'What's wrong with you? Why don't you know how to talk to me! My God, do you think it's easy to die? [...] Why do you just stand there? Why do you just listen to me! [...] Do something for me!' (p. 233).

Flirtatious Behavior
She'd put on lipstick and a hair ribbon; and her face, which had been twisted up, was half all right: the lines were pretty much up and down and not crooked; and my heart began to beat sadly for myself – she was going to try to be nice for a little while; she was going to ask me to stay (p. 234).

Discussion

In this explorative chapter, we used three literary products (two novels, one autobiographical story) to analyze how 'hysteria' is depicted in literature. We found that the elements of the – disputed – diagnosis 'hysteria' are relatively easily traceable in the three literary works. This in itself is not a major finding as we selected the three works precisely because they turned up in a literature search for books on 'hysteria'. What we feel is important is that our study shows that literary works can be used as a source of data in order to analyze a certain concept (i.e. hysteria), which in its turn allows enriching a (psychological) theory (in our case, the Common Sense Model), which may shed additional light on living with hysteria and even on psychotherapeutic suggestions for adjusting to hysteria.

Earlier work led to comparable findings. We ourselves described how *Cancer Ward* by Solzhenitsyn is a beautiful source of material when analyzing illness perceptions in people with cancer [17]. Similarly, the autobiographical novel *The Breath* by Thomas Bernhard served as a very useful illustration of models of patient-physician interaction [18]. Even the Bible has been used to analyze how neurological disorders are depicted in a literary, albeit religious, work [20]. The same goes for classical sources such as Homer [21], and even a comic book like *Asterix*, analyzing wounds in Roman warriors [22].

The context of medical humanities allows extending the source of data from novels to also poems, music, paintings, and movies. In the case of hysteria, the website of Columbia University (New York) lists, for instance, *American Beauty* as an example of a movie where 'hysteria' is a prominent feature. The painting of Hedda Gabler by Bleken in this chapter reflects various 'hysterical features' (the exuberant colors reflect emotionality, as does the handing over of a pistol with the implicit invitation to commit suicide) [23]. A new chapter might be devoted to analyzing how movies, paintings, poems, and music contain elements that may be characterized as 'hysterical'. Earlier, we published a paper on how these five art forms (movies, paintings, poems, and music along with literature) may reflect important phenomenological and experiential themes resultant from asthma, chronic obstructive pulmonary disease, cystic fibrosis, and lung cancer [24].

A limitation of our chapter is a methodological issue. We set out to find elements in the sources we used that reflect elements of our operationalization of the concept 'hysteria'. This is like looking for white swans in a pool full of white swans – in order to 'prove' that all swans are white. At the same time, the concept of 'hysteria' is elusive, and in literary theory there is hardly consensus on how literary works can and should be analyzed for various purposes: 'simply put, at this juncture, rehabilitation researchers and clinicians would appear to lack both the vocabulary and the methodology to systematically study and report on the narrative nature of illness, injury, disability, and related phenomena' [16, p. 401]. A method that is used quite often in literary research pertains to defining elements of the core concepts (which we did) and then taking 'chunks' from these sources [15]. A method used by psychologists is the linguistic inquiry and word count which uses all of the text of a novel to analyze characteristics of specific word usage, such as the proportion of self-focused language (e.g. first-person pronouns) or negative emotion words [25]. Future researchers could use this technique to analyze the three literary works that we analyzed in our method.

Additional suggestions for further research pertain to refinements in the methodology, for instance extending the number of raters of the 'chunks' in the books used, refining the operationalization of the 'hysteria' concept, and using novels and autobiographic material that are written on characters that are generally agreed to be very un-hysteric and/or by authors who are known to exhibit no hysteric behavior at all.

Clinically, the chapter also tries to show how reading novels may help clinicians increase their sensitivity to persons with certain diagnostic labels. Medical students and students in other health-related fields may benefit from reading novels on various illnesses – in both works that pertain to 'psychiatric' or more 'physical' diseases. Beveridge gives strong arguments to say 'yes' to his question in his paper: 'Should psychiatrists read fiction?', namely [26, p. 385]:

We can explore the lives and inner worlds of a wide variety of individuals by imaginatively engaging with them in novels. A purely bioscientific model offers a limited view of human beings. Reading literature helps to develop empathy. Aesthetic approaches to the medical study of literature lead to the development of complex interpretive skills. Ethical approaches teach ethical reflection [it should be mentioned that Beveridge also gives arguments to say 'no' to his question].

As detailed in an earlier paper of ours, novels can also be employed as a means of impacting on the health and behavior of readers, and, finally, literary sources do represent valid and useful material to study health, illness, and illness behavior. MRI, blood tests, and various other 'objective' methods in medicine are not the only way to do research in healthcare. Medical humanities deserves a safe and solid position in medical curricula [27–29].

Lewis [30, p. 12] summarizes much research on 'hysteria' and concludes: 'a tough old word like hysteria dies very hard. It tends to outlive its obituarists.' Recently, Julien Bogousslavsky (the editor of this volume) expressed similar views in his analysis of the concept of 'hysteria', entitled: 'Hysteria after Charcot: back to the future' [31]. It will be exciting to see whether and how 'hysteria' is discussed in future publications.

Acknowledgment

The author is grateful to Joshua M. Smyth, PhD, Biobehavioral Health and Medicine, Pennsylvania State University, University Park, Pa., USA, for helpful feedback on structure and content of an earlier version of the chapter.

References

1 Diagnostic and Statistical Manual of Mental Disorders, ed 5. Washington, American Psychiatric Association, 2013.
2 Scull A: Hysteria – The Biography. Oxford, Oxford University Press, 2009.
3 Gilman CP: The Yellow Wall-Paper. New York, The Feminist Press at CUNY, 1996.
4 Smyth J, Arigo D: Recent evidence supports emotion regulation interventions for improving health in at-risk and clinical populations. Curr Opin Psychiatry 2009;22:205–210.
5 Smyth J, Nazarian D, Arigo D: Expressive writing in the clinical context; in Denollet J, Nyklicek I, Vingerhoets A (eds): Emotion Regulation: Conceptual and Clinical Issues. New York, Springer, 2008, pp 215–233.
6 Barsky AJ, Ahern DK, Bauer MR, Nolido N, Orav EJ: A randomized trial of treatment for high-utilizing somatizing patients. J Gen Intern Med 2013;28:1396–1404.
7 Petrie KJ, Weinman J: Patients' perceptions of their illness: the dynamo of volition in health care. Curr Dir Psychol Sci 2012;21:60–65.
8 Leventhal H, Leventhal EA, Breland JY: Cognitive science speaks to the 'common-sense' of chronic illness management. Ann Behav Med 2011;41:152–163.
9 Hagger MS, Orbell S: A meta-analytic review of the Common-Sense Model of illness representation. Psychol Health 2003;18:141–184.
10 Owens C, Dein S: Conversion disorder: the modern hysteria. Adv Psychiatr Treat 2006;12:152–157.
11 Moss-Morris R, Spence MJ, Hou R: The pathway from glandular fever to chronic fatigue syndrome: can the cognitive behavioural model provide the map? Psychol Med 2011;41:1099–1107.
12 Flaubert G: Madame Bovary. French Classics in French and English (translated by E. Marx; critical introduction by F. Brunetière), Ithaca, NY, Cornell University Press, 1904.
13 Ibsen H: Hedda Gabler (English version by D. Hughes). New York, Dramatists Play Service Inc., 2001.
14 Brodkey H: A story in an almost classical mode; in: Stories in an Almost Classical Mode. New York, Vintage Books, 1988, pp 219–265.
15 Altieri JL: Children's contemporary realistic fiction portraying dyslexic characters: an examination of the issues confronted and the gender of the characters. Reading Res Instruct 2006;45: 161–178.
16 Albright KJ, Duggan CH, Epstein MJ: Analyzing trauma narratives: introducing the narrative form index and matrix. Rehab Psychol 2008;53:400–411.
17 Kaptein AA, Lyons AC: The doctor, the breath and Thomas Bernhard. J Health Psychol 2009;14:161–170.
18 Kaptein AA, Lyons AC: Cancer ward: patient perceptions in oncology. J Health Psychol 2010;15:848–857.
19 Nabokov V: Lectures on Literature. London, Picador, 1980.
20 Budrys V: Neurology in Holy Scripture. Eur J Neurol 2007;14:1–6.
21 Konsolaki E, Astyrakaki E, Stefanakis G, Agouridakis P, Askitopoulou H: Cranial trauma in ancient Greece: from Homer to classical authors. J Craniomaxillofac Surg 2010;38:549–553.

22 Kamp MA, Slotty P, Sarikaya-Seiwert S, Steiger HJ, Hänggi D: Traumatic brain injuries in illustrated literature: experience from a series of over 700 head injuries in the Asterix comic books. Acta Neurochir 2011;153:1351–1355.
23 Bondevik H: La donna è mobile – om hysteridiagnosen i Norge på 1800-tallet. Tidsskrift for Den norske legeforening 2007;127:3254–3258.
24 Kaptein AA, Meulenberg F, Smyth JM: Do art lovers make better doctors? Lancet Respir Med 2013;1:769–770.
25 Pennebaker JW, Booth RJ, Francis ME: Operator's Manual. Linguistic Inquiry and Word Count: LIWC2007. Austin, University Texas Austin, 2007.
26 Beveridge A: Should psychiatrists read fiction? Br J Psychiatry 2003;182:385–387.
27 Tomorrow's Doctors. London, General Medical Council, 2009.
28 American Society for Bioethics and Humanities (ASBH): ASBH Task Force on Ethics and Humanities Education in Undergraduate Medical Programs. Glenview, ASBH, 2009.
29 Raamplan Artsenopleiding 2009 (Framework Medical Education). Utrect, NFU, Utrecht, 2009.
30 Lewis A: The survival of hysteria. Psychol Med 1975;5:9–12.
31 Bogousslavsky J: Hysteria after Charcot: back to the future. Front Neurol Neurosc 2011;29:137–161.
32 The New Yorker, 5 Feb 1995, p 12.

Ad A. Kaptein, PhD
Professor of Medical Psychology
Leiden University Medical Centre
PO Box 9600, NL–2300 RC Leiden (The Netherlands)
E-Mail a.a.kaptein@lumc.nl

Bogousslavsky J (ed): Hysteria: The Rise of an Enigma. Front Neurol Neurosci. Basel, Karger, 2014, vol 35, pp 99–108
DOI: 10.1159/000360063

Traces of Hysteria in Novels

Joost Haan[a, b] · Peter J. Koehler[c]

[a]Department of Neurology, Rijnland Hospital Leiderdorp, Leiderdorp, [b]Department of Neurology, Leiden University Medical Centre, Leiden, and [c]Department of Neurology, Atrium Medical Centre Heerlen, Heerlen, The Netherlands

Abstract

There have been many descriptions of presumed 'hysterics' in fiction, many appearing in French literature, but also in a number of other languages. It is clear that contemporary medical ideas and insights about hysteria had a major influence on its depiction in novels. This is particularly true for naturalistic literature, which has been the subject of previous reviews. Here, we focus on a more recent novel: *Human Traces* by Sebastian Faulks (2005). What is special about the depiction of hysteria in this work is that the presumed 'hysteric' turns out not to be hysteric at all. In the novel, as well as in this chapter, the diagnosis of hysteria is discussed in the light of theories about hysteria of around 1900. For comparison, we present some examples of true 'hysterics' as they occur in fiction. Since it has become clear that severe nonpsychiatric diseases such as an ovarian teratoma can lead to bizarre phenotypes, the association of 'hysteria' with the womb has to be seen in another light.

According to her doctor, Katharina von A. is a textbook case of hysteria with 'interesting complications'. The doctor wrote a paper on her disease and intends to read this as a 'case' at the autumn meeting of the Psychiatric Association in Vienna. Here is a summary of his findings:

Fräulein Katharina von A.

In the early summer of 189-, a patient was referred to me by a physician in a private clinic in Vienna. A young woman, aged twenty-five years had been complaining of severe lower abdominal pain, accompanied by infrequent vomiting. She also suffered from intermittent amenorrhea. As a child, she had a tendency to infections of the throat, but further her childhood had been apparently uneventful. In addition to abdominal pain, she reported chronic joint pain in the shoulders, elbows and fingers. She had also spasms in the shoulders, hips and face. Since the age of seventeen, she had suffered from right-sided occipital headaches, ascribed to astigmatism. She had complained of complete aphonia on two occasions.

Her father was a businessman of considerable means. She had a younger brother and sister. Her mother appeared to have been an indolent and rather foolish woman. There was no obvious neuropathic heredity in the family. The patient especially expressed a most natural and pleasing affection to her father, who treated her more as a sister than a daughter and appeared to rely on her for a level-headedness and equanimity sometimes absent in her mother.

At physical examination she had a fine epidermis with a scattering of reddish-brown maculae on legs, arms and lower back. The areolae were unusually thin and her pelvis appeared fairly narrow. Further examination was normal, although there was a minor irregularity of the pulse and a temperature elevated a degree above normal. The pupils did not show the Argyll Robertson sign.

The patient was clearly distressed by her pain, spoke of it in a cool manner which rose the suspicion that her attention was in fact more passionately engaged elsewhere, on issues of which the pain in her joints and lower abdomen might be little more than representations. I attributed this to what Charcot called the *belle indifference* of the hysteric. The picture was complicated by a state of superficial anxiety, chronic insomnia, a tendency to low spirits and a somewhat morbid fear of animals.

When Katharina was twenty-one years old, her father had fallen ill with a heart complaint. The task of nursing him fell to her, since her mother declared herself too distraught and was not in good health herself. During her father's sickbed, he was often visited by Herr P, a business partner. On such occasions, Katharina would go to the kitchen or to her bedroom to let the men conduct their business in private. For almost two years she had nursed her dying father. Then, one day at lunchtime, she left her father with the doctor. He died in her absence. At the moment she heard of his death, she became violently sick and vomited her lunch over the tray. The present abdominal complaints began at that time. Her mother was engaged to be married again within a year – with Herr P.

As I concluded that it was hysteria that was now conducting the orchestra, I started some massage, electrotherapy and supervision of diet and exercise regimen. Furthermore, I massaged her back and shoulders and stroke the parts of the lower abdomen that had most troubled her. Hereafter, I decided to hypnotize the patient. As I applied mild pressure on her forehead, she confessed that she craved attention and had Sapphic fantasies about the older girls at school and had occasionally masturbated at night in her bed. When she was twelve, she played with a girlfriend in the woods and felt excited when she discovered that her brother was spying on them. Later, her father's secretary had seduced her to touch herself. Around this time she felt lonely and vulnerable and fell in love easily with young men.

I felt that a fairly clear picture of the trauma that had precipitated her hysteria was now available to me. A traumatic incident had been deliberately suppressed by her conscious mind because she found the implications of it intolerable. Her suppressed ideas had turned pathogenic. I explained to her: 'When you are anxious about your clothing you wish to be naked. You wish your mother dead and wish to marry Herr P. The vomiting after the news of your father's death revealed a revulsion at what the future had in store for you. The intermittent pains in the abdomen are a mnemic symbol or *aide-mémoire* of that distressing emotion.

Having explained to Fräulein Katharina the genesis of all her symptoms, I warned her that it might be some time before she felt a full remission from them. Just as it took some time for the conversion of trauma to manifest itself in the production of hysterical phenomena (Charcot called this the 'period of working out' or 'elaboration'), so the reverse was also true: some time was required for the catharsis to work through the system.

Traces of Hysteria

Katharina von A. is not a real person, nor is her doctor. They are both characters in the novel *Human Traces* (2005) by the English author Sebastian Faulks [1]. It is one of the most recent novels of a long series, in which hysteria (and Charcot) plays an important role. In Faulks' novel, the diagnosis of a 'textbook case of hysteria' (p. 292) and the description of Katharina's disease (pp. 294–309), summarized above, is made by the French neurologist Jacques Rebière. His main motivation to specialize in diseases of the mind was the severe mental disease of his older brother, Olivier, who despite normal early development, developed severe behavioral problems between puberty and adulthood, including violent behavior and hallucinations. His mind went 'little by little, like smoke beneath the door' (p. 7). Olivier had to be kept permanently chained to a wall in the stable with the horses and sometimes was even put away with the pigs (p. 23). Rendering the historical terminology applied to the disease, the diagnosis given to Olivier was 'degeneration' (p. 104), 'hebephrenia' (p. 104), or 'dementia praecox' (p. 493). Also Bleuler's proposal to call such a disease 'schizophrenie' is mentioned, but not taken very seriously (p. 493), as Jacques Rebière keeps calling it 'Olivier's disease' (p. 102). He has studied medicine in Paris and trained as a 'specialist in nervous disorders' at Salpêtrière under Charcot. In addition, he spent some time in Nancy with Bernheim.

Another protagonist of the novel, the Englishman Thomas Winterbottom, is also fascinated by the human mind and its abnormalities. At first, he wanted to 'study Shakespeare and some of the other English poets' (p. 38), but followed his sister's advice to study medicine instead, as she says: 'You are fascinated by illness. You love those long medical words even if you don't know what they mean' (p. 43). Indeed, his love of words and interest in philosophy inspired Thomas to study medicine and become an alienist. At the end of his studies, his bookcase contains: *On Insanity* by Vincenzio Chiarugi, *Rhapsodies of the Psychological Method of Cure in Mental Alienation* by Johann Reil, Pinel's *Traité médico-philosophique sur l'aliénation mentale*, *Observations on Insanity* by John Haslam, three volumes of *Des maladies mentales* by Jean-Etienne Esquirol and *Die Pathologie und Therapie der psychische Krankheiten* by Wilhelm Griesinger (pp. 101–103). These are his heroes, but most of all he is influenced by the philosophical ideas of John Hughlings Jackson, 'the father of English neurology' (p. 506).

Jacques and Thomas meet during a holiday in Deauville, at the Normandy coast, when they both have just started their medical training. They immediately realize that they have the same passion. As 'blood brothers' they swear to keep in touch and collaborate on what they would see as their dream: to '...somehow try to understand the meeting point between thought and flesh', '...understand and cure those whose sickness is in the mind and determine its causes...' (p. 55), '...intend to establish beyond doubt how the mind works...', and '...show what makes us human' (p. 236).

Thomas is trained in Cambridge, and has spent some time in Edinburgh and at St. Bartholomew's (London) (p. 71). After completing his studies, he works in an asylum, where more than 2,000 patients are cared for and receive so-called 'moral treatment' (p. 73). This basically means that they are not put away in a stable or cellar (like Olivier), but are allowed to be among other patients, now and then in free air, and even in the garden and the laundry to do some simple work. Thomas' senior colleague describes the work in the asylum in Pinel's words: 'We use the ways of gentleness' (p. 75). This, however, has not made him very enthusiastic:

> Now, thirty years later, I have cured almost no one. The most common ailments in this asylum are idiocy, which is inherited and incurable, and epilepsy which may have some source in the activity of the brain, though we know not where. Then there is general paralysis of the insane, the result of which I have observed post-mortem when the brain is severely damaged. But we have no idea what causes it. My own suspicion is that it is somehow connected with syphilis, but we have no way of demonstrating this. And finally there is a kind of dementia, hearing voices and so on, which appears to begin in young people and to intensify. We are far from agreeing even a description, let alone a cure for that. Some forms of mania and melancholia do seem to improve, but whether that is because of hot baths and cascarilla or whether they have just run their course, I could not say. It is a damnable state of affairs (pp. 170–171).

Simultaneously, in Paris, Jacques attends many of Charcot's public lectures.

> There was nothing triumphant in Charcot's manner of speaking, which remained clipped, reluctant and packed with meaning. No word escaped him that did not bend each syllable to work. 'In Parkinson's disease, long-established', he said, 'we have a complete clinical picture of the symptom, but our microscopes and our

best endeavors have yet to locate its lesion. Other conditions in this pregnant state include Huntington's disease, epilepsy and hysteria (p. 161).

In one of the lectures, Charcot presents a woman with hysteria (to Jacques' slight disappointment it is not Blanche Wittmann, the famous hysterical patient fainting in the arms of Babinski on the well-known Brouillet painting *Leçon clinique à la Salpêtrière* 1887).

'Hysteria, as you know', said Charcot, 'was once thought of as an ailment only of the uterus. Indeed that is how it gained its name, from the Greek word for the womb. [...] Hysteria is a bridesmaid, like Parkinson's, though one of my distinguished colleagues will doubtless find its lesion within the next few years – or months. Hysterics suffer from fits similar to, but less severe than, those endured by epileptics. The classic attack has four parts which we shall shortly demonstrate to you. A predisposition to hysteria is inherited. In this respect, as in almost all the others, it is a standard neurological disorder. The fascination of hysteria, the aspect that makes it *sui generis*, is the way that it offers a bridge between the physical and mental function of the patient. [...] Let me recap: a standard neurological illness. Lesion, nervous malfunction, motor disorder with hereditary predisposition. Yet we note also the persistence of some ovarian element. A hysterical attack can be arrested by a doctor applying pressure to the ovaries (p. 162).

Charcot explained how he discovered that 'all hysterical patients can be hypnotized, whereas those who do not suffer from this condition can under no circumstances' be hypnotized (pp. 162, 163) (thereby referring to the famous controversy between the Salpêtrière school and the Nancy school of Liébault and Bernheim, who believed that anyone could be hypnotized). The patient with hysteria was demonstrated by Charcot's staff. A hysterical attack began after the sound of a gong a few inches from her ear. Charcot commented on parts of the different stages: the aura, globus hystericus ('the sensation that her uterus has risen in her abdomen'), a subepileptic seizure, acrobatic clownism, burbling vocalization, and a protracted delirium. After manual pressure on the abdomen, the attack ended. After the demonstration, Charcot thrust his notes at the chest of his chief assistant Pierre Marie and said: 'Arrange all this for publication' (p. 165).

Jacques takes his wife Sonia (Thomas's sister) to the next demonstration, persuading her to come as 'half the audience are not medical people' (p. 194). This lecture is called 'Traumatic hysteria. Three cases'. One of the cases is a man. Charcot: 'Some of you will be surprised that a man can suffer from what used to be a woman's ailment, especially a man who is not in himself effeminate. In this instance, the hysterogenic action of the womb itself is absent, though we may surmise that there has been some testicular influence in its place' (p. 196).

After having worked in the asylum for some years, Thomas joins Jacques and his sister Sonia in Paris, where they open a practice. Their clientele mostly consists of young women, 'impressed by its proximity to the Boulevard St. Germain and strong enough to make the climb' (to the 3rd floor) (p. 188) (Charcot lived at Boulevard St. Germain 217 in his 'hôtel'). Both young doctors are heavily under the influence of Charcot, 'the Napoleon of the medical sciences' (p. 258) (a critical term which was among others used by Charcot's former student Léon Daudet, son of novelist Alphonse), and mainly look for ovarian disorders in their patients (p. 189). After a while they open a clinic in the mountains of Carinthia (Austria): 'Schloss Seeblick. Sanatorium and Clinic for Nervous Disorders' (p. 249). Here, 'Thomas took more of the severe psychiatric cases and Jacques more of the neurasthenic' (p. 253) (at that time, neurasthenia was a relatively new disease popularized by the American George Beard and explained by enfeeblement of the nervous force). The clinic offers a 'rest cure' with intensive nursing, baths, massage, electrical treatments, and diets (p. 238). Here, Katharina von A., the 'textbook case of hysteria', is one of Jacques' patients.

Hysteria or the Womb?

Jacques asks Thomas to look critically at his paper, which he intends to read at the Austrian Psychiatric Meeting (p. 291). Immediately after Thomas reads the text he sends Katharina to a surgeon. Two cysts are removed from one of her ovaries. 'One was the size of a hen's egg, the other about as large as a Seville orange. The larger one had twisted on its pedicle, cutting off its own blood supply' (p. 311). Her intermittent fevers are explained by rheumatic fever.

After surgical treatment, Katharina recovers completely from her abdominal complaints. Thomas considers Jacques' wrong diagnosis of hysteria as 'the result of intense and lewd speculation which has transpired to have no basis in reality' and 'a desire to supply a sensational cure for an ailment it had partially invented' (p. 316). 'Jacques and he had not been able to cure madness, so they had fabricated something that they could cure' (p. 316). His main accusations towards Jacques include separating the symptoms and dismissing the ones that are not of interest to him (p. 332), concluding that Katharina's apparent sanity is a symptom of insanity ('belle indifférence' of the hysteric) (p. 333), not examining her throat at any stage (p. 333), not speaking to her family (p. 334), and solving the puzzle with limited information (p. 335). In his opinion, Jacques had to understand 'the dangers to a patient of a theory that is too rigid' (p. 341). Jacques does not agree:

> Fräulein Katharina presented a case of hysteria which has been cured by the techniques of psychophysical resolution. I told you at the outset that I believed it was not quite a classical case and that there were some complications. And so there were. You discovered them. Well done. But it takes more than two invisible sacs full of benign fluid to destroy the work of a decade (p. 326).

Thomas' anger rises: 'I sincerely doubt that the disease entity of hysteria will continue to be recognized in ten years' time.' Jacques: 'That is an absurd thing to say. It is one of the most completely described neurological-.' 'For God's sake, Jacques, do you not read the papers and journals? Do you not see how Charcot's heirs are respectfully trying to distance themselves from him (p. 326)? Thomas realizes that he and Jacques have gone separate ways in their profession: 'We are in the same room, but we are looking from different windows (p. 320)'; 'His guiding light is Charcot and mine is Darwin (p. 321)'.

Katharina and Thomas fall in love and marry. Despite the quarrel, Jacques and Thomas keep on working together and open a new sanatorium. As soon as Olivier, Jacques' brother, is transferred to this new place he commits suicide. So, where Jacques failed in his diagnosis and treatment of Katharina, Thomas does so in the case of Olivier. Some years later, due to World War I, Jacques and Thomas are forced as foreigners to leave the sanatorium, which is on Austrian territory. They go their own way with their families. Back in England, Thomas starts to have memory complaints, diagnosed by 'various distinguished gentlemen at the hospital in Queen Square' (p. 596) as presenile dementia. His disease is one of the first in which structural lesions can be seen in the brain 'under a Zeiss lens without staining' (p. 596). Jacques keeps on working, but this becomes increasingly difficult as he becomes obsessed with the death of his only son in the trenches of the First World War.

Some More 'Hysterics' in Fiction

'Hysteria' has always been a difficult diagnosis. Today, it no longer exists [2]. The diagnosis concerned the mind-body dualism and the dichotomy of organic versus psychogenic disorders [2, 3]. In the time of Charcot, it was considered a 'névrose', i.e. a neurological disorder of which the pathological substrate was expected to be found in the brain (like in Parkinson's disease, chorea, and migraine). In the current psychiatric criteria, hysteria as a diagnosis has been replaced by other diagnoses, such as 'somatization disorder, conversion disorder, pain disorder, hypochondriasis, body dysmorphic disorder, undifferentiated somatoform disorder and somatoform disorder not otherwise specified' [3].

There have been many descriptions of presumed 'hysterics' in fiction [4–7]. The question is why hysteria has inspired so many authors of fiction. As described elsewhere [7], many descriptions of hysterical attacks (often referring to Charcot) can be found in French naturalistic literature, particularly in that of Emile Zola [to whom Thomas refers in *Human Traces* – with respect to 'degeneration' and 'accumulated inheritance' (p. 498)]. An accurate description of all aspects of society, including diseases, was considered important by naturalistic authors. After Zola and his school, descriptions of hysteria can be found in naturalistic novels from several other European countries including Russia, the Scandinavian countries, Spain, Italy, Germany, and the Netherlands. As nicely illustrated in *Human Traces*, the demonstrations at Salpêtrière and descriptions of hysterical patients in medical books and journals aroused much interest at that time and resounded throughout Europe for decades. As can also be found in *Human Traces*, heredity (Darwin, the hero of Thomas) and degeneration were two main topics in medical science in the fin-de-siècle times (the latter particularly in psychiatry, along the theories of Morel and Magnan, but also applied by Charcot and his student Féré in neurology; see e.g. Féré [8]). These themes can easily be recognized in most naturalistic novels [7]. The influence of the demonstrations at Salpêtrière (where laymen such as Thomas' sister in *Human Traces* were also allowed to attend; several novelists actually visited the demonstrations, e.g. Guy de Maupassant) [9] and more particularly the very extensive descriptions in *Iconographie photographique de la Salpêtrière* was probably of great importance for the spread throughout Europe. Zola's novels may have been an intermediary in this respect. *Iconographie photographique* provided reports of observed 'hysterical' attacks, including therapeutic measures, such as ovarian compression. There are also biographical details of the patients, many of whom had been sexually abused. Several of the women became well known, including Blanche Wittmann, Augustine, Geneviève, Rosalie, and Justine. Comparing the descriptions in *Iconographie photographique* (including the many photographs of the women in several phases of their attacks) with those in novels, it becomes clear that many authors were inspired by them.

Here, we mention only a few examples of novels in which hysteria has played a role. Next to the French novels discussed previously [9], we add: *Germinie Lacerteux* (1864, de Goncourt and de Goncourt), *La fille Elisa* (1877, Edmond de Goncourt), *La dévouée* (1878, Léon Hennique), *La conquête de plassans* (1874, Zola), and *Possession* (1887) and *Soeur Marthe* (1890, both by Charles Epheyre, the pseudonym for the well-known physiologist Charles Richet, Nobel Prize winner for his studies on anaphylaxis, who influenced Charcot to study hypnosis) [10–12].

In *En rade*, one of Huysmans' novels, Louise gets an hysterical attack: 'Suddenly she uttered a short cry and threw the right foot forward. [...] Jacques carried her to the bed, where the kicking forward continued... preceded by a cry, aches similar to electric shocks flowing off in the legs... recurring, roaming along her thighs, bursting out again in abrupt discharges' [13, p. 117].

In another of Huysmans' novels, *Là-bas*, hysteria is discussed: 'My mother's housemaid had a daughter who suffered from paralyzed arms and legs, severely suffering from the chest, roaring when she was touched...' [14, p. 418]. She had been suffering for 2 years. 'Dismissed from the Lyon hospitals as being incurable, she came to Paris, followed a treatment at the Salpêtrière, she went without anybody knowing what she had and without any drug giving relief' [14, p. 418]. At last she was brought to abbé Johannès, an exorcist, who had cured persons as disabled as she (the character of abbé Johannes was probably based upon the satanist abbé Boullan 1824–1893). 'Miss, you're a victim of the evil of consanguinity' [14, p. 419]. He reminded her of the quarrel she had with her aunt 2 years earlier, when the paralysis started, and cured her without touching her or prescribing drugs.

The Dutch naturalistic author Marcellus Emants had read several scientific and medical books, including those published by Charcot. In several of his novels hysteria can be recognized. An example may be found in *Fanny* (*Drie Novellen*, 1879), where Emants describes hysterical hemiplegia and an '*arc-de-cercle*' [15, pp. 294–295]:

> Then, the first anxious scream escaped her mouth, a dark red blush rushed over her face. She attempted to rise, yet fell backwards again, rotated in the bed, frenetically squeezed the pillows with her healthy arms, ripped off and flung away the blankets, rose in the air like an arch on the back of the head and turned her eyes, screamed and laid about herself, such that Jan believed it was a nervous attack.

As was noted in *Human Traces*, Charcot was one of the first to recognize hysteria in men. The Dutch novelist Louis Couperus is among the few in literature to portray hysteria in a man in *De Berg van Licht (Mountain of Light)*, a historical novel on the Roman Emperor Helegabalus (218–222 AD) [16]. The emperor is described to be as hysterical as his mother and has feminine traits. He has a sexual preference for men and often behaves like a 'hysterical woman'.

In Russian literature, hysteria as well as references to Charcot are found in the work of Leo Tolstoy, for instance in his *Kreutzer Sonata* [17]:

> All the hospitals are full of hysterical women who violate the laws of Nature. The epileptics and Charcot's patients are the complete wrecks, whereas the world is full of half-maimed women… . Charcot, I am sure, would have said that my wife was hysterical, and of me he would have said that I was an abnormal being, and he would have wanted to treat me.

From the Scandinavian countries, August Strindberg is perhaps the best known author from this period. In analogy to Zola, he wrote several naturalistic books (but unlike Zola, these included many drama's), including *Fadren* (*The Father*; 1887), *Fröken Julie* (*Miss Julie*; 1888), and *Fordringsägare* (*Creditors*; 1889). The influences of heredity and environment are visible in *Fröken Julie*, who may be considered a hysteric. Strindberg read about Charcot's and Bernheim's opinions with respect to hypnosis, and possibly visited Charcot's demonstrations [18–20].

From Spanish literature, we wish to mention Emilia Pardo Bazán, a naturalist writer. In the novel *Doña Milagros* (1894), Argos experiences a convulsion after her mother's death. She shows distorted movements and throws her body into a vibrating arch, with the spine of a snake, while 4 persons are unable to control her. An '*arc-de-cercle*' and epileptiform aura may be recognized in the description. Maurice Hemingway, in his biography of Bazán (1983), argued that Bazán was probably inspired by Charcot for this scene [21]. Smith [22] discusses two other Bazán novels in which hysteria plays a role. In one of these, *La novia fiel*, Amelia shows signs of hysteria, including a full-blown hysterical attack with a sensation of a knot in her throat that gradually strangles her, an outburst in laughter, and a horrible and persistent convulsion.

Several writers of the Verismo movement, the Italian version of naturalism, described hysteria. A hysterical attack is depicted in Matilde Serao's (1856–1927) first novel, *Fantasia* (1883). A 3-hour convulsive hysterical attack including the classical phases is described in a later novel [23, p. 220]:

> …she fell down in the frightful convulsions to which she had been subject from her childhood. Her arms beat the air, and her head rebounded on the floor. […] Andrea grasped her wrists, and felt them stiffen like iron in his hands; her teeth chattered as if from ague, and the pupils of her eyes disappeared under her lids. She stammered unintelligible words… . […] When

Andrea called her, her face became more livid, and the convulsions redoubled in intensity. [...] Then, tired, worn out, with aching bones and joints, incapable of moving away, she fell asleep on the sofa, wrapped up in a shawl.

Hysteria in Fiction after the Naturalism Movement

Many descriptions of hysteria have also been included in fiction in subsequent periods, but it seems that the motivation to include these was different. In contrast with 'objective descriptions' of the naturalism period, criticism on the diagnosis of hysteria became the motivation for using Charcot and his teachings on hysteria in novels and plays. An example is Anne Furse's play *Augustine* (1997) [24], which critically depicts the story of one of Charcot's famous patients. Furse studied the archives at Salpêtrière and presents the story with Augustine as 'focalisator'. The four phases of hystero-epileptic attacks and projected historical photographs of Augustine's hysterical fits, probably taken from the *Iconographie photographique*, are shown on the stage. During the play, Augustine begins to reject the doctors' attempts to direct her behavior as she becomes more and more aware of the fact that they abuse her as an instrument to affirm their theories. Augustine's violator is called 'Monsieur C'. A recent French movie is also entitled Augustine (2012).

Another example of a modern novel is the one by Per Olov Enquist (b. 1934) *Bogen om Blanche og Marie* (2004; translated as *The Book about Blanche and Marie* in 2006). Partly based on historical facts – the boundary between history and fiction is not sharp – Enquist introduces Marie Curie (1867–1934), Blanche Wittmann (1859–1913), and Jane Avril (1868–1943, the famous dancer of the Moulin Rouge, who was portrayed many times by Henri de Toulouse-Lautrec and stayed at the Salpêtrière) [25].

Finally, although not a novel, we would like to mention Aragon's and Breton's paper in *La Révolution Surréaliste* of March 1928, *Le cinquantenaire de l'hystérie* [26, 27], as it may cast light upon the question of why hysteria has inspired so many authors: 'We surrealists, wish to celebrate here the fiftieth anniversary of hysteria, the most significant poetic discovery of the end of the 19th century, and that at the very moment that the fragmentation of the concept of hysteria appears to have been accepted.' They concluded the paper by proposing a new definition of hysteria, the last sentence of which reads: 'Hysteria is not a pathological phenomenon and may, in all respects, be considered a supreme means of expression'. This fascination by Aragon and Breton must be related to the interest so many authors have shown to describe hysteria and hysterical (mainly) women. Perhaps it is related to the fascination the doctor at the beginning of our story, Jacques Rebière, had for his patient, Katharina von A., whom he considered a 'textbook case of hysteria', although that was at least mixed with his fascination for Charcot.

When compared with these descriptions of 'hysterics', *Human Traces* offers the reader a much more subtle description of presumed 'hysteric' symptoms. The patient does not show an *'arc-de-cercle'*, epileptiform aura, or paralysis. Nevertheless, the argumentation of Jacques to call her hysteric is based on his careful application of Charcot's teachings. In conformity with the historical perspective, the book does not offer a standpoint in the discussion about organic/psychic. What makes the novel different from other novels on the topic is that it elaborates upon the different ideas on hysteria, by presenting a 'hysteric' patient, who seems not to be hysteric at all. Hysteria is not the only disease discussed in the book. Another main theme of the book is 'Olivier's disease' (schizophrenia), which is explained by Thomas from an evolutionary perspective as a natural result of evolving human consciousness and the origin of language [28, 29]. In fact, Faulks carefully follows the evolution of neuropsychiatry around the turn of the century, mentioning many of the milestones in this area.

It is clear that contemporary medical ideas and insights about hysteria enormously influenced its depiction. 'Hysterics' were seen as subjects that were haunted by the past; they unconsciously repressed memories of psychic trauma through physical symptoms and used a corporeal discourse to articulate 'what is otherwise unspeakable' [4]. After centuries of misogynistic theorizing about an association of hysteria and the womb, it has become clear that probably some of those so-called 'hysterics' suffered from severe nonpsychiatric diseases that were not known at the time, such as an ovarian teratoma with can lead to a bizarre phenotype [30].

The First World War has an important place in *Human Traces*. Thomas and Sonia are English, Jacques is French, Katharina is German (Prussian), and Jacques' 'maitresse' is Russian. The sanatoria are in Austria and have to be left because of the political tension. At first, Jacques' son Daniel is injured near Ypres [Faulks suggests from shell shock (p. 550), which was previously considered as male hysteria and traumatic neurosis, but did not elaborate on the concept] and finally killed in battle (in Italy). The real origins of the First Word War still are an enigma [31]. A fascinating theme of *Human Traces* is the striking parallel between this enigma that shook the world and the neurology/psychiatry struggle around hysteria that did so as well, and still does. This parallel is beautifully illustrated by Sebastian Faulks: 'They [Jacques and Thomas] have fought to a standstill and now they cannot quite remember what the argument was about' [31, p. 588].

References

1 Faulks S: Human Traces. London, Vintage, 2006.
2 Micale MS: On the 'disappearance' of hysteria. A study in the clinical deconstruction of a diagnosis. Isis 1993;84: 496–526.
3 Scheurich N: Hysteria and the medical narrative. Perspect Biol Med 2000;43: 461–476.
4 Parker E: A new hystery: history and hysteria in Toni Morrison's *Beloved*. Twentieth-Century Literature 2001;47.1: 1–19.
5 Hobbs C: Reading the symptoms: an exploration of repression and hysteria in Mary Shelley's *Frankenstein*. ProQuest 1993;25:152–169.
6 Walusinski O: Hysteria in fin the siècle French novels; in Bogousslavsky J, Diegez S (eds): Literary Medicine: Brain Diseases and Doctors in Novels, Theater, and Film. Basel, Karger, 2013, vol 31, pp 35–43.
7 Koehler PJ: Charcot, La Salpêtrière and hysteria as represented in European literature; in Finger S, Stiles A, Boller F: Neurology and the Arts (Progress in Brain Research). New York, Elsevier, 2014.
8 Féré C: La famille névropathique. Théorie tératologique de l'hérédité en de la prédisposition morbide et de la dégénérenscence. Paris, Alcan, 1894.
9 Koehler PJ: About medicine and the arts. Charcot and French literature at the fin-de-siecle. J Hist Neurosci 2001; 10:27–40.
10 Marquer B: Les romans de la Salpêtrière. Genève, Droz, 2008.
11 Kemperink M: Gedeelde Kennis. Literatuur en Wetenschap in Nederland van Darwin tot Einstein (1860–1920). Antwerpen, Garant, 2011.
12 Bogousslavsky J: Following Charcot: A Forgotten History of Neurology and Psychiatry. Basel, Karger, 2011.
13 Huysmans JK: En rade. Paris, Gallimard, 1887.
14 Huysmans JK: Là-bas, ed 11. Paris, Tresse & Stock, 1895.
15 Emants M: Een Drietal Novellen. Haarlem, De Graaff, 1879.
16 Couperus L: De berg van licht. Amsterdam, Veen, 1905–1906.
17 Tolstoy N: Kreutzer Sonata (from chapters 13 and 17, translation by Louise and Aylmer Maude, distributed by the Tolstoy Library and Project Gutenberg). http://great-authors.albertarose.org/leo_tolstoy/kreutzersonata/index.htm.
18 Lane H: Strindberg, August; in Banham M (ed): The Cambridge Guide to Theatre. Cambridge, Cambridge University Press, 1998, pp 1040–1041.
19 Meyer M: Strindberg: A Biography, Lives. Oxford, Oxford University Press, 1985.
20 Micale MS: Approaching Hysteria. Disease and Its Interpretations. Princeton, Princeton University Press, 1995.
21 Hemingway H: Emilia Pardo Bazán (Cambridge Iberian and Latin American Studies). Cambridge, Cambridge University Press, 1983, pp 107–132.
22 Smith J: Reinterpreting hysteria under patriarchy in Emilia Pardo Bazán's 'La novia fiel' and 'Error de diagnóstico'. Decimonónica 2012;9:92–106.
23 Serao M: Fantasy, a Novel (translated by Henry Harland and Paul Sylvester). London, Heinemann, 1891.

24 Furse A: Augustine. Big Hysteria. Amsterdam, Harwood Academic Publishers, 1997.
25 Bonduelle M, Gelfand T: Hysteria behind the scenes: Jane Avril at the Salpêtrière. J Hist Neurosci 1999;8:35–42.
26 Aragon L, Breton A: The quinquagenary of hysteria (1878–1928). Translator and editor Patrick Waldberg. Surrealism. London, Thames and Hudson, 1997.
27 Haan J, Koehler PJ, Bogousslavsky J: Neurology and Surrealism: André Breton and Joseph Babinski. Brain 2012;135:3830–3838.
28 Crow T: Is schizophrenia the price that *Homo sapiens* pays for language? Schizophr Res 1997;28:127–141.
29 Brüne M: Schizophrenia – an evolutionary enigma? Neurosci Biobehav Rev 2004;28:41–53.
30 Pollak TA: Hysteria, hysterectomy, and anti-NMDA receptor encephalitis: a modern perspective on an infamous chapter in medicine. BMJ 2013;346:f3756.
31 Clark C: The Sleepwalkers. How Europe Went to War in 1914. New York, HarperCollins, 2012.

J. Haan, MD, PhD
Department of Neurology, Leiden University Medical Centre
PO Box 9600
NL–2300 RC Leiden (The Netherlands)
E-Mail J.Haan@lumc.nl

Bogousslavsky J (ed): Hysteria: The Rise of an Enigma. Front Neurol Neurosci. Basel, Karger, 2014, vol 35, pp 109–125
DOI: 10.1159/000360244

Sigmund Freud and Hysteria: The Etiology of Psychoanalysis?

Julien Bogousslavsky[a] · Sebastian Dieguez[b]

[a]Center for Brain and Nervous System Diseases, GSMN Neurocenter, Clinique Valmont, Glion/Montreux, and [b]Laboratory for Cognitive and Neurological Sciences, Unité de Neurologie, Département de Médecine, Université de Fribourg, Fribourg, Switzerland

Abstract

Sigmund Freud developed a specific interest in hysteria after his stay with Professor Jean-Martin Charcot during the winter of 1885–1886, although his previous activity mainly consisted of neuropathology and general medical practice. Most of his initial studies on hysteria (hysteria in men, influence of subconscious ideas, role of traumas, and psychological and sexual factors) were indeed 'borrowed' from Charcot and his immediate followers, such as Pierre Janet and Paul Richer. Subsequently, Freud developed with Breuer a theory of hysteria which encompassed a mixture of Janet's 'fixed subconscious ideas' with the 'pathological secret' concept of Moriz Benedikt. After their book *Studies on Hysteria* (1895), Freud interrupted his collaboration with Breuer and developed the concept of conversion of psychological problems into somatic manifestations, with a strong 'sexualization' of hysteria. Firstly, he believed that actual abuses had occurred in these patients (the 'seduction' theory), but then blamed them for having deceived him on that issue, so that he subsequently launched a 'fantasy' theory to explain the development of hysterical symptoms without the necessity of actual abuses. Like many of his contemporaries, and contrary to his claims, Freud did not follow a scientific process of verified experiments, but rather adapted his theories to the evolution of his own beliefs on psychological conditions, selectively emphasizing the aspects of his 'therapies' with patients which supported his emerging ideas, with often abrupt changes in theoretical interpretations. While it remains difficult to get a clear, synthetic vision of what was Freud's definite theory of hysteria, it is obvious that hysteria really was the origin of what would become Freud's psychoanalytical theory. Indeed, psychoanalysis appears to have been initially developed by him largely in order to absorb and explain his many changes in the interpretation of hysterical manifestations.

While psychoanalysis has endured continuous attacks ever since the 'talking cure' began to be developed by Sigmund Freud (1856–1939; fig. 1) and Joseph Breuer, it has recently witnessed a reemerging interest, including an unlikely fascination by prestigious nonclinician neuroscientists [1, 2]. At about the same time, hysteria and hypnosis made a noticeable comeback in brain sciences, thus addressing in new terms the very origins of psychoanalysis [3, 4].

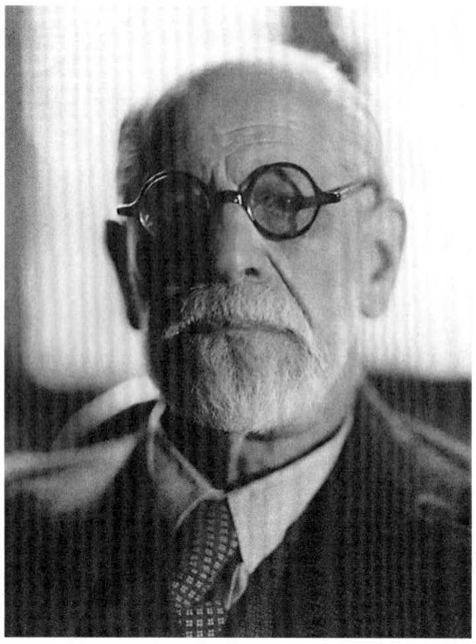

Fig. 1. Rare photographic portrait of Freud. Philippe Helaers library, with kind permission.

Hysteria can be considered as the first significant clinical topic studied by Freud, and it really introduced him into the field of psychology. Indeed, before his 1885–1886 stay with Jean-Martin Charcot at La Salpêtrière, Freud was mainly a neuropathologist with scarce clinical experience. Freud had started his medical studies in Vienna in 1873 and obtained his diploma in 1881. During the last part of these usually long studies, he worked with Carl Claus in anatomy and then with Ernst Brücke in physiology and histology, where he also met Josef Breuer, who was also involved with clinical practice. It is possible that this encounter stimulated Freud to leave a purely basic science career, and he indeed started work with Hermann Nothnagel in surgery, before going in 1883 to the service of Theodor Meynert, who was mainly involved in neuroanatomy, along with clinical activity with patients with nervous system disorders. He did some work on cocaine and also spent some time in the medical service of Scholtz, before he obtained his 'Privat-Dozent' title and a travel grant with the support of Brücke and Meynert. This is when he decided to go to Paris to study with Professor Jean-Martin Charcot, who was famous internationally. His stay there was rather short (he met Charcot on October 20, 1885 and left on February 23, 1886), but was critical for his career. Indeed, it is striking that a look at Freud's library shows that before coming to Paris, he had virtually no books on hysteria, hypnosis, or other psychological topics, while the stay with Charcot was the trigger of a tremendous series of acquisitions of works in these fields [5].

For Freud, hysteria really became the entry door to neuropsychiatry. On the other hand, paradoxically, it is striking that there is no simple way to find out what Freud's views of hysteria were. Imagine a curious reader completely unacquainted with the subtleties of psychoanalytic tenets and history, who nevertheless would like to find out what the famous man exactly said on the matter. This reader might think that *Studies on Hysteria* [6], published in 1895 with Breuer, would be an appropriate start. However, he might be surprised then to find almost no hint of sexuality in that book. Or this reader might read Freud's later writings aimed at the general public, then learning about the tripartite structure of the mental apparatus, hidden and opposing forces fighting back in a dark corner of our minds, about an analytical technique that cures apparently incurable ailments, and about the discovery of deep and universal laws of human sexual and mental development, yet he would only get the most cursory information about the hysterical symptoms which Freud examined several decades earlier in a handful of patients. Again, in most books on the history of psychoanalysis, the reader might also learn that hysteria was first explained by repressed shameful or harmful experiences, subsequently uncovered by a therapeutic cathartic process involving hypnosis, pressure on the forehead, or the free association of words; then by actual early experiences of sexual abuse, and then not, after all, by actual abuses, but by a process of fantasy involving the imagining of seduction scenes as an attempt to solve a universal conflicting experience through which all normal infants have to go.

So What Is the Place of Hysteria in Freud's Work and Theory?

When one reads Freud's work in chronological order, one sees that like in many of his contemporaries, there are no actual 'studies' with an experimental paradigm, which could then be submitted to confirmation or disproval, as in what we now consider as scientific activity. Rather, Freud reported cases from his (or Breuer's, initially) practice, where his 'findings' seemed to coincide with the evolution of his own concepts, so that it is indeed difficult to guess what was first: the concepts or the observations? Freud has always remained elusive on his 'method', never really explaining how he actually went about making his discoveries on 'curing' people [7]. It is particularly telling that his 1908 project to publish *General Methodology of Psychoanalysis* never saw completion. Indeed, it appears that there never was such a 'method', with details and technical specifics, which one could for instance publish in a scientific methodology section. Contemporary reviews of Freud's works clearly pointed to the vague nature of Freud's assertions and the impossibility to replicate his results. Even his former colleague and friend, the otorhinolaryngologist Wilhelm Fliess (whom he had met in 1887), famously accused him of 'reading his own thoughts into the minds of his patients'. While the absence of a clear method, the evolving character of Freud's attitude towards therapy and theory, the retrospective revisions of these views, and the inherently subjective, intuitive, and private nature of the practical aspects of his 'technique' may now look controversial and underline what we can now call an exploratory, nonscientific, approach, at the time they effectively made him immune to criticism and created a legendary aura of secretiveness. This would contribute to the institutional diffusion of psychoanalysis, while at the same time building up his own legend of the isolated avant-garde scientist. In fact, as Wittgenstein put it quite plainly, he merely had 'given up one way of thinking and adopted another'. It is not that Freud gave up scientific practice and discourse to create psychoanalysis, but rather that psychoanalysis *was* the direct result of the evolution of his concepts, where patients were at least as much used as confirmation as 'origin' of these concepts.

Put simply, it may seem that Freud's case histories were never really meant to adduce evidence for his methods and ideas. Indeed, they were mostly 'fragments' or 'notes' mixed with theoretical speculations, incomplete or unsuccessful analyses, becoming increasingly contradictory as years went by, along with the changes in Freud's concepts. In parallel, we are now unable to retrieve information on the exact method that was being used. Also, because Freud commonly acknowledged his previous 'mistakes' along the evolution of his concepts, he acquired a flavor of modesty associated with a concern for truth, which fitted well with the progressive nature of a scientific endeavor.

Freud's Beginnings in Hysteria: A Charcot Sequela

Freud's conception of hysteria is inseparable from his larger intellectual legacy. The very idea of the (Freudian) unconscious was derived from the observation of some obstacles in the treatment of a handful of hysterical patients.

One knows the famous words of Freud [6, p. 42]: 'Our hysterical patients suffer from reminiscences. Their symptoms are the remnants and the memory symbols of certain (traumatic) experiences.' While Freud had heard of the case of Anna O. through Breuer already in November 1882, it is obvious that his interest for hysteria was built around his stay with Jean-Martin Charcot during the winter of 1885–1886. At that time, the great French neurologist was developing his studies on hysterics at La Salpêtrière, initially upon the stimulation from his former 'interne' Désiré Bourneville, and subsequently with other collaborators, such as Paul Richer, then followed by Joseph

Babinski and Georges Gilles de la Tourette. Freud met all of them during his short stay in Paris, and even reported to his fiancée Martha Bernays the 'décolleté' of Madame Richer and the rivalry he had with Babinski. Freud's Parisian correspondence shows his ambition to become important in a field opened by Charcot, and as we already mentioned, he acquired a conspicuous amount of books devoted to hysteria and hypnosis [5].

At the time, Charcot devised the concept of 'dynamic lesions' and recognized the role of traumatic events, physical or psychological, in the triggering of hysteria. However, he also maintained a strong emphasis on the role of heredity, and confided these traumatic events to that of mere '*agents provocateurs*' (triggering factors). Yet the focus on heredity, which in due time Freud would strongly oppose, would lead Charcot and his colleagues to collect extraordinarily careful and detailed personal and familial case histories, an investigation not much different from the information Freud would subsequently strive to gain in psychoanalytical sessions. Combined with the practice of hypnosis, in order to demonstrate the suggestible nature of the symptoms presented by these patients, the grounds for psychotherapy were indeed well laid down during those early years at La Salpêtrière.

The influence of Charcot on Freud has led to endless discussions. That the young neuropathologist was greatly impressed by the Parisian master is undeniable, although in the first place, he counted on his visit to advance his career. Shortly thereafter, he translated a volume of Charcot's work into German and even named his first son Jean-Martin.

In 1886, upon his return from Paris, Freud made two presentations on hysteria [8, 9, pp. 458–464]. The first one was never published, but its content could be fairly well reconstructed from several reports on the event. The second one concerned a case report of male hysteria [10]. The first lecture took place on October 15, 1886: Freud presented Charcot's views on male hysteria and its traumatic (physical) etiology, and introduced a case he had seen at La Salpêtrière, which was part of the lectures he translated into German, a bricklayer named 'Pin'. The presentation was coldly received: the audience saw it as unoriginal (ideas on hysteria and male hysteria were already widely discussed in Vienna, and Freud may simply not have been aware of the large amount of previous and ongoing works on the matter) or simply wrong to link a physical trauma to hysterical symptoms. Perhaps a certain chauvinism was at play, where the Austrian medical audience was unhappy with Charcot's ideas, that seemed to contradict the widely held organic view of hysteria. In addition, 'Pin' turned out to present only mild symptoms and certainly was not an example of 'grande hystérie'.

The second lecture was held on November 26, 1886 [10]: Indeed, in the month following the first lecture, Freud was able to find a new case of male hysteria. Interestingly, this case of hysterical hemianesthesia in a male did not seem to be directly associated to a physical trauma. Rather, the trauma involved a violent and frightful dispute with the patient's brother, who threatened the patient with a knife. This was followed by a 'ringing' in the head and an episode of violent spasms involving loss of consciousness. The fear itself, rather than the specific event leading to the fear, was the key etiological feature of the 'trauma', which fitted well with Charcot's theory and would subsequently also adapt to Freud's further elaborations on the etiology of hysteria. However, at age 8, the patient was involved in an accident, in which he was run over in the street. At this point, Freud did not consider the possible link between both events, i.e. the old accident and the more recent dispute with the brother. The paper also contained clinical data predating Freud's subsequent elaborations on the distinction between organic and hysterical paralysis, thereby foreshadowing the notion of 'conversion hysteria'. Most notably, the clinical findings did not follow the laws of anatomy, a point which he would develop in his 'Hysteria' entry in the Villaret medical encyclopedia in 1888 (*Handwörter-*

buch der gesamten Medizin) [11] and in a paper commissioned by Charcot which was published only in 1893 (after Charcot's death).

At the time, and still in the encyclopedia entry, Freud defended rather forcefully the hereditary views of Charcot, which he would subsequently criticize [11, p. 50]:

> The etiology of the status hystericus is to be looked for entirely in heredity: hysterics are always disposed to disturbances of nervous activity, and epileptics, psychical patients, tabetics, etc., are found among their relatives. Direct hereditary transmission of hysteria, too, is observed, and is the basis, for instance, of the appearance of hysteria in boys (from their mother). Compared with the factor of heredity, all other factors take a second place and play the part of incidental causes, the importance of which is as a rule overrated in practice.

But in his Charcot obituary (1893) [12], Freud took some distance from the master's ideas: 'As for the etiological theories which Charcot defended in his doctrine of the "famille névropathique" and made the cornerstone of his whole conception of nervous disease, they too will probably soon need to be probed into and corrected'. Freud's footnotes in his translation of Charcot's lessons also make clear that he did not fully subscribe to the hereditary approach.

That the hysterical symptoms did not respect anatomical constraints was suggestive of a nonphysiological mechanism at work. Indeed, in the Villaret entry [11], Freud made the argument that there *cannot* be an organic lesion at work in hysteria precisely because its symptoms do not match the laws of anatomy. What is, then, this nonphysiological, functional, dynamical principle at work? Not mere malingering, but something like the 'idea' of a disease stored in the mind and engaged unconsciously in the production of symptoms. The concept was very close to Pierre Janet's ideas on dissociation, which Freud indeed acknowledged. During hysterical paralysis of an arm, for instance, what happens would be that the concept, the idea of the arm, cannot be integrated with the rest of the ideas constituting the conscious ego. The concept of the arm would not be destroyed or damaged, but merely be inaccessible. The reason why an idea may become inaccessible and separated from other ideas is that it is affectively overcharged and the patient currently is unable to deal with the emotion associated with a certain body part. In other words, the representation of an organ becomes linked to a traumatic memory, and both end up buried deep under and apart from the rest of conscious bodily representations. It is striking that this theory is more or less identical with the one delineated by Charcot in newly discovered archives material [13].

Also striking is that within a single month separating both 1886 lectures, Freud moved from the older Charcot-Oppenheim view of male hysteria as being prominently linked to physical trauma (Hermann Oppenheim was famous for his physical trauma theory, which he developed in the context of train accidents), to a picture closer to the simultaneously developing views of Charcot, in which hysteria depended foremost on the psychological consequences, especially the unconscious ones, of a psychical trauma. Physical and psychical traumatic events could then have the same pathological effects. From an epistemological point of view, it is fascinating that this turn in Freud's views could very well be entirely due to the urgent need to find a new case of male hysteria, and thus perhaps of stumbling on an unsatisfying one (provided so to speak at the last minute by laryngologist Dr. von Bergszászy, as Freud was denied access to the wider population of the general hospital), while at the same time retaining some ambiguity since the case still could be interpreted as linked to an early physical trauma perhaps revived by the newer one. Sexuality, by the way, played no role at all at this stage.

The Invention of Freud's Hysteria

Back in Vienna from Paris, Freud heard again of Josef Breuer's work on hysteria and the two set out to work on a paper advancing new conceptions of the condition [14]. With the adjunction of a series of case reports and theoretical and clinical developments, the paper later became a full book, *Studies on Hysteria* [6].

Indeed, Freud followed-up on his interest for Breuer's cathartic method during his 'analyses' of the patients provided by him. Progressively, thus, hysterical symptoms became associated neither with a hereditary predisposition nor with the emotional impact per se of a physical or even psychical trauma, but with the affect *connected* to an unpleasant idea or memory and effectively aiming at its suppression from conscious thought. Charcot's concept of an 'agent provocateur', in his mind a physical trauma activating the *idea* of a physical impairment and ultimately leading, through self-directed suggestion, to hysterical paralysis, was thus expanded to include purely psychical events that could directly lead to similar effects. The trend seemed to follow-up on Charcot's progressive turn from neurology to psychology to explain hysteria.

In 1892, Freud and Breuer published their first paper on 'traumatic hysteria', in which a hypnoid state was emphasized, along with a dissociation of consciousness. The latter concept, again, was very close to the ideas of Pierre Janet, who was preparing his medical doctorate under the supervision of Charcot. In his published thesis (1893), Janet indeed quoted the present work, although he misspelled Breuer's name into 'Brener'. Freud and Breuer underscored the symbolic role of emotional trauma, with two rules: the strength of the trauma, and its close link with the symptoms.

The psychologization of hysteria is the topic of the celebrated 'preliminary communication' by Freud and Breuer, 'On the psychical mechanism of hysterical phenomena' [14], in which, as in the subsequent book *Studies on Hysteria*, heredity is almost altogether absent. He and Breuer still held to the notion that hysterical patients had a certain 'proclivity' to express the disorder, although such 'proclivity' and its features were said to remain mysterious. The short preliminary communication is indeed a landmark because it is a concentrate of the psychological mechanisms that Freud would develop at large during the following years, and which can grossly be summarized into the association of the concept of the pathological secret of Moriz Benedikt with that of the 'idées subconscientes fixes' (fixed subconscious ideas) of Pierre Janet. Benedikt, who by the way had supported Freud's 1885 trip to Paris with a letter to Charcot, had developed the concept of private secrets invading the life and behavior of patients at the origin of their mental dysfunction. On the other hand, Pierre Janet already had a significant experience with the management of hysterical patients before he joined Charcot's service in 1889, and his first reports of cathartic cures allowing subconscious ideas to emerge into consciousness dated back to 1886 in Le Havre. Thus, while the preliminary communication was a brilliant synthesis, none of its individual concepts could be qualified as new.

A few months later in 1893, Freud published an article in French in the *Archives de Neurologie*, an earlier assignment from Charcot, where he showed the differences in organic versus hysterical paralyses [15, 16]. Here, he quoted Janet about the lack of respect of anatomical rules in hysterical paralysis. One year later, Freud introduced the term 'Abwehr' (defense), which he had borrowed from his Austrian mentor Theodor Meynert, in order to focus on psychological mechanisms designed by patients to protect their own functioning. And then came the important 1895 book *Studies on Hysteria*, which included several case presentations, some of which would become famous, such as Anna O. or Emmy von N. These case descriptions have been discussed at length, along with criticisms on the authenticity of certain features [9], such as the cure of Anna O. by Breuer. Indeed, Freud himself declared years later that the cathartic cure of Anna O. (Bertha Pappenheim, 1856–1936) never happened, although it was reported to have taken place in 1882 (but published 13 years later). This case was particularly strange, and to our knowledge a similar patient has never been reported again. Among other peculiar symptoms, she displayed a time switch of 365 days between her present hallucinations and what she had actually lived a year earlier, with impeccable memory of all the details of her life during the corresponding time. The cure supposedly occurred when the patient was able to revive retrospectively each day of the whole year. The patient herself coined the process a 'talking cure' and a 'chimney sweeping', obviously sarcastically, in English (as one of her symptoms was being deprived of the use of her mother tongue, German). On the other hand, Freud spoke of 'cleansing of the soul' to describe Breuer's cure with Anna O. In any case, the fact that the cure report seemed fraudulent, along with the fact that the actual publication dated from 1895, clearly confirms that Pierre Janet was right in claiming priority of the cathartic cures of hysterics. While Janet and Freud had never met (when Freud went to Paris, Janet was still in Le Havre), they remained lifelong rivals. In 1913 at the International Congress of Psychiatry, Janet strongly criticized Freud, and when Janet went to Vienna two decades later, Freud refused to receive him.

These reports with Breuer would make Freud pinpoint at an intrapsychic conflict of representations. In their work, they also emphasized the 'Nachträglichkeit' or deferred action of the trauma: an initial trauma becomes a symptom only at a later stage of development, when a second trauma reactivates the earlier one, which at the time could not be reacted to adequately. It is also in *Studies on Hysteria* that the term 'la belle indifférence' first appeared to describe a patient, Elisabeth von R., and was later attributed by Freud to Charcot [17]. The exact meaning of this symptom has been disputed, but it refers to an apparent serene cheerfulness in the face of an underlying disturbance, obvious to anyone but the patient. It is noteworthy that Freud would mention 'la belle indifférence' again only in 1915, in his paper on repression [18], only a few months after Babinski presented his cases of anosognosia and the concept of anosodiaphoria at the Société Neurologique [19]. It was in *Studies on Hysteria* that Freud and Breuer wrote their well-known aphorism, 'hysterics suffer mainly from reminiscences', by which they sought to describe a 'commemoration of events by symptoms' [20].

It is also interesting to mention that during this period (the last decade of the 19th century), Freud also pursued some works on classical neurological topics, such as aphasia and agnosia (he even coined the latter term), or infantile palsy and hemiplegia, fields which he would soon abandon. It seems as if Freud initially wanted to keep a strong organic/neurological basis in his work, as was clearly evident in his ambitious 1895 uncompleted and unpublished *Project for a Scientific Psychology* [21], before he definitively and completely switched to psychology, the unconscious, and sexuality.

Conversion, Repression, and Abreaction as Embodied Metaphors

In 1895, Freud and Breuer published *Studies on Hysteria* and an article on anxiety neurosis. With reference to mechanisms of hysteria, three main types were put forward by Freud and Breuer during the years 1894–1895. 'Abwehrhysterie' (defense hysteria) corresponded to a protective reaction against unpleasant representations. 'Retentionshysterie' (retention hysteria) corresponded to affects which were not 'abreacted', i.e. lacking the emotional discharge which would have freed the subject from clinical manifestations. 'Hypnoidhysterie' (hypnoid hysteria) was associated with hypnoid states, which lead to unconscious representations developing during such states, usually in connection with fear. However, these categories were subsequently abandoned by Freud without much explanation, probably because they no longer fit with the new evolutions of his thinking and theories.

The term 'conversion', which has had an incredible success in the 20th century, first appeared in 1894 in Freud's article on defense psychoneuroses, and it was subsequently used in *Studies on Hysteria* for the cases of Emmy von N. and Cäcilia M. It implied a transposal of the intrapsychic conflict with a resolution attempt through somatic manifestations.

The metaphorical origin of the symptoms of conversion has understandably raised some eyebrows, to say the least. Yet the notion, as explained by Freud while discussing the case of Cäcilia M. is most interesting in light of current developments in embodied cognition research [22]. The patient, for instance, would suffer from facial neuralgia traceable, according to Freud, to an instance where her husband had made a remark that felt 'like a slap in the face'. Likewise, through a process of 'associative reverberations' she would complain of a shooting pain in her right heel, apparently due to the fact that at some point, she did not 'find herself on a right footing' with some strangers. A penetrating pain in her forehead would be due to the 'penetrating look' of her grandmother, which she remembered 'had gone right into her brain'. And so forth. Freud offered an evolutionary explanation, and alluded to Darwin's *The Expression of the Emotions* [6, p. 223]:

> All these sensations and innervations belong to the field of 'The Expression of the Emotions', which, as Darwin (1872) has taught us, consists of actions which originally had a meaning and served a purpose. These may now for the most part have become so much weakened that the expression of them in words seems to us only to be a figurative picture of them, whereas in all probability the description was once meant literally; and hysteria is right in restoring the original meaning of the words in depicting its unusually strong innervations. Indeed, it is perhaps wrong to say that hysteria creates these sensations by symbolization. It may be that it does not take linguistic usage as its model at all, but that both hysteria and linguistic usage alike draw their material from a common source.

While the term 'conversion' thus appeared early in Freud's work, it is striking that this was not the case for 'conversion hysteria'. Indeed, Freud first coined the term in a discussion on the 'Little Hans' case (published in 1905) in 1909, in order to distinguish it from 'anxiety hysteria' presented by the patient. Anxiety (or fear) hysteria ('Angst Hysterie') had been introduced by Wilhelm Stekel in 1908 to express a phobia, in which a substitute object focuses anxiety. This was different from Freud's 1895 'anxiety/fear neurosis' ('Angst Neurosis'), where no substitute object is present. In both conversion hysteria and anxiety hysteria, the term 'hysteria' was justified in Freud's view since in both instances repression tends to dissociate representations from their corresponding affect.

The Sexualization of Hysteria

Studies on Hysteria almost completely lacked explicit sexual issues and explanations. According to Freud himself, this was so because of Breuer's unease with the sexual matter, but this a posteriori claim may more accurately reflect Freud's own evolution after his split from Breuer. In putting together the second edition of the book in 1908, Freud indeed distanced himself from the initial work with Breuer. The development of psychoanalysis was by then well under way, and Freud sought to introduce a wealth of new ideas into his views of hysteria. This restructuring already took place in his study of the Dora case in 1905.

Therein, Freud's belief of the sexual origins of *all* hysterical symptoms was made explicit. And revisiting his early cases, Freud noted in the fourth chapter of *Studies on Hysteria* ('The psychotherapy of hysteria') that they all must have been marked by sexual traumas. He put forward the thesis that at the bottom of every case of hysteria there are one or more occurrences of premature sexual experience, occurrences which belong to the earliest years of childhood.

Moreover, as Allison and Roberts [23, pp. 255–256] underscored, Freud would then generalize his sexual theory of hysteria to all cases of neurosis:

> In the early writings on hysteria, Freud had focused on the importance of memory, trauma, and the therapeutic use of hypnosis, to help diagnose his patients. By the time of his major case studies, he was equipped with a remarkably well developed theoretical apparatus. During the intervening years – preceding the celebrated Dora case – he had elaborated the mechanics of the unconscious and repression, the dynamics of the dream-work, the theory of infantile sexuality, the oedipal complex, etc. This would permit him to engage in a far more complex analysis of what he examined early on in his professional career, namely, hysteria. In the Dora case, e.g., he would explicitly identify neurosis in general with a sexual etiology, and hysteria in particular would be equated with the inability to deal successfully with the erotic drives on a conscious level.

These papers, beyond the 'seduction theory' per se (see below), argued for a new nosological approach to the neuroses. Freud's ambition was to find a specific etiology for each specific ailment (anxiety, hysteria, obsession, paranoia, etc.), whereby he could establish a proof of a special etiological relationship between the nature of the sexual influence and the pathological species of the neurosis. This is somewhat contradictory with the meticulous efforts made in *Studies on Hysteria* to track back the very specific symbolic elements derived from singular traumatic events that would each find their way in their own particular 'innervation' pathway to be expressed as symptoms. The new formula – repressed early abuse inevitably leading to hysteria after having been reactivated by a similar event – suddenly seems much more generic and vague, while at the same time ruling out countless possibilities merely because they do not involve a sexual element. The patients would 'reproduce' in therapy, to the request of Freud, their early abuse. Now, what Freud meant by 'reproduce' was not made exactly clear. In any case, the patients would thoroughly deny ('resist') Freud's proposal that they must have been abused.

In 1895, these repressed 'memories' of childhood abuse were nowhere to be found in *Studies on Hysteria*. Yet in 1896, Freud now claimed evidence for 16 cases (none of which, by the way, involved fathers as assailants; fathers would become involved first in a later letter to Fliess). These three papers of 1896, presented and published in Paris, Berlin, and Vienna [24–26], make no ambiguity about the fact that Freud believed these patients had been abused, but he was more mysterious about the way he obtained that information, not to mention just how far he verified it. In the 'Aetiology' paper [26], he wrote that 'in a few instances the accumulation of sexual experiences coming from different quarters was truly amazing', including quite explicitly 'all the abuses known to debauched and impotent persons, among whom the buccal cavity and the rectum are misused for sexual purposes'. In the 'Further remarks' paper, he noted that the cases were all 'of a severe kind' involving 'grave sexual injuries; some of them [...] positively revolting'. In the paper 'Heredity and the aetiology of the neuroses' [24], where we can find the first mention of the word 'psychoanalysis', he referred to these infantile scenes as 'a brutal assault'.

Again, none of that had ever seen light in *Studies on Hysteria*, despite the fact he had been using more or less the same 'technique', supposed now to uncover a universal and unmistakable truth about the origins of hysteria. However, as we will see, all of it would be forgotten and negated a year later anyway.

The 'Seduction' (Abuse) Theory

How did Freud argue for the reality of the early sexual abuse while avoiding providing clinical evidence? He assured the reader that [see 27]:

(1) the patients relived vividly and intensely those events (and they most vehemently

denied any *remembrance* of the event, unlike other types of recovered forgotten memories);
(2) all the patients reacted independently in the same fashion;
(3) the memories fitted nicely with the rest of the clinical history, and
(4) the symptoms disappeared thanks to the unveiling of the early memory.

The possibility that he may have suggested or forced the memories appeared 'untenable' to him because, as he claimed, he generally failed to induce or force such memories when he tried so. Moreover, Freud claimed (in the Vienna paper [26]) to have obtained corroborating evidence of sexual abuse for 3 patients (one brother confirming that a patient was abused; and 2 patients accusing a common abuser). Nevertheless, the 'pressure technique', 'insistence', and suggestion may look like a very effective way of getting patients to say what the therapist wanted to hear, whether or not these patients believed what they were saying.

In any case, in a mere 4 months after having first stated the seduction theory [28], Freud claimed, in two articles, to have found 16 patients in which he could trace back their symptoms (13 hysterics and 3 'pure obsessionals') to infantile sexual abuse experiences. Such experiences, using a similar clinical method, had never appeared even shortly before, and thus, Freud's patients could not have been selected on the basis of having been abused. So, assuming that the patients were truly victims of early sexual abuse, either his new theory was correct and he had somehow failed to find memories of sexual abuse in his prior patients despite considerable efforts at tracing back symptoms to their causes, or the theory was wrong and by sheer coincidence *all* his subsequent patients turned out to have been abused. Obviously, it makes more sense to consider the possibility that these 'memories' were simply new interpretations by Freud, conveniently fitting his new theory, just as he did prior to the seduction theory when all his interpretations fitted the 'innervation' approach to the traumatic theory of conversion. In *A Short Account of Psychoanalysis* (1924), Freud candidly reported that his patients, at the time, 'did not bring up what had actually been forgotten', but 'with the help of a certain amount of supplementing and interpreting, *the doctor was able to guess (or reconstruct) the forgotten material from it* [italics added]' [28, p. 196].

In a way, it seems that whatever 'evidence' Freud needed at any developing stage of his views, he managed to obtain it. When he no longer needed it, he simply forgot about it and obtained new confirmatory facts for his newer views. Freud evolved as a 'thinker', or even a philosopher, whose aims were to develop new ideas and theories, rather than the scientist he claimed to be. One should of course remember that at the time, this attitude was not uncommon among many of his colleagues completely outside the field of psychoanalysis, when facts were often retained mainly if they corroborated beliefs.

Were the memories of abuse really 'recovered', were they 'unconscious'? In describing his 'technique' in *Studies on Hysteria*, Freud admitted that this was not always the case. It seems that the arduous process of uncovering repressed thoughts sometimes merely corresponded to a confession of something that was accessible to conscious awareness all along, but which the patient was reluctant to share [6, p. 324]:

> The patient then adds: 'I could have told you that the first time.' 'Why didn't you say it?' [Freud asks]. 'I couldn't believe it could be that. It was only when it came back every time that I made up my mind to say it.' Or else 'I hoped it wouldn't be that of all things. I could well do without saying that. It was only when it refused to be repressed that I saw I shouldn't be let off...'. Thus, after the event the patient betrays the motives for a resistance which he refused to admit to begin with.

While it is commonly said the 'discovery' of infantile abuse came to Freud as a 'surprise', in *Studies on Hysteria* it was made clear by Freud himself that his habit was to indicate to patients what he expected them to produce. In any case, it seems obvious that the 'theory' came to him before the 'discovery'.

'I No Longer Believe in My Neurotica', September 21, 1897

In this famous letter to his friend and colleague, Wilhelm Fliess, Freud confessed that he did not believe anymore in the fact that his patients had actually been sexually abused. From that point on, he built a new theory based on 'phantasmatic' seduction and 'abuse' to replace his previous hypotheses. Among the reasons stated to give up his 'seduction theory', Freud pointed out that a high incidence of sexual abuse would be required in order to account for the high incidence of hysteria, whereas such a distribution of perversion against children seemed very unlikely to Freud. Also, Freud acknowledged that in the unconscious there is no necessary sign allowing phantasms to be distinguished from actual reality, so that one cannot differentiate between the truth and a fiction invested with feelings. And Freud, who looked rather distressed, ended his letter to Fliess [quoted in 35, p. 177]:

> … in the deepest psychoses the unconscious memory does not force its way through, so that the secret of experiences of childhood would also not reveal itself in the most confused delirium. When one sees that the unconscious never overcomes the resistance of the conscious, then the expectation that in treatment the opposite has to happen, to the point of the complete taming of the unconscious by the conscious, also sinks. I was so struck by this that I was ready to give up two things: complete resolution of a neurosis and the certain knowledge of its etiology in childhood. Now I have no idea where I stand… .

Thus, after much fanfare about his revolutionary theory, Freud shortly thereafter silently abandoned it. The idea that there was a smooth shift from the abuse theory to the fantasy theory only later contributed to the Freudian legend, being mainly fostered by Ernest Jones and Ernst Kris [29].

By 1906, almost 10 years after his private abandonment of the seduction theory, Freud started providing retrospective accounts of this episode, essentially blaming his patients in order to explain his 'mistake' [30]. They were the ones who produced the false 'memories' after all! The method by which the private information was 'obtained', the fact that this information remained unconscious and that patients often disagreed with the 'finding', were now firmly buried in the past. As Esterton [30] reports:

> ...perhaps because he had recently reread the seduction theory papers, Freud's 1925 account is particularly revealing. He wrote that he was obliged to recognize that the 'scenes of seduction' were 'only phantasies which my patients had made up *or which I had perhaps forced on them*' (emphasis added). He went on to say: 'I do not believe even now that I forced the seduction phantasies on my patients, that I "suggested" them', but remarkably, given the 'overwhelming importance' he accorded his discovery of the supposed infantile phantasies, he gave no *reason* why he rejected this possibility.

For several authors this corresponded to a 'same-method-same-errors' problem, as Cioffi summarized: 'Freud could not bring himself to recognize the reasoning by which he had persuaded himself of the authenticity of the seductions because it was the same sort of reasoning which, for the rest of his career, he was to employ in his reconstruction of infantile fantasy life and of the content of the unconscious in general' [quoted in 31].

Now, of course, to make matters even more complicated, it should be noted that the element of fantasy was not altogether absent from the seduction theory. To the contrary, Freud held that fantasies were invented precisely to disguise or replace the traumatic events [see 32, fn 25].

The fact remains that once Freud privately abandoned the theory that actual infantile abuse leads to the delayed appearance of hysterical symptoms, he had a problem. Either he had data to substantiate his earlier theory, or he simply did not. In the first case, if he was misled by his patients, he could have reported evidence of the forged nature of these accounts of abuse, for example by further investigation of the files or actual interrogation of the involved parties, in addition to the explicit admission of such accounts by his patients (as opposed to merely inferring that the patients had made up the accounts). However, if the accounts were true, in addition to the aforementioned explicit admission and factual documentation of the abuses, he would have had to report that his theory was based on the coincidental finding that *his* patients somehow all had in common the unfortunate, but irrelevant, experience of having been abused. Now what if he simply had no evidence whatsoever for the 'actual abuse theory'? In this case, of course, he would have to admit that his theory was a product of his imagination, that he recanted it, and in fact that his previous scientific and medical publications on the matter were mainly hypotheses. And what about the *new* theory, that of 'seduction fantasies' which in fact never happened other than in his patients' imagination? Did he actually have newly found evidence? Freud realized that he could no longer sustain the abuse theory when the theory 'broke down under the weight of its own improbability', as he put it himself in 1914 *(History of the Psycho-Analytic Movement)*. But why was it improbable in the first place? Freud never explained. In a way, he *had* to come up with something else, but he did not give specific evidence leading to the change, except that he simply did not believe his previous concepts anymore. In a way, leaving the older theory was a good move since the new 'discovery', in fact, covered exactly the realization that the previous findings were untrue. That the theory of actual abuse was unfounded indeed became a major discovery – if not the most seminal event in the history of psychoanalysis, certainly its most iconic origin. Epistemologically, it marked a revolutionary turn from reality-based life to a parallel, self-sustaining, and extremely intrusive universe of fantasies, hidden mechanisms, and deep secrets in symbolic disguise. In fact, none of it would have been possible without the early revelatory missteps.

Jeffrey Masson is among the few but influential scholars claiming that Freud was wrong to recant, as his patients really had been abused and his change of views thus was a betrayal to them [see also 27]. According to Masson, Freud's 'cover-up' of the seduction 'findings' could be associated with an attempt to escape the subversive and isolating consequences, among his male colleagues, of this theory of widespread incest and pedophilia (the 'loss of courage' hypothesis). However, the fact is, sexual perversions were nothing new in Freud's intellectual environment, and accusations of incest could hardly shock scholars. Furthermore, that Freud's 'discovery' of the fictional content of his patient's 'claims' was nothing new either is clear from the writing of his 'colleagues' in the field of sexual medicine. Krafft-Ebing, as Freud himself reported, saw the seduction theory story as a 'scientific fairy tale', and Löwenfeld, wrote in 1899 [quoted in 32, p. 24]:

> By chance, one of the patients on whom Freud used the analytic method came under my observation. The patient told me with certainty that the infantile sexual scene which analysis had apparently uncovered was pure fantasy and had never really happened to him.

As we have seen, it would take many years for Freud to publicly admit the very same thing. The fact is Freud's 1896 claims were received coldly not because of their sexual contents, but because of their background theory and method. Unsurprisingly, authors hinging on the constitutional (hereditary, endowment) theory of hysteria were unconvinced by Freud's new etiology. But mostly, critics were dismayed by the way Freud obtained his material, namely by suggestion [33].

The 'overestimation' hypothesis, in essence stating that it just so happened by coincidence that cases of actual abuse were overrepresented in Freud's early sample population, implies that far from being wrong, dishonest, or misled by his patients, Freud was correct about the recovered memories of 'seduction' being real. This is stated explicitly in his first published detailed account acknowledging his mistake, in 'My views on the part played by sexuality in the etiology of the neuroses' (1906) [34]:

> At that time my material was still scanty, and it happened by chance to include a disproportionately large number of cases in which sexual seduction by an adult or by older children played the chief part in the history of the patient's childhood. I thus over estimated the frequency of such events (though in other respects they were not open to doubt).

Yet he immediately attempts to have it both ways, admitting the following:

> 'Moreover, I was at that period unable to distinguish with certainty between falsifications made by hysterics in their memories of childhood [die Erinnerungs-täuschungen der Hysterischen über ihre Kindheit] and traces of real events'.

He continued [34]:

> Since then I have learned to explain a number of phantasies of seduction as attempts at fending off memories of the subject's *own* sexual activity (infantile masturbation). When this point had been clarified, the 'traumatic' element in the sexual experiences of childhood lost its importance and what was left was the realization that infantile sexual activity (whether spontaneous or provoked) prescribes the direction that will be taken by later sexual life after maturity.

Did he overestimate the importance of abuses in infancy and mistakenly consider them as necessary for hysteria? Or could it be that he simply had no means to distinguish real from fantasized (or forcibly extracted, or plainly suggested) abuses? Note also that in 1906, Freud seemed to imply that while *then* (in 1896) he was unable to distinguish with certainty between falsifications and real events, he could *now*. But how? Freud remained silent on this point [35, p. 179]. Was Freud 'blind' in believing the stories his patients told him? In his *Autobiographical Study* (1925) he stated that 'this was at a time when I was intentionally keeping my critical faculty in abeyance so as to preserve an unprejudiced and receptive attitude towards the many novelties which were coming to my notice every day' [36].

Retrospectively, several questions remain, but it appears that Freud's change of views was more associated with the private evolution of his own theories than with experimental facts or reproducible observations. According to Triplett [29], the seduction theory anyway was a 'misnomer' and a 'historical distortion'. Indeed, the seduction theory would have been more appropriately referred to as the 'infant genital trauma theory' in the first place. Besides, in his retrospective accounts of his abandonment of the seduction theory, Freud would focus specifically on the role of *fathers*. This is remarkable insofar as fathers were not mentioned in the seduction papers of 1896. It makes little sense to claim that Freud *chose* to disguise fathers as other adults in 1896. Rather, it seems that Freud, in light of his new Oedipal theory, would distort his earlier theory to make the continuity smoother. Freud blamed fathers, but no fathers or repressed memories, instances of actual 'seduction', or even any success with the cathartic method for that matter were presented in his writings. His correspondence with Fliess, on the other hand, indicated in many instances that Freud, in fact, was short of cases and did not 'complete' any at this time. It appears that he had a theory without data, a fact on which he spent a great deal of his career trying to somehow accommodate.

'Dora' and Further Developments

'Dora', the first psychoanalytic case study was written in 1901 and published in 1905 (fig. 2). It included the application of Freud's new ideas

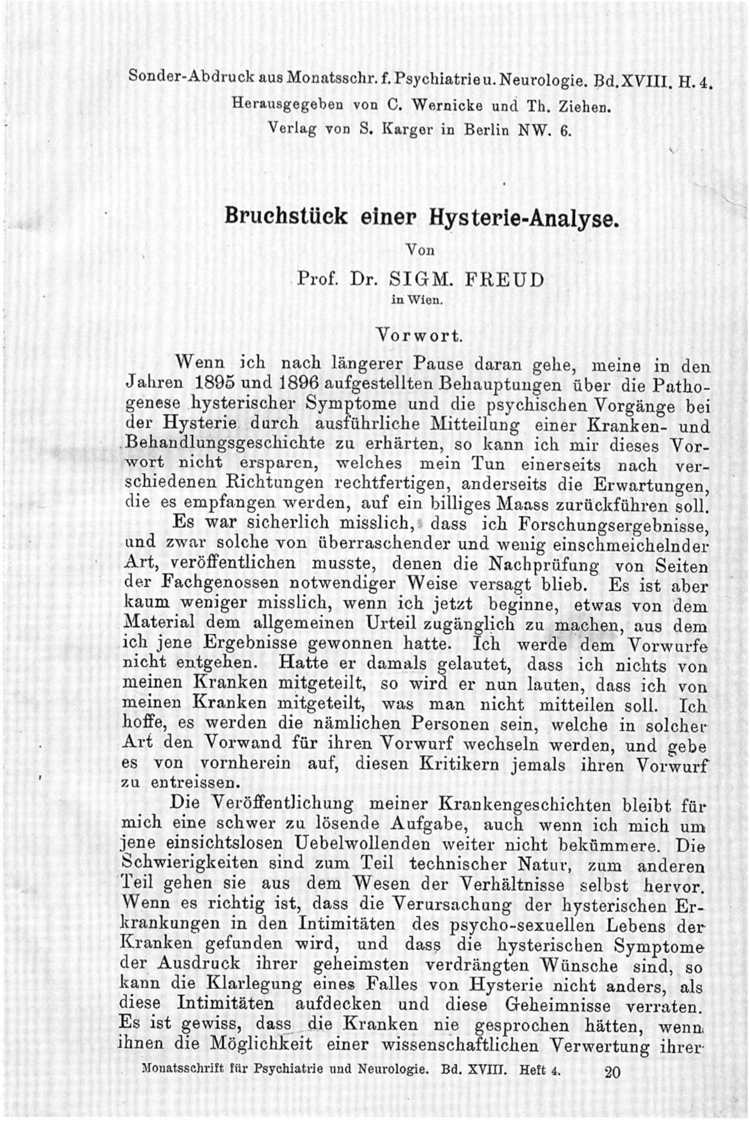
Sonder-Abdruck aus Monatsschr. f. Psychiatrie u. Neurologie. Bd. XVIII. H. 4.
Herausgegeben von C. Wernicke und Th. Ziehen.
Verlag von S. Karger in Berlin NW. 6.

Bruchstück einer Hysterie-Analyse.

Von

Prof. Dr. SIGM. FREUD

in Wien.

Vorwort.

Wenn ich nach längerer Pause daran gehe, meine in den Jahren 1895 und 1896 aufgestellten Behauptungen über die Pathogenese hysterischer Symptome und die psychischen Vorgänge bei der Hysterie durch ausführliche Mitteilung einer Kranken- und Behandlungsgeschichte zu erhärten, so kann ich mir dieses Vorwort nicht ersparen, welches mein Tun einerseits nach verschiedenen Richtungen rechtfertigen, anderseits die Erwartungen, die es empfangen werden, auf ein billiges Maass zurückführen soll.

Es war sicherlich misslich, dass ich Forschungsergebnisse, und zwar solche von überraschender und wenig einschmeichelnder Art, veröffentlichen musste, denen die Nachprüfung von Seiten der Fachgenossen notwendiger Weise versagt blieb. Es ist aber kaum weniger misslich, wenn ich jetzt beginne, etwas von dem Material dem allgemeinen Urteil zugänglich zu machen, aus dem ich jene Ergebnisse gewonnen hatte. Ich werde dem Vorwurfe nicht entgehen. Hatte er damals gelautet, dass ich nichts von meinen Kranken mitgeteilt, so wird er nun lauten, dass ich von meinen Kranken mitgeteilt, was man nicht mitteilen soll. Ich hoffe, es werden die nämlichen Personen sein, welche in solcher Art den Vorwand für ihren Vorwurf wechseln werden, und gebe es von vornherein auf, diesen Kritikern jemals ihren Vorwurf zu entreissen.

Die Veröffentlichung meiner Krankengeschichten bleibt für mich eine schwer zu lösende Aufgabe, auch wenn ich mich um jene einsichtslosen Uebelwollenden weiter nicht bekümmere. Die Schwierigkeiten sind zum Teil technischer Natur, zum anderen Teil gehen sie aus dem Wesen der Verhältnisse selbst hervor. Wenn es richtig ist, dass die Verursachung der hysterischen Erkrankungen in den Intimitäten des psycho-sexuellen Lebens der Kranken gefunden wird, und dass die hysterischen Symptome der Ausdruck ihrer geheimsten verdrängten Wünsche sind, so kann die Klarlegung eines Falles von Hysterie nicht anders, als diese Intimitäten aufdecken und diese Geheimnisse verraten. Es ist gewiss, dass die Kranken nie gesprochen hätten, wenn ihnen die Möglichkeit einer wissenschaftlichen Verwertung ihrer

Monatsschrift für Psychiatrie und Neurologie. Bd. XVIII. Heft 4. 20

Fig. 2. First page of the original report of 'Dora', the first psychoanalytic case, published in 1905 by Karger Publishers in the 'Monatsschrift für Neurologie und Psychiatrie'. This journal was founded 1897 by Wernicke and Ziehen and changed later its name into 'European Neurology'. Philippe Helaers Library.

on dreams and the unconscious to a hysteric patient. It is somewhat ironic that Freud would be confronted by a patient that was, unquestionably, *actually* 'seduced' at a time when he had not yet repudiated publicly his 'seduction theory', but about 3 years after he did privately. This was Freud's first effort to relate the Oedipus complex to an individual patient.

However, the interpretation of that case was also criticized. For example, Huopainen [37, pp. 100–101] stated about the Dora case:

> In his thought, Freud was unable to integrate contemporary traumas explaining Dora's hysteria, such as a child's naturally felt horror and repulsion towards pedophilic sexuality and her background of traumatic interaction experiences in childhood, and

was thus unable to understand the frailty of Dora's ego. Freud's bypassing of his patients' real emotional difficulties prevented not only Dora's integration but also the resolution of her libidinal conflicts and the continuation of her treatment, and together these factors most likely served to further aggravate Dora's difficulties.'

On the other hand, it could be argued that Freud was well aware of these facts, but was simply paid to silence a turbulent young girl that was getting in the way of her family's libertine whereabouts. Indeed, it can be questioned whether Dora was 'ill' at all, let alone 'hysteric' [38].

From Hysteria to Psychoanalysis

Critics of psychoanalysis often point out the numerous 'Freudian lies'. In fact, psychoanalysis was born precisely out of the attempt *not* to lie. The 'seduction theory' put Freud in such an uncomfortable situation that he had to resort to an unfalsifiable alternate reality positing the existence of an invisible world of conflicts that would secure the 'progress' of the theory while at the same time immunizing it against all attacks, and in the progress, actually indicting the very attacks as symptoms and 'resistance' [39]. Rhetorically, the stroke of genius was, retrospectively and smoothly, to link the unfortunate episode of the abuse theory to the 'discovery' of the Oedipus complex. It was fathers all along! This is the place that hysteria occupies in the history of the psychoanalytic movement: an embarrassing condition, which Freud, however, managed to integrate in his developing theories of libido, finally to obtain an initially unexpected success.

Before the emergence of a scholarly Freudian critique, the retrospective accounts of Freud's change of mind were typically interpreted as a sign of scientific guarantee, which of course helped to propagate and solidify the legend. Others have tried to account for this period's events through psychoanalytic or psychological lenses, for instance analyzing the meaning of Freud's dreams of that period and pointing to the emotional and professional turmoil he endured at that time, shortly following his father's death, even by postulating a 'creative illness' [9]. As we have seen, such accounts still do not account for how exactly he came up with the seduction theory in the first place, what became of his early 'data', what changed in his 'method' afterwards, and so forth. The chronological developments as well as the nature of the changes in Freud's theory may in fact suffice to state that Freud in fact found the answers he was looking for 'in himself'.

Freud used hysteria to build a reputation and develop his new psychological theory. In the process, hysteria per se was in fact hardly addressed, much less explained, solved, or cured. The very same processes that would in time explain 'conversion symptoms', which required (as we have seen) revising, ignoring, and somewhat distorting previous explanations, would end up as the all-purpose neuropsychoanalytic package still in use today. With intelligence and intuition, Freud would subsequently apply in all matters of human existence his purportedly universal discoveries about the human psyche. It is truly remarkable that his failure to document and test his early ideas about hysterical symptoms would progressively transform, without the benefit of any actual new scientific research, into a mechanism that could likewise explain everything from dreams, jokes, art, and culture, not to mention mental disorders.

That hysteria is intrinsically linked to the emergence of psychoanalysis, to the extent that without this specific condition it would probably never have seen light, is not a new idea:

> Analysts today believe that psychoanalysis could only have evolved out of work with hysterics because hysterics formed strong, explicit transferences to their doctors and thus provided examples of projection and sexual conflict. Kurt Eissler has hypothesized that 'the discovery of psychoanalysis would

have been greatly impeded, delayed, or even made impossible if in the second half of the nineteenth century the prevailing neurosis had not been hysteria' [40, p. 44].

Likewise, du Preez stated that 'one might, in fact, argue that it was from the "wandering wombs" identified in hysterical patients of the late nineteenth and early twentieth centuries that psychoanalysis and the discovery of the unconscious emerged' [41, p. 47].

But perhaps one could go a step further and submit that hysteria really was the cause, the *etiology* of psychoanalysis. Indeed, let's imagine that Freud was right about the seduction theory, or that he had stumbled upon some causal mechanism that would resolve the mystery of hysteria once and for all. There would have been no subsequent need to develop psychoanalysis because there would be no error to justify retroactively. Imagine, likewise, that Freud had never proposed the seduction theory in 1896, but instead continued struggling with the cathartic method, trying to uncover the deepest strata of unconscious traumatic memories that led to the symptoms. There would have been no need to posit some universal and all-encompassing mechanism to rationalize the errors and failure to cure the patients in the long term. As a clinician he would have simply followed, like everybody else, the course of medical discomfort with conversion and dissociative disorders (indeed, it is not as if these are well understood even today, not to mention easily curable). Psychoanalysis seemed to have developed within a context in which the patients always confirmed any pre-established theory. They may have led to psychoanalysis as a mirror of their suggestibility, malleability, and sheer mysteriousness. The rest is history, of course, with the need for psychoanalysis to insulate itself further, not unlike a 'secret society', as Ernest Jones put it. Using Pierre Janet's terms, psychoanalysis thus became the new clothes of hysteria.

References

1 Carhart-Harris RL, Friston KJ: The default-mode, ego-functions and free-energy: a neurobiological account of Freudian ideas. Brain 2010;133:1265–1283.
2 Kandel ER: Biology and the future psychoanalysis: a new intellectual framework for psychiatry revisited. Am J Psychiatry 1999;156:505–524.
3 Halligan PW, David S: Conversion hysteria: towards a cognitive neuropsychological account. Cogn Neuropsychiatry 1999;4:161–163.
4 Oakley DA, Halligan PW: Hypnotic suggestion: opportunities for cognitive neuroscience. Nat Rev Neurosci 2013;14: 565–576.
5 Bogousslavsky J: Sigmund Freud's evolution from neurology to psychiatry: evidence from his La Salpêtrière library. Neurology 2011;77:1391–1394.
6 Breuer J, Freud S: Studies on Hysteria. New York, Avon Books, 1895/1966.
7 Sulloway FJ: Reassessing Freud's case histories. Isis 1991;82:245–275.
8 Libbrecht K, Quackelbeen J: On the early history of male hysteria and psychic trauma: Charcot's influence on Freudian thought. J Hist Behav Sci 1995;31:370–384.
9 Ellenberger HF: Histoire de la découverte de l'inconscient. Paris, Fayard, 1970.
10 Freud S: Observation of a severe case of hemianesthesia in a hysterical male (1886); in The Standard Edition of the Complete Psychological Work of Sigmund Freud. London, Hogarth Press and The Institute of Psycho-Analysis, 1966, vol I, pp 23–31.
11 Freud S: Hysteria. The Standard Edition of the Complete Psychological Works of Sigmund Freud, vol I (1886–1899): Pre-Psycho-Analytic Publications and Unpublished Drafts, 1888, pp 37–59.
12 Freud S: Charcot. The Standard Edition of the Complete Psychological Works of Sigmund Freud, vol III (1893–1899): Early Psycho-Analytic Publications, 1893, pp 7–23.
13 Bouchara C: Jean-Martin Charcot 1825–1893: did he anticipate Freud's first topology? Am J Psychiatry 2010;167:387.
14 Breuer J, Freud S: On the psychical mechanism of hysterical phenomena: preliminary communication (initially published in Neurol Zentralbl 1893;XII:4–10, 43–47); in The Standard Edition of the Complete Psychological Work of Sigmund Freud. London, Hogarth Press and The Institute of Psycho-Analysis, 1966, vol II, pp 13–17.
15 Freud S: Quelques considérations pour une étude comparative des paralysies motrices organiques et hystériques. Arch Neurol (Paris) 1893;26:29–43.
16 Koehler PJ: Freud's comparative study of hysterical and organic paralyses: how Charcot's assignment turned out. Arch Neurol 2003;60:1646–1650.
17 Stone J, Smyth R, Carson A, Warlow C, Sharpe M: La belle indifférence in conversion symptoms and hysteria: systematic review. Br J Psychiatry 2006;188: 204–209.

18 Freud S: Repression (1915); quoted in Laplanche J, Pontalis JB: Vocabulaire de la psychanalyse. Paris, PUF, 1967.
19 Babinski J: Contribution à l'étude des troubles mentaux dans l'hémiplégie organique cérébrale (anosognosie). Rev Neurol 1914;27:845–848.
20 de Marneffe D: Looking and listening: the construction of clinical knowledge in Charcot and Freud. Sign 1991;17:71–111.
21 Freud S: Project for a Scientific Psychology (1895); quoted in Ellenberger HF: Histoire de la découverte de l'inconscient. Paris, Fayard, 1970.
22 Lakoff G, Johnson M: Philosophy in the Flesh: The Embodied Mind and Its Challenge to Western Thought. New York, Basic Books, 1999.
23 Allison DB, Roberts MS: On the constructing of the disorder hysteria. J Med Philos 1994;19:239–259.
24 Freud S: Heredity and the aetiology of the neuroses (published originally in French in Revue Neurologique, March 1896); in The Standard Edition of the Complete Psychological Work of Sigmund Freud. London, Hogarth Press and The Institute of Psycho-Analysis, 1966, vol III, pp 143–156.
25 Freud S: Further remarks on the neuro-psychoses of defence (published originally in Neurol Zentralbl 1896); in The Standard Edition of the Complete Psychological Work of Sigmund Freud. London, Hogarth Press and The Institute of Psycho-Analysis, 1966, vol III, pp 162–185.
26 Freud S: The aetiology of hysteria (published originally in five weekly installments, May-June, 1896, in Wien Klin Rundsch); in The Standard Edition of the Complete Psychological Work of Sigmund Freud. London, Hogarth Press and The Institute of Psycho-Analysis, 1966, vol III, pp 191–221.
27 Gleaves DH, Hernandez E: Recent reformulations of Freud's development and abandonment of his seduction theory: historical/scientific clarification or a continued assault on truth? Hist Psychol 1999;2:324–354.
28 Esterson A: Misconceptions about Freud's seduction theory: comment on Gleaves and Hernandez (1999). Hist Psychol 2002;5:85–91.
29 Triplett H: The misnomer of Freud's 'seduction theory'. J Hist Ideas 2004;65: 647–665.
30 Esterson A: The mythologizing of psychoanalytic history: deception and self-deception in Freud's accounts of the seduction theory episode. Hist Psychiat 2001;12:329–352.
31 Esterson A: Jeffrey Masson and Freud's seduction theory: a new fable based on old myths. Hist Hum Sci 1998;11:1–21.
32 Borch-Jacobsen M: Neurotica: Freud and the seduction theory. October (MIT Press) 1996;76:15–43.
33 Esterson A: The myth of Freud's ostracism by the medical community in 1896–1905: Jeffrey Masson's assault on truth. Hist Psychol 2002;5:115–134.
34 Freud S: My Views on the Part Played by Sexuality in the Aetiology of the Neuroses (1906 [1905]). The Standard Edition of the Complete Psychological Works of Sigmund Freud, vol VII (1901–1905): A Case of Hysteria, Three Essays on Sexuality and Other Works, 1906, 269–279, p 274.
35 Ahbel-Rappe K: 'I no longer believe': did Freud abandon the seduction theory? J Am Psychoanal Assoc 2006;54:171–199.
36 Freud S: An Autobiographical Study. The Standard Edition of the Complete Psychological Works of Sigmund Freud, vol XX (1925–1926): An Autobiographical Study, Inhibitions, Symptoms and Anxiety, The Question of Lay Analysis and Other Works, 1925, 1–74, p 33.
37 Huopainen H: Freud's view of hysteria in light of modern trauma research. Scand Psychoanal Rev 2002;25:92–107.
38 Stadlen A: Was Dora 'ill'? in Spurling L (ed): Freud: Critical Assessments. London, Routledge, 1989, vol 2, pp 196–203.
39 Boudry M, Braeckman J: Immunization strategies and epistemic defense mechanisms. Philosophia 2011;39:145–161.
40 Showalter E: Hystories: Hysterical Epidemics and Modern Culture. New York, Columbia University Press, 1997.
41 du Preez A: Putting on appearances: mimetic representations of hysteria. De Arte 2004;69:47–61.

Julien Bogousslavsky, MD
Center for Brain and Nervous System Diseases
GSMN Neurocenter, Clinique Valmont
CH–1823 Glion/Montreux (Switzerland)
E-Mail jbogousslavsky@cliniquevalmont.ch

Bogousslavsky J (ed): Hysteria: The Rise of an Enigma. Front Neurol Neurosci. Basel, Karger, 2014, vol 35, pp 126–138
DOI: 10.1159/000360056

Paul Sollier, Pierre Janet, and Their Vicinity

Olivier Walusinski

Olivier Walusinski Family Physician, Private Practice, Brou, France

Abstract

Paul Sollier (1861–1933) and Pierre Janet (1859–1947) shared the same fate: achieving fame during their lives, then slipping into obscurity. However, their work is highly relevant for describing and explaining hysteria in the tradition of Jean-Martin Charcot (1825–1893). Both men had their teacher's clinical perspicacity, which enabled them to accumulate detailed clinical and psychological descriptions. These were published in books that achieved success in their day. From his descriptions, Sollier deduced a pathophysiology of hysteria in which a psychic inhibition led to a functional deficit in sensory-motor areas. This is partially confirmed by current functional brain imaging techniques. As for Janet, he developed concepts which are still valid today, involving personality dissociation, what he referred to as 'fixed ideas', and the subconscious. Sollier and Janet both saw hysteria as a response to the trigger of an emotional shock, specific to certain personalities. While the fundamental work by Joseph Babinski (1857–1932) on hysterical paralysis did much to enrich neurological semiology, Sollier contributed a novel description of the pathophysiology of hysteria, and Janet elucidated its psychopathological mechanisms.

Most often, medical history books that cover hysteria suggest that the great neurologist Jean-Martin Charcot (1825–1893) lost his way in his work on hysteria. As early as 1907, Paul Hartenberg [1] (1871–1949) wrote: 'Who could have foreseen, when Charcot was developing his concept of hysteria, that one day this laborious edifice would be victoriously attacked, that perhaps little or nothing would remain standing?' Henri Cesbron [2] (1879–1952), grandson of Charles Lasègue (1816–1883) and student of Joseph Babinski (1857–1932), whose theories he passionately defended, wrote in his 1909 thesis: 'Charcot's genius built a powerful conception of hysteria that was perfectly consistent; newly acquired knowledge has toppled that edifice.' More recently, in 1965, Ilza Veith dealt another blow: 'The collapse of his hypotheses cost him much of the renown and respect that his earlier work had earned him.' Veith drew on the words of Pierre Marie (1853–1940), who on the occasion of the 100-year anniversary of Charcot's birth in 1925 'spoke with indulgence of the unfortunate hypnotism experiments of his teacher as "a few errors"' [3, 4].

Should such peremptory judgments still be accepted? More than anyone else, Charcot, whose integrity is beyond reproach, helped pull hysteria from the swamp where alienists focused on degeneration and the first neurologists had left it to drown [5] (see Bogousslavsky [this vol., pp. 44–55]). According to Veith [3]: 'the extent of his influence is clear in light of the fact that three of his most remarkable students – Janet, Babinski and Freud – devoted several years of their lives to the very subject that had so intensely absorbed Charcot during his last ten years.' The concepts developed by Babinski and Sigmund Freud (1856–1939) are analyzed in other chapters of this book (see Bogousslavsky and Dieguez [this vol., pp. 109–125] and Poirier et al. [this vol., pp. 139–148]).

Overlooked by Veith and all the other historians, Paul Sollier (1861–1933), also one of Charcot's disciples, may be considered as the first neuropsychologist. He also proved to be the most innovative. Following the example of Jean Lhermitte (1877–1959) and Georges Guillain (1876–1961), who brought Charcot back from disrepute in the 1950s, we will show here why the concepts developed by Sollier should be released from purgatory. Current functional brain imaging tools (see LaFrance [this vol., pp. 198–204]) have made his work relevant once again, and it should be situated parallel to the psychopathology of hysteria developed by Pierre Janet (1859–1947), who rivalled but was eclipsed by Freud [6, 7].

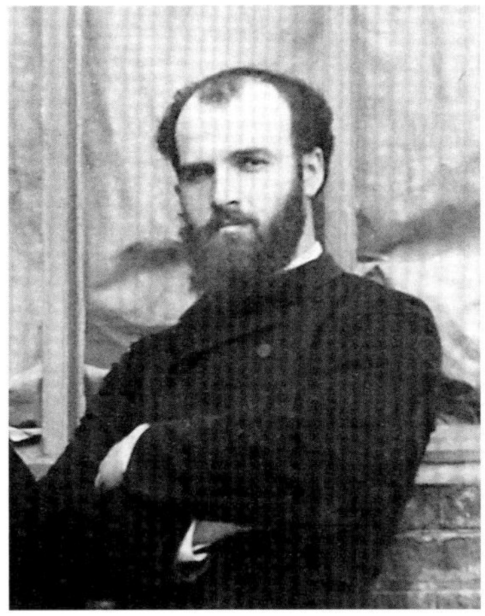

Fig. 1. Paul Sollier, House Officer at La Salpêtrière 1886. Private collection of the author.

Paul Sollier

Sollier's work, forgotten for nearly 75 years, has recently returned to the fore in the history of neuropsychology and the history of literature: 'Everything would suggest that an extraordinary meeting took place when Marcel Proust sought out care from Doctor Sollier' [8]. Born on August 31, 1861 in Bléré in the Indre-et-Loire Department of Central France, Sollier grew up in Le Mans in the Sarthe Department and began his medical studies in Paris in 1881. Brilliantly achieving the 5th best score on the competitive exam for an 'interne' (house officer) position in 1886, he went on to study nervous system diseases at Bicêtre Hospital and La Salpêtrière Hospital, where he was a contemporary of Babinski (fig. 1). He studied under Désiré-Magloire Bourneville (1840–1909), who gave him this evaluation: 'Excellent student, very devoted, very intelligent, broad-minded with a healthy understanding of his obligations, which is an increasingly rare quality in hospitals.' He was also a student of Jules Dejerine (1849–1917), Auguste Voisin (1829–1898), and Victor Cornil (1837–1908). Sollier attended the lessons of Charcot, building solid neurological and psychiatric foundations [9]. In 1891, he became 'Chef de Clinique des Maladies Mentales' under Voisin. He clearly explained his ideas in his first book, written in 1889 during his time as an 'interne'. The book, prefaced and published by Bourneville, was entitled *Du rôle de l'hérédité dans l'alcoolisme*: 'For us, mental pathology and nervous pathology form a single entity; they cannot be separated into two subspecialties' [10]. In 1890, Sollier [11] defended his thesis, inspired by Bourneville, with

Psychologie de l'idiot et de l'imbécile. His teacher Cornil, who presided over his defense, called him an 'alienist of the future' [9]. This thesis is one of the first works on child psychiatry ever written. It was published as a book the following year and immediately became very well known, remaining so for over 40 years. German and Polish translations were also published [11–13].

Sollier shared Bourneville's progressive ideals and helped him in his campaign to secularize the hospitals. In 1889, still an 'interne', he wrote: 'We hope that under a Republican regime, we will find more Republicans willing to accept this reform and cease fighting against it' [14]. Apparently, later on Sollier had to treat Edouard Drumont (1844–1917) at his hydrotherapy center, a journalist and politician who in 1892 founded *La Libre Parole*, an anti-Dreyfusard, nationalistic, and anti-Semitic paper. He wrote to a friend: 'Anti-Semitism is a very curious psychic manifestation which is only one episode of a highly characterized mental state, accompanied by numerous defects indicating intellectual degeneration. It is a particular way of thinking which corresponds to a particular brain configuration. [...] One is predisposed to it as one is to insanity' [15]. Sollier was qualified as an 'uncompromising materialist' by Léon Daudet (1867–1942), who referred to him in the most complimentary terms [16]:

> He had always been considered by everyone to have a brilliant future. I can still see him, next to Brissaud and Babinski, in the courtyards of La Salpêtrière. [...] Brissaud's contributions related to the pyramidal tract, Babinski's to the patellar reflex and Sollier's to the 'syncope de la trentième heure' [syncope after 30 h of wakefulness, a humorous reference to neurosis]. He was very quick to untangle, in what was then called hysteria, drowsiness and 'awakening' by motor stimulation, from the attack which, in his view, released the subject from a numbness that had lasted days, weeks and months. His clinical curiosity was boundless, and he was incredible when, speaking masterfully, he only accepted what he had personally observed. Above all, he sought to heal, whereas Charcot, Brissaud and even Marie and Ballet were content to observe.

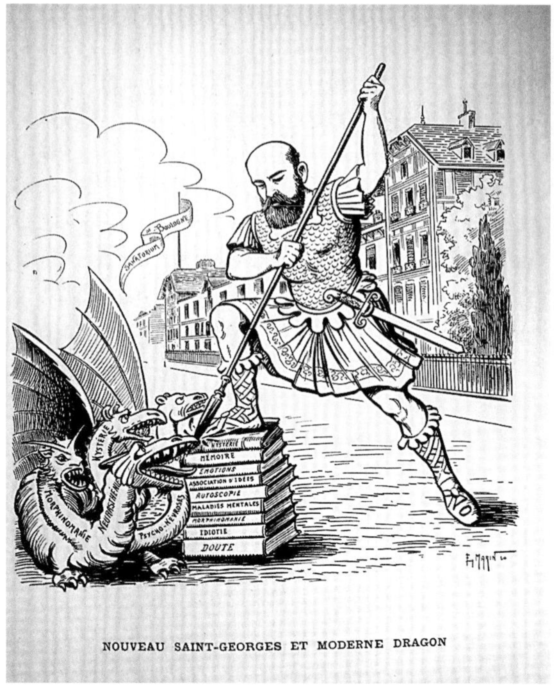

Fig. 2. Paul Sollier. Cartoon by E. Marin. Album Le Rictus 1911. Private collection of the author.

In 1897, Sollier founded the Boulogne-Billancourt Hydrotherapy Center with his wife Alice Mathieu-Dubois (1861–1942), who was also a physician, on the edge of the Bois de Boulogne to the west of Paris. There he initiated new therapeutic methods – precursors to current cognitive-behavioral methods [17]. His most famous patient was Marcel Proust, who came to him at the end of 1905.

Sollier was a prolific author, who was widely read and translated until World War II. He covered a multitude of subjects, including doubt, psychic energy, conscience, morality, addiction to gambling, anorexia nervosa, and morphine withdrawal (fig. 2). He became a professor of psychology at Université Nouvelle de Bruxelles in 1898, but never held this position in France. He became president of the Medical Psychological Society in 1926. On several occasions before and after World War I, he was a candidate for entry

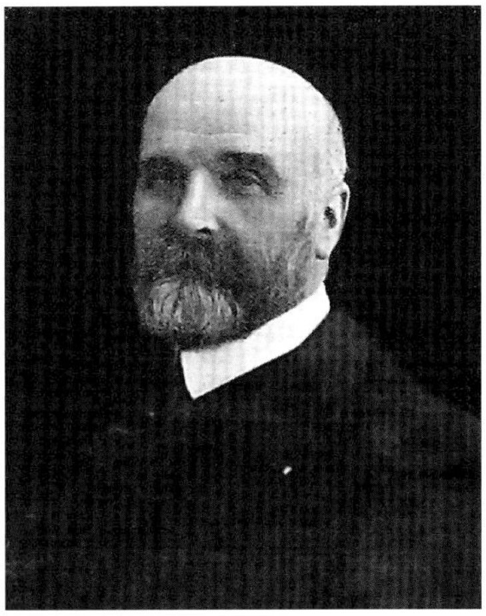

Fig. 3. Paul Sollier around 1930. Private collection of the author.

into the French Academy of Medicine, but was never elected [18, 19].

As director of the neurological center of the 14th military district during the war, Sollier coordinated the preparation of a wartime clinical neurology treaty, published in 1918. The word 'clinical' in the title reveals how Sollier was thinking at the time and distinguishes him from other authors. In particular, he took special interest in victims of explosions, experimenting on and autopsying rabbits. He was thus the first to describe the multiple subcortical microhemorrhages resulting in comas that had previously been considered hysterical in nature. His psychotherapeutic treatment of 'war psychoneuroses' was distinctly different from the more violent method using 'persuasion by faradic currents', which soldiers referred to as 'le torpillage' (torpedoing) and which was advocated by Clovis Vincent (1879–1947) and Gustave Roussy (1874–1947) [20, 21]. At the end of his career, he devoted himself to mental health in the workplace and occupational therapy, which he named 'la psychotechnique' (fig. 3). This orientation reveals how profoundly impacted Sollier was by his extensive work with the war injured [22, 23].

Because of its modernity, his thinking in three domains is familiar to us: emotions, memory, and hysteria. A contemporary of William James (1842–1910), Sollier studied emotions with an emphasis on the cenesthetic sensation, which is similar to the current concept of interoception, or the capacity to perceive functional modifications in the body that result in cognitive emotional sensation [24–26]. In 1900, Sollier published *Le problème de la mémoire* in which he presented a novel conception of memory from an anatomical viewpoint, and with a cellular substrate, thus challenging the philosophical ideas of the time. Although he used other terms, he distinguished procedural from semantic memory, declarative from involuntary memory, and introduced the term 'reviviscences' with reference to involuntary memory, especially affective involuntary memory, a concept Janet would develop 30 years later in his book *L'évolution de la mémoire et la notion de temps* [27]. Reviviscences are the keystone in Proust's *A la recherche du temps perdu,* published beginning in 1913. This shows the degree to which Proust integrated the ideas of Sollier on emotional memory without ever openly recognizing his influence, except in his 1908 notebook in which Sollier's name appears next to the first mention of involuntary memory [28–30].

Genesis and Nature of Hysteria According to Sollier

The theme of the 17th Conference of French Alienists and Neurologists, held in Geneva and Lausanne in August 1907, was 'Definition and Nature of Hysteria'. In their report, Henri Claude (1869–1945) and Louis Schnyder (1868–1927) from Bern included the ideas of Albert Pitres (1848–1928), faithful student of Charcot; Hippolyte Bernheim (1840–1919) from the Nancy school; Joseph Grasset (1849–1918), who borrowed from Janet; Fulgence Raymond (1844–

1910), who spoke of modifications to cortical and subcortical reflexes, and Babinski, who explained his notion of 'pithiatism' [31]. The two most novel presentations were given by Édouard Claparède (1873–1940) from Geneva and by Sollier.

Something of an ethologist, Claparède established a phylogenetic parallel between hysteria and protective behavioral inhibition in response to a predator in the animal world: 'Hysterical reactions are defence reactions or phenomena symbolising a defence. But for the most part, these reactions are used in the normal individual only in the rudimentary state; some of them may only be the reviviscence of ancestral reactions whose biological utility is only evident in animals that manifest them' [31].

As for Sollier, he noted from the start: 'What causes the current confusion in the study of hysteria is the introduction of philosophical, psychological, moral and even metaphysical concepts. We must limit ourselves to anatomy and physiology to avoid Scholastic discussions on words we cannot define, such as consciousness, idea, image, representation, etc.' [31]. Sollier added to this idea at the beginning of the book he devoted to hysteria in 1897: 'I have arrived at a new conception of the genesis and nature of hysteria, which I will say immediately that I consider not as a purely psychic condition, as is commonly thought today, but as a physical condition, albeit a solely functional one' [32].

Sollier's novel conception is based on a notion of sleep, and in particular partial sleep, limited to certain brain regions [32]:

> The fundamental fact is that totally anaesthetic hysterics are asleep; they are in a state of vigilambulism from which they can be awakened by any means, thereby putting an end to all the hysterical stigmata and accidents. [...] Thus, it now appears that hysteria is essentially a special state of the brain affecting a greater or lesser number of its centres, similar to a drowsiness, to a sort of sleep. [...] Each brain centre affected by this sort of sleep stops functioning, which leads to more or less marked disturbances in the organic sphere functionally linked to it, depending on the degree of sleep, such that hysteria is actually composed of an aggregation and a combination of local hysterias.

Note that at the beginning of the 20th century, virtually nothing was known about sleep physiology, as Sollier himself explained: 'As to the nature of the cerebral sleep leading to hysteria, the fact that I offer no hypotheses will hopefully be overlooked, as we do not yet understand natural sleep and what causes it' [32].

Currently, functional brain imaging shows reduced activity in sensory parietal areas and increased activity in ventral frontal regions, especially on the right side, with a hypoactivation of the thalamus, caudate nucleus, and putamen on the side opposite the hysterical deficit. This suggests that the basal ganglia block access to sensory-motor cortical areas under the influence of frontal inhibition originating in the limbic system (amygdala). The patient, convinced of the resulting deficiency, would be unable to consciously move or feel given that the blockage is subcortical, outside the field of consciousness (see LaFrance [this vol., pp. 198–204]). If we replace Sollier's 'partial sleep' by functional hypoactivation, his concept aligns with current theories [32, 33].

Once he had provided a pathophysiological explanation for the symptoms, Sollier proposed an etiopathogenesis: 'Emotion plays a fundamental role. The anaesthesia depends on emotion and not on the trauma.' Sollier distinguished himself from Babinski by evoking an idea, an interpretation, or self-suggestion, rather than 'considering the nervous shock' as the trigger. Sollier explained that 'the idea itself is merely the interpretation of the motor disturbance. The subject, referring to her feelings, builds an explanation that seems very probable to her, which in all honesty she believes to be exact and aligned with reality.' Sollier continued [32]:

> Clinical experience shows us that subjects suffering from hysterical accidents that are absolutely identical, have ideas that are absolutely different. Isn't it

surprising that different ideas can lead to identical reactions? [...] My argument is that by itself, an idea never directly provokes hysteria. It must first result in an emotion, an emotional state. [...] It is thus the emotional state which is fundamental. The emotional state in turn produces the anaesthesia from which paralysis develops.

Sollier went on to explain hysteria as follows: 'Brain centres stop functioning, drowsiness and sleep occur in these centres as a result of exhaustion produced by the emotion, whether this emotion is justified or not' [32].

Sollier was arguing against false reasoning, notably that of Freud [32]:

A tendency which has intensified in recent years is to consider nothing but the psychic manifestations of hysteria, which has led to deeming it a mental illness, and to give ideas a primordial role in its general development and in the forms it adopts. The result of considering only the mind is that the brain and nervous system are completely neglected. The organ of thought and its physiology has been neglected through focusing solely on one manifestation of its function.

Once again showing great foresight, Sollier distinguished 'an organic brain' (i.e. sensory-motor) from 'a psychic brain' which he situates in the frontal area [32]:

In hysteria, the disturbances are purely functional. There is no physical lesion. The pathways of transmission are not cut off. The nerve impulse can thus be propagated. Since the receptive centres of the organic brain are in a very reduced state of function and react very little to the excitation that reaches them, the excitation they transmit to the psychic brain centres is also extremely reduced.

It is clear that working at the turn of the 20th century, Sollier could not have been aware of an inhibitive frontal hyperactivity. He went on to conclude by comparing his theory with 'the dynamic lesion' proposed by Charcot 20 years prior: 'I thus agree with Charcot and Marie, who consider hysteria not so much an illness, in the ordinary sense of the word, as a particular way of sensing and responding' [32].

Pierre Janet

Janet provided his own introduction in his lecture on March 11, 1892 at La Salpêtrière, which was attended by Charcot [34]:

You know that Mr. Charcot has demonstrated the moral and psychological nature of hysterical paralyses, that he has had the audacity of presenting certain flaccid paralyses which appeared entirely physical as simple thought phenomena. He thereby laid out the path for studying the other symptoms of hysteria in the same way. It is thus only natural that Mr. Charcot would wish to hear presented, in the clinic's auditorium, new studies on the mental state of hysterics, studies that continue his own work. Personally, I am very proud that Mr. Charcot chose me to present you with questions of such interest to him. I am especially proud that he had enough confidence in me to trust that my psychological analyses would not depart from medical truth, and from clinical truth, to which everything here must be subjected. I am also happy to have this opportunity to express my gratitude to him. Ten or twelve years ago, when I was a philosophy teacher in the provinces, I came to Mr. Charcot, lacking any qualifications, to ask for advice on the experimental psychology studies I wanted to undertake. Mr. Charcot has undoubtedly forgotten, but I still remember his kind welcome and the precious suggestions he made. I am one of his students, more so than he knows. Later, when I came to work in his department, everyone's kindness and friendship endeared me to them, and if my humble work might add some small detail to the wonderful research carried out here, I would be happy.

Pierre Janet was born in Paris on May 30, 1859 to a family of modest means. His uncle was philosopher Paul Janet (1823–1899). At the École Normale Supérieure, he began preparing in 1878 for the competitive exam to become a philosophy teacher, along with Henri Bergson (1859–1941), Emile Durkheim (1858–1917), and Jean Jaurès (1859–1914). At the same time, he worked as an assistant to Albert Dastre (1844–1917), a physiology professor at La Sorbonne. This is key to understanding Janet's interest in medicine. Passing his test in 1882, he went to Le Havre where he

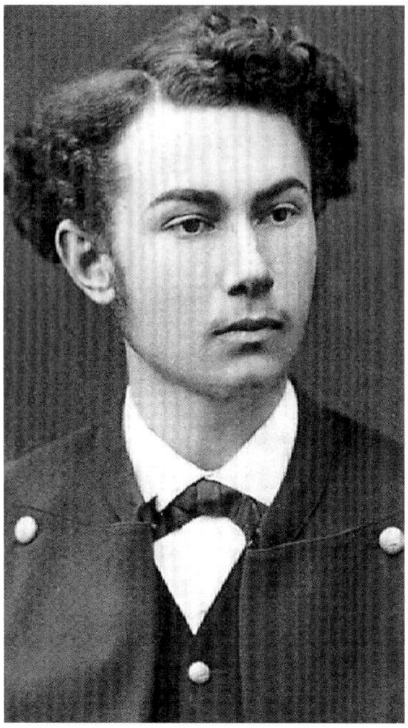

Fig. 4. Pierre Janet 1878. Private collection of the author.

taught for 7 years (fig. 4). One of his students was the son of a hospital alienist, Joseph Gibert (1829–1899), who was a friend of Félix Faure (1841–1899), President of France, and who also actively supported Captain Dreyfus during the famous turn-of-the-century case, which was marked by anti-Semitism. Gibert, who founded the journal *La Normandie Médicale*, published seven articles describing attacks of hysteria between 1891 and 1893, and employing expressions such as 'passionate attitude'. This led to his nickname, 'The Norman Charcot', but more importantly revealed that he saw hysteria as secondary to sexual disorders. He and Janet became friends. Influenced by the teachings of Théodule Ribot (1839–1916), Janet began spending time at the hospital in order to study hypnosis for his thesis. This led to a decisive meeting; Gibert and his colleague Léon-Jean Powilewicz (1852–1932) presented Janet with a patient, the 'clairvoyant and magnetist' Léonie Leboulanger, a servant in her 40s and a 'somnambulant hysteric' with whom the region's magnetists had been familiar since 1860 [35]. Observations concerning Leboulanger, which Janet collected in 1885 and 1886, were one of the main sources for his humanities thesis, defended in 1889 and generating considerable interest. The work was dedicated to Gibert 'with gratitude and affection'; its title translates as *Psychological Automatism; Experimental Psychology Essay on the Inferior Forms of Human Activity* [36, 37]. Janet was probably influenced by Jules Baillarger (1809–1890) who spoke in 1845 of the 'involuntary exercise of memory and intelligence' resulting in the 'independence of faculties removed from personal control', and who built a theory of psychic automatism. In his thesis, Janet focused on diseases of personality, especially multiple personalities, and tried to reconcile the phenomena of consciousness with the notion of a subconsciousness, 'which lies under consciousness, but is of the same nature'. Janet expressed his ideas through the phenomenon of double personality, and his perspective was clearly philosophical rather than medical, as his thesis jury's commendations confirm [38–40].

Janet met Charcot in Le Havre in 1885. Charcot came with future Nobel Prize winner Charles Richet (1850–1935) and other members of the Physiological Psychology Society, created with Ribot and Richet in 1868, to examine Léonie. Janet began spending time at La Salpêtrière shortly thereafter. Charcot founded a 'psychology laboratory' for him in 1890, combining scientific philosophy and medicine, in the positivist tradition of August Comte (1798–1857). Charcot brought into being what he had mentioned to his students on January 17, 1888: 'We must create a field of psychology reinforced by our pathological studies. We are doing so with psychologists who, this time, are willing to consider not only what is known as interior observation' [41]. Janet was one such psychologist, but not Ribot, though he had been previously singled out by Charcot, who included him in the famous 1887 portrait by André Brouillet (1857–1914), *Leçon clinique à La*

Salpêtrière [42]. Janet remained the director of this laboratory until 1910, when Dejerine, Charcot's second successor, dismissed him and blocked his election to the French Academy of Medicine. Dejerine, who held a Lutheran moral ideology, could not accept Janet's obstinate refusal to mix medicine, which treats and sometimes heals, with morality, which condemns. After his dismissal, the neuropathologist and alienist Jean Nageotte (1866–1948) gave Janet a small room so that he could continue working at La Salpêtrière. Probably out of nostalgia, Janet continued all his life to publish his major works under the auspices of the psychology laboratory of La Salpêtrière, even though it had ceased to exist [43, 44].

Janet defended his doctoral thesis in medicine on July 29, 1893. Along with the thesis defended the same day by the 'interne' Henri Lamy (1864–1909), it was the last defense presided by Charcot, who died on August 16, 1893 [45]. Charcot wrote in the commercial edition of Janet's thesis: 'The studies of my student Janet confirm the thinking often expressed in our lessons, namely that hysteria is largely a mental illness. This is one aspect of the disease that we must never neglect if we wish to understand and treat it' [46].

Janet practiced as a clinical psychotherapist in Le Havre and at La Salpêtrière. He failed in his first attempt to enter the Medical Psychological Society in November 1893, being neither a former 'interne' in the hospitals nor an alienist. His medical career was simply too atypical. Furthermore, he defended a concept of psychic trauma as the cause of hysteria in a small circle that since Bénédict Augustin Morel (1806–1873) had been won over by ideas of 'degeneration' and 'hereditarism'. Janet often attended the dinners at the Vanves asylum, run by Jules Falret (1824–1902), during which the guests mingled with patients. The support of Falret, who was the rapporteur for his candidature to the society, helped him get admitted in 1895; he went on to become president in 1929. In 1897, he was appointed to the Experimental Psychology Chair at La Sorbonne. He took over from Ribot at the Collège de France, where he occupied the Experimental and Comparative Psychology Chair from 1902 to 1934. Janet founded the Psychology Society in 1901 and the *Journal de Psychologie Normale et Pathologique* in 1904. Janet never founded a movement, but his influence is evident in the work of the psychiatrists Gaëtan Gatian de Clérambault (1872–1934), Karl Gustav Jung (1875–1961), Henry Wallon (1879–1962), Eugène Minkowski (1885–1972), Jean Piaget (1896–1980), Henri Ey (1900–1977), Jacques Lacan (1901–1981), and Jean Delay (1907–1987). Although he covered nearly all domains of normal and pathological psychology, and his publications included some 20 volumes and nearly 300 articles or contributions to collective volumes, Janet was largely forgotten after World War II due to the success of psychoanalysis (fig. 5). Might another factor be his intense dislike of publicity? Did certain enmities, notably on the part of Alfred Binet (1857–1911), play a role? Undoubtedly, but there is also the fact that Janet, in keeping with his initial training, often published psychiatric observations in the *Revue Philosophique*, which did not help their dissemi-

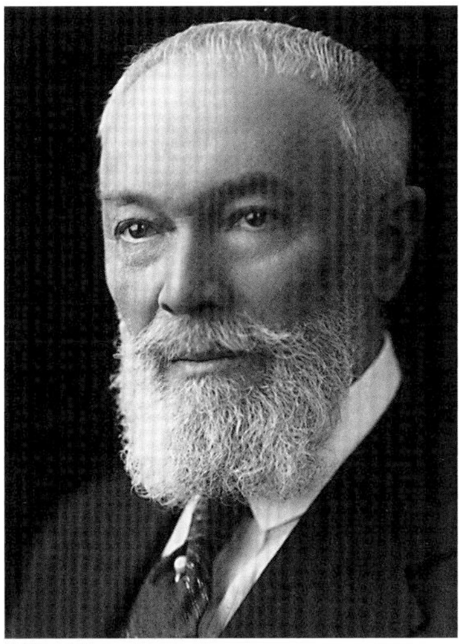

Fig. 5. Pierre Janet around 1930. ©BIU Santé Paris, with kind permission.

nation among physicians. Because his discoveries were largely forgotten, many others took credit for his results. Already in his 1889 thesis, he wrote: 'A banished idea, like a psychic parasite, causes all accidents stemming from physical and mental diseases.' Janet's tribute to Charcot could very well apply to Janet himself: 'Thanks to the considerable authority of his name, he was able to elucidate facts which until then had been observed in the shadows and bring science to bear in areas previously surrounded by mystery and superstition' [47, 48].

Definition and Nature of Hysteria According to Janet

Janet assumed that hysteria was not a result of organic lesions, but was instead psychological in nature, i.e. 'related to the highest functions of the brain, but we wish to avoid any metaphysical speculations on unknown damage to brain cells' [49]. His approach was purely clinical, based on examination of the patients. He began in 1892 with anesthesia, which became the prototype for his conception. In contrast to the philosopher-psychologists for whom sensation is a state of consciousness, Janet associated perception with a more complex idea, specific to the subject's personality at a given time, i.e. personal memories and imagination. Thus, sensation forms through the synthesis of perception and its interpretation, which varies according to affective state. He qualified this process as subconscious, drawing on the work of philosopher Pierre Maine de Biran (1766–1824), a forerunner already interested in sleep and somnambulism.

Incidentally, Janet wanted to combine the influences of Maine de Biran and Charcot in founding a scientific psychology, which the La Salpêtrière neurologist named in wishes formulated during his January 17, 1888 lesson: 'What I call psychology is the rational physiology of the cerebral cortex' [34, 41, 50].

To return to the above-mentioned synthesis, when it is absent, a deficit such as anesthesia or paralysis results, secondary to a 'reduction in the field of consciousness' [49]. The mechanisms of hysterical amnesia are identical; perceptions are no longer aligned with the whole personality, especially the affective aspects [49]:

> Despite all the complications that this symptom can present, the fact that the subject forgets everything that happens during the somnambulism when she returns to the normal state seems to us to be the only constant and essential character of somnambulism. [...] It is always the result, the manifestation, of a doubling of personality.

For Janet, the ecstasies, catalepsies and fugues are only 'various degrees or forms of somnambulism' and the main explanation is that 'the psychological phenomenon on which these accidents depend is amnesia' [46]. He then extended his reasoning: 'The attack is caused by a psychological phenomenon associated with the emotional state, the fixed idea, and also dreams, which constitute a second existence' [49]. We see here Janet's own concept of 'fixed ideas', i.e. during hysterical manifestations, certain ideas distinguish themselves from others by taking on abnormal importance, like a parasitic thought becoming similar to an involuntary automatism, occurring outside the subject's knowledge: 'This state of natural and perpetual distraction prevents the subject from appreciating any other sensation outside that which currently occupies her mind'. An organized system of old images is reproduced, develops, and perpetuates itself; the subject has no control over it, having lost her capacity for synthesis [51]. Janet noted that Charcot had already written: 'Due to the dissociation of the mental unit, certain centres may be activated without the other regions of the psychic organ being informed or called to take part in the process' [52].

Suggestion, a concept of minimal importance according to Janet, involves a similar mechanism, but is not a parasitic idea introduced into the sub-

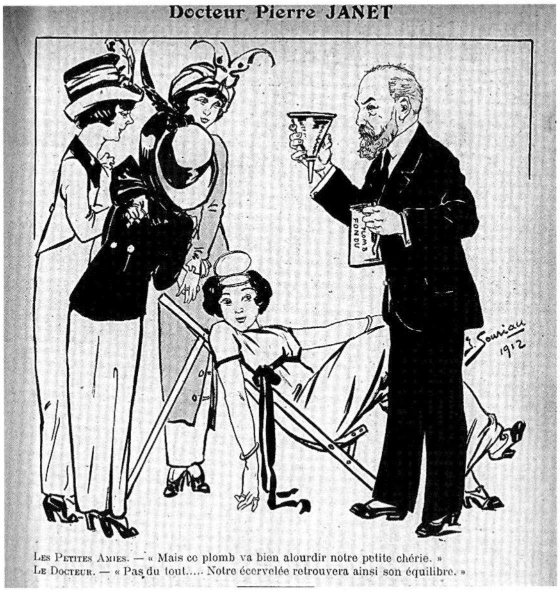
Docteur Pierre JANET
J. Sourniau 1912
Les Petites Amies. — « Mais ce plomb va bien alourdir notre petite chérie. »
Le Docteur. — « Pas du tout..... Notre écervelée retrouvera ainsi son équilibre. »

Fig. 6. Pierre Janet. Cartoon from Jacques Sourniau. Le Rictus. 1912. ©BIU Santé Paris, with kind permission.

ject's mind unbeknownst to her. Unlike obsession, the subject is unaware of the system of fixed ideas. Janet argued that an original psychic trauma, emotional in nature, reappears later in somatic expressions (anesthesia, paralysis, ecstasy, delirium, agitation, ticks, shaking, and contractures). Hysterics seem caught up in an incident in their lives that they cannot overcome (fig. 6).

Paul-Oscar Blocq (1860–1896), a former Charcot 'interne' and creator of a reflex hammer, presented in his name by Babinski during a meeting of the Société Médicale des Hôpitaux de Paris in 1892, summarized Janet's concepts as follows [53, 54]:

> One of the most significant psychological consequences of reducing the field of consciousness is a number of sensations and images that are not assimilated with the subject's personality. Although these sensations and images are unconscious perceptions, they persist nonetheless in the subject's mind. These phenomena may subsist only in simple form, or they may combine and organise themselves, like their counterparts in the conscious mind, so as to constitute a new psychological system, a personality independent from the first. This new personality may at times acquire such importance that it momentarily dominates the old personality; at other times, the two may simply coexist. Most hysterical accidents or attacks correspond to these various forms of damage to the personality.

Why Read Sollier and Janet Today?

The words of Marcel-Marie Riser (1891–1975), written in 1952, are accurate but incomplete [55]:

> Working almost entirely alone, Babinski built up a critical body of work that impresses with its precision and force and serves as the basis for our current semiology. He introduced an exact method of examination, which is taught and used throughout the world. It is based on rigorous observation, limited to a few signs, and has no influence on the observed.

Janet and Sollier also furthered the ideas of Charcot in decisive ways. Both wanted to encompass all psychological phenomena: perception, emotions, memory, language, belief, personality, etc., while at the same time offering a new interpretation, especially for the psychopathology of hysteria.

Janet clearly originated novel concepts such as 'fixed ideas' and 'the subconscious' as well as 'a reduction in the field of consciousness', which led to the idea of 'disaggregation of the personality'. After much back and forth due to translation, this idea became 'dissociation', which was amplified by Freud, Josef Breuer (1842–1925), and Eugen Bleuler (1857–1939) in the description of the pathophysiological mechanisms of psychoses, but was also abusively borrowed and extrapolated throughout the 20th century by psychoanalysis, which Janet never adhered to. Jung declared in 1907: 'The theoretical bases for the conceptualisation of Freudian research lie primarily in the results of Janet's research. The observation of psychic dissociation and unconscious psychological automatism gave rise to the first formulation of the problem of hysteria by Breuer and Freud' [56, 57]. Janet was close to Sollier in seeing hysteria as a 'deficit' resulting in anesthesia on a physical level, and amnesia on a mental level. It is regrettable that Janet's cautiousness prevented him from ever proposing a pathophysiology for hysterical manifestations; he only went so far as to state: 'The stigmata take the form of weakness and loss (at least apparent) of sensation, memories and movements. This is evidence of reduced nervous functions and an exhaustion of the organs' [46]. Janet was influenced by the notion of exhaustion developed by Charles Féré (1852–1907): 'Hysterics are in a permanent state of psychic fatigue which results in weakened exercise of the will' [58]. In consequence, Janet simply attributed hysteria to 'a manifestation of general brain exhaustion', which caused the weakened subject to be 'incapable of assembling and condensing psychological phenomena, and of assimilating them into her personality' [50]. However, his concept of the subconscious as relating to involuntary sensory perception has become relevant once again. It is being confirmed to the extent that Freud's 'unconscious' is losing its validity, as shown by the recent work of Lionel Naccache [59].

We found no trace of direct contact between Sollier and Janet, and it is unclear whether they knew each other personally. In his writings, Sollier frequently cited Janet (Janet rarely cited Sollier), with whom he shared several conceptions on the psychology of hysterics. He compared their viewpoints thusly: 'Where Mr. Janet sees a simple question of automatism and consciousness, I see the effect of a sensitivity disorder, whose automatism and unconsciousness are but consequences and serve as intermediaries between the two phenomena without being the primary cause' [32]. Sollier virulently opposed Babinski, who caricatured Sollier's conclusions in a way that was understandable, given what was known and accepted at the time and the rigor Babinski applied in his reasoning: 'This supposed disturbance would seem to involve a numbing of the brain. This is simply a mental construct that is very imprecise. There is no way to prove its accuracy' [60].

However, the theory defended by Sollier now appears grounded and his refutation of Babinski's pithiatism justified. Sollier denied the notion of self-suggestion, denied that hysteria alone could be cured by persuasion and opposed Babinski's refusal to allow a central role to a causal emotion [61]. Sollier provides the best summary of his theory of hysteria [62]:

> Due to a state of inhibition [...] Given that cortical centres have a double sensory-motor and psychic function, this state manifests itself by sensory, motor or visceral disturbances depending on its location, and also by disturbances in perception, representation and association. Anything that produces this state in the cortex – from traumatic shocks to emotions and mental representations – causes the same disturbances.

The statement Sollier wrote for his candidacy to the French Academy of Medicine is a precious hand-written testimony that, to date, has never been published. It was read on February 20, 1912. Sollier presented his method for treating hysteria, amongst other neuroses, referring also to his theory, Janet's concepts and his opposition to Babinski [63]:

> When motor function is addressed through appropriate excitation, using special gymnastics, the lost or diminished sensitivity in the relevant regions reappears parallel to the restored movements. [...] The excitation caused by the peripheral gymnastics moves to other brain centres and determines the appearance of psychic reactions in the form of representations and affective or emotional states. Consequently, as the sole result of peripheral mechanical excitation, the physical disturbances disappear at the same time as sensitivity and motor function return; secondarily, the related psychic, intellectual or moral disturbances in the form of fixed ideas and persistent affective states disappear. Without any suggestion, persuasion, psychological treatment or moral treatment whatsoever, a

purely mechanical action can return not only the subject's physical personality but also her moral personality to a normal state.

Janet provides us with a good conclusion [49]:

The word hysteria must be preserved. It would be difficult today to change it, and this word has such a long and beautiful history that it would be overly complicated to give it up. Should the etymology prove too awkward, it would be better to change the word 'uterus' rather than 'hysteria', as Charcot said so rightly. But because each era has given it a different meaning, we should seek out what it means for today's authors.

An excellent reason to read this book.

References

1 Hartenberg P: Les nouvelles idées sur l'hystérie. La Presse Médicale 1907;15: 469.
2 Cesbron H: Histoire critique de l'hystérie. Thèse No. 133. Paris, Asselin & Houzeau, 1909.
3 Veith I: Hysteria: The History of a Disease. Chicago, University of Chicago Press, 1965.
4 Marie P: Eloge de J.-M. Charcot, centenaire de naissance de Charcot. Rev Neurol (Paris) 1925;1:731–745.
5 Wildlöcher D, Dantchev N: Charcot et l'hystérie. Rev Neurol (Paris) 1994;150: 490–497.
6 Lhermitte J: L'École de la Salpêtrière, J.-M. Charcot, psycho-physiologiste. L'Encéphale 1950;4:297–310.
7 Guillain G: J.-M. Charcot, sa vie son œuvre. Paris, Masson, 1955.
8 Bizub E: Proust et le Docteur Sollier: les 'molécules impressionnées'. Bulletin de la Société des Amis de Marcel Proust 2006;56:41–51.
9 Sollier P: Fiche administrative No. 314. Paris, Archives AP-HP, 1883.
10 Sollier P: Du rôle de l'hérédité dans l'alcoolisme. Paris, Lecrosnier et Babé, 1889.
11 Sollier P: Psychologie de l'idiot et de l'imbécile (Essai de psychologie morbide). Thèse No. 66. Paris, Alcan, 1890.
12 Sollier P: Psychologie de l'idiot et de l'imbécile. Paris, Alcan, 1891.
13 Dumas G: Allocution prononcée à l'occasion du décès de M. Paul Sollier le 26 juin 1933. Bull Soc Médico-Psychologique 1933;14:67–68.
14 Sollier P: Réformes. L'Année Médicale. Aux Bureaux du Progrès Médical (Paris) 1889;11:393–397.
15 Sollier P: Lettre manuscrite, non datée, destinataire non identifié. Collection privée de l'auteur.
16 Daudet L: Paul Sollier. Le Progrès Médical 1933;10:1162–1163.
17 Le Maléfan P: La psychothérapie naissante au sanatorium du Dr Sollier (1861–1933). A propos de Cam. D., délirante spirite. Bull Psychol 2011;6:559–571.
18 Sollier P: Titres et Travaux scientifiques. Paris, Alcan, 1912.
19 Bogousslavsky J, Walusinski O: Paul Sollier: the first clinical neuropsychologist. Front Neurol Neurosci 2011;29: 105–114.
20 Sollier P, Chartier M, Rose F, Villandre C, Baratte D: Traité de neurologie clinique de guerre. Paris, Alcan, 1918.
21 Bogousslavsky J, Tatu L: French neuropsychiatry in the Great War: between moral support and electricity. J Hist Neurosci 2013;22:144–154.
22 Sollier P: Titres et travaux scientifiques. Paris, Alcan, 1912.
23 Sollier P, Drabs J: La psychotechnique, introduction à une technique du facteur humain dans le travail. Comité Central Industriel de Belgique (Bruxelles). Paris, Alcan, 1935.
24 Sollier P: Le mécanisme des émotions. Paris, Alcan, 1905.
25 James W: What is an emotion? Mind 1884;9:188–205.
26 Craig AD: How do you feel? Interoception, the sense of the physiological condition of the body. Nat Rev Neurosci 2002;3:655–666.
27 Janet P: L'évolution de la mémoire et la notion de temps. Paris, Chahine, 1929.
28 Sollier P: Le problème de la mémoire. Essai de psycho-mécanique. Paris, Alcan, 1900.
29 Bougousslavsky J: Memory after Charcot. J Neurol Neurosur Psychiatry 2007; 78:1373–1374.
30 Bougousslavsky J: La mémoire de Proust. Vevey, Le Cadratin, 2009.
31 Claude H, Schnyder L: XVIIè congrès des médecins aliénistes et neurologistes de France et des pays de langue française. La Presse Médicale 1907;15:532–534.
32 Sollier P: Genèse et nature de l'hystérie. Recherches cliniques et expérimentales de psycho-physiologie. Paris, Alcan, 1897.
33 Cojan Y, Waber L, Carruzzo A, Vuilleumier P: Motor inhibition in hysterical conversion paralysis. Neuroimage 2009; 47:1026–1037.
34 Janet P: L'anesthésie hystérique. Arch Neurol 1892;23:323–352.
35 Janet P: Note sur quelques phénomènes de somnambulisme. Rev Philos 1886;21: 190–198.
36 Carroy J: Le docteur Gibert ou le 'Breuer' de Pierre Janet; in Félida P, Villa F (eds): Le cas controverse. Paris, Presses Universitaires de France, 1999, pp 213–230.
37 Pichon-Janet H: Pierre Janet, quelques notes sur sa vie. L'Evolution Psychiatrique 1950;15;345–355.
38 Quercy P, Quercy D: Pierre Janet, l'hypnotisme, la suggestion, l'hystérie (1886–1892). Ann Med Psychol (Paris) 1948;106:257–280.
39 Baillarger J: Recherches sur les Maladies Mentales. Paris, Masson, 1845.
40 Carroy J, Plas R: How Pierre Janet used pathological psychology to save the philosophical self. J Hist Behav Sci 2000;36: 231–240.
41 Charcot JM: Leçons du Mardi à La Salpêtrière. Policliniques 1887–1888. Paris, Aux Bureaux du Progrès Médical, 1888.
42 Signoret JL: 'Une leçon clinique à La Salpêtrière' (1887) par André Brouillet. Rev Neurol (Paris) 1983;139:687–701.

43 Couchet JL: Janet à La Salpêtrière. L'Evolution Psychiatrique 1950;15:357–364.
44 Allilaire JF: Pierre Janet et La Salpêtrière. Ann Med Psychol (Paris) 2008;166:185–190.
45 Janet P: Contribution à l'étude des accidents mentaux chez les hystériques. Thèse No. 432. Paris, Rueff, 1893.
46 Janet P: Etat mental des hystériques, les stigmates mentaux. Paris, Bibliothèque Charcot-Debove, Rueff, 1893.
47 Janet P: J.-M. Charcot, son oeuvre psychologique. Rev Philos Fr étran 1895;39: 569–604.
48 Minkowski E: Pierre Janet, essai sur l'homme et l'œuvre; in: Centenaire de Théodule Ribot. Jubilé de la Psychologie scientifique française. Agen, Imprimerie Moderne, 1939.
49 Janet P: Quelques définitions récentes de l'hystérie. Arch Neurol 1893;25:417–438.
50 Postel J, Quetel C: La psychasthénie et Pierre Janet. Pierre Janet, un philosophe à la Salpêtrière in Nouvelle histoire de la psychiatrie. Paris, Dunod, 2009.
51 Janet P: L'automatisme psychologique. Paris, Alcan, 1889.
52 Charcot JM: Œuvres complètes. Paris, Bureaux du Progrès Médical, 1886–1894, vol 3.
53 Blocq PO: L'état mental des hystériques. Gazette des Hôpitaux Civils et Militaires 1893;66:1273–1280.
54 Berrios GE: The History of Mental Symptoms: Descriptive Psychopathology since the Nineteenth Century. Cambridge, Cambridge University Press, 1996.
55 Riser MM: Pratique neurologique. Paris, Masson, 1952.
56 Ellenberger HF: The Discovery of the Unconscious. New York, Penguin Press, 1970.
57 Mueller FL: Histoire de la psychologie. Paris, Payot, 1960.
58 Féré Ch: Sensation et Mouvement. Paris, Alcan, 1887.
59 Naccache L: Le nouvel inconscient: Freud, le Christophe Colomb des neurosciences. Paris, Odile Jacob, 2009.
60 Babinski J: Quelques remarques sur l'article de M. Sollier, la définition et la nature de l'hystérie. Archives Générales de Médecine 1907;198:271–283.
61 Société de Neurologie présidée par M. Klippel: discussion sur l'hystérie, Séance du 14 mai 1908. Rev Neurol (Paris) 1908;16:375–404/494–519.
62 Sollier P: La définition et la nature de l'hystérie. Archives Générales de Médecine 1906;197:2585–2600.
63 Dossier Sollier: Paris, Archives à la Bibliothèque de l'Académie de Médecine, 1912.

Olivier Walusinski, MD
Family physician, Private practice
20 rue de Chartres
FR–28160 Brou (France)
E-Mail walusinski@baillement.com

Bogousslavsky J (ed): Hysteria: The Rise of an Enigma. Front Neurol Neurosci. Basel, Karger, 2014, vol 35, pp 139–148
DOI: 10.1159/000360058

Criticism of Pithiatism: Eulogy of Babinski

Jacques Poirier • Christian Derouesné

Faculté de Médecine Pitié-Salpêtrière, L'Hôpital de la Salpêtrière, Paris, France

Abstract

Babinski, 'Chef de Clinique' of Charcot from 1885 to 1887, fully supported the ideas of his teacher on hysteria and thought that a dynamic brain cortical lesion is the cause of the disease. After Charcot's death in 1893, Babinski gradually revised his position. In a first step, he described many neurological signs in order to clearly distinguish hysterical manifestations from the organic disorders of the central nervous system. The most famous one bears his name, the Babinski sign, an inversion of the plantar cutaneous reflex, testifying to a lesion of the pyramidal tract. In a second step, he defined what remained of hysteria and proposed in 1901 to abandon the term 'hysteria' in favor of the neologism 'pithiatism', defined as a pathologic state resulting in disorders which can be very accurately reproduced by suggestion, and can disappear by persuasion. Babinski therefore retained the exclusive etiological role of suggestion and refuted, unlike Dejerine, the role of emotion. He also sought to separate pithiatism from simulation, but ambiguously he made pithiatics 'semi-malingerers'. During the Great War, with Froment, he described physiopathic disorders and separated them from pithiatic disorders and simulation. After being accepted by many French neurologists, pithiatism, the word as well as the concept, gently died out. There remained little more than a few philosophical uses (especially by Jean-Paul Sartre and Maurice Merleau-Ponty) or metaphorical ones. What remains of the work of Babinski in the field of hysteria is not so much the creation of pithiatism as the masterly description of neurological signs to formally exclude an organic lesion of the nervous system or simulation before looking like hysteria disorders.

Certain affections have
an unfortunate destiny. [1]

Joseph Babinski's (1857–1932; fig. 1) major contribution to hysteria is not the concept of 'pithiatism', which did not last long, but to clear out the old hysteria of organic disorders, simulation, and physiopathic disorders, which currently remains valid. Pithiatism can thus be considered as a side effect of the dismembering of Charcot's hysteria [2–4].

The Dismembering of Hysteria and the Creation of Pithiatism

Babinski himself described the two-step process by which he developed pithiatism [5].

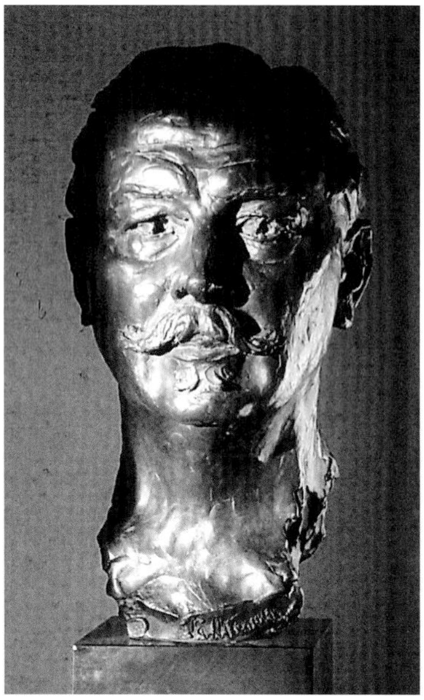

Fig. 1. Joseph Babinski's bust. Courtesy of Bernard Ferval, Dr. Henri Parinaud's grandson.

First Step

In a first step, Babinski's main aim, which began before his definition of pithiatism, was to establish a clear distinction between hysterical phenomena and organic disorders [5, 6].

In 1896, he described the 'toe phenomenon', which was later termed the 'Babinski sign'. When the plantar foot is pin-pricked in a hemiplegic patient, the big toe on the paralyzed side, instead of going to ventral flexion (as normal), performs a dorsal flexion, indicating an organic lesion of the pyramidal system. In 1903, Babinski described two varieties of the toe abduction sign, as a complement to the toe sign.

In 1897, he described three other signs: hypotonia of the members on the affected side in organic hemiplegia, the trunk-thigh test (the patient lying supine in his bed is asked to sit up holding his arms crossed across the chest; if an organic hemiparesis is present, the hip flexes and there is an involuntary elevation of the leg on the affected side), and the platysma sign (during resistance to flexion of the chin against the chest, the platysma on the normal side contracts, whereas it does not on the affected side).

In 1900, in *Diagnostic différentiel de l'hémiplégie organique et de l'hémiplégie hystérique* Babinski summarized the semiology and claimed once more that hysteria never modifies tendinous reflexes, nor cutaneous, pharyngeal and pupillar reflexes. He also affirmed the absence of clonus, amyotrophy, and sphincterian troubles in hysteria.

In 1907, Babinski described the pronation sign. In an organic hemiplegia, the hand of the affected side is generally in pronation; if, by a passive movement the examiner places it in supination and leaves it in this position, it will return to pronation, demonstrating the organic nature of the hemiplegia. In 1912, once more, in his four lessons on reflexes, Babinski claimed the normality of the reflexes in hysteria. Thus, the diagnosis of hysteria became primarily a diagnosis of exclusion. In the obituary he wrote for Babinski, the famous American physiologist John Farquhar Fulton (1899–1960) recognized the paramount importance of this first step: 'Perhaps his most important contribution lays in establishing satisfactory criteria for differentiating hysterical manifestations from those caused by organic lesions of the nervous system' [7].

Second Step

As senior resident of Jean-Martin Charcot (1825–1893), Babinski entirely supported Charcot's ideas on hysteria, and published many contributive papers. However, he progressively departed from Charcot's ideas, and, in a 1909 paper, he made clear that they were to be challenged, despite his admiration for his teacher [8].

> Beginning my neurological career at the Salpêtrière School where I had the honor to be senior resident of Charcot from 1885 to 1887, I was at first imbued with the ideas on hysteria that were taught there at that time, and which were, until recently, almost unanimously accepted. I first agreed with these ideas without reservation, but later, struck by some findings that I considered difficult

to conciliate, I gradually began to doubt their accuracy and decided that henceforth, I would monitor the exactitude of all facts with a rigorous analysis, without any preconceived opinion. If the results of my research resulted in departing from the doctrine of my famed Master, I do maintain my feelings of deep admiration for the great neurologist, who, despite some errors has provided important insights on hysteria, which moreover constituted a small part of his impressive work.

In a second step, Babinski divided the hysterical symptoms into two distinct groups [8–10]. The first group [seizures, paralysis, contractures, tremor, choreic movements, disorders of speech, breathing, sensitivity (anesthesia, hyperesthesia), and sensory disturbances] was characterized by the possibility to be reproduced by suggestion and disappear 'under the influence of persuasion or counter suggestion alone'. The second group included disorders that cannot be reproduced by suggestion and disappeared by countersuggestion, such as dermographism and overstated emotive reactions. These phenomena might be observed in healthy subjects and therefore cannot be considered hysterical.

Babinski proposed in 1901 to abandon the term 'hysteria' in favor of the neologism 'pithiatism', 'from *peitho* persuasion and *iatos* curable, that is to be cured by persuasion'. He defined hysteria-pithiatism as 'a pathologic state resulting in disorders which can be very accurately reproduced by suggestion in some subjects, and can disappear by persuasion (or counter suggestion) alone' [9].

The main consequence of these ideas was the quite complete disappearance of hysteria from hospital departments, recognized by Babinski [10], Philippe Chaslin (1857–1923), Édouard Brissaud [11], and many other physicians, such as Alfred Binet (1857–1911) and Théodore Simon (1872–1961), who wrote in 1909 [12]:

Since Babinski and his pupils only consider these seizures as the result of vulgar suggestion and unimportant phenomena, seizure frequency remarkably decreased, and they were no more observed in some departments.

Professor Anatole Chauffard (1855–1932) in 1912 also remarked [13]:

By a remarkable change, hysteria nearly disappeared in our departments in women as well as in men. Personally, I believe that I have no more observed a serious case of hysteria for more than 10 years in my wards. The explanation is that our ideas have been deeply modified since Charcot, on account, in a major part, of the objective criticism of hysteria by M. Babinski.

Finally, Doctor Noir commented in 1932 [14]:

...seizures of major hysteria, so frequent in the past, have totally disappeared. [...] Doctor Babinski played a major role in this kind of mental health sanitation....

The Role of Suggestion and Emotion

In a lesson at Salpêtrière, given at Charcot's invitation, on June 25, 1891 [15], Babinski pointed out the crucial role of suggestion in hysteria as well as in hypnotism: 'exaltation of suggestibility may constitute, from a psychological point of view, the most distinctive feature of hysteria'. For Babinski, suggestion by the physician or by the patient himself (autosuggestion) was indeed the crucial factor of hysterical disorders, which can be cured by persuasion (countersuggestion). Later, Babinski, on many occasions – being obsessive – drew a core distinction between suggestion (innuendos) and persuasion (reasonable statements). Nevertheless, if the role of suggestion, particularly under the influence of physicians, was clearly highlighted by Babinski, the mechanisms of autosuggestion, on the contrary, remained vague and ill-defined. However, in 1912, he wrote [16]:

In hysteric, suggestion is only being active when it is of interest for her, and would appear to some extent like necessary by circumstances... . Similarly, hysteric grasp a pathologic idea which becomes effective when the idea is of special interest for her; it focuses her attention, and is imposed by her feelings, arousing abnormal desire to amaze and attract attention, lastly infinitely diverse motives which may engage the easy to be influenced will of these subjects.

However, be careful! Babinski was not alone and not the first to highlight the role of suggestion in hysteria. Hippolyte Bernheim (1840–1919) and the Nancy school, for several years, had stated that hysterics were highly suggestible and that medical suggestion, conscious or unconscious, played a major role in initiating their manifestations. However, unlike Babinski, they thought that suggestibility was a common fact not reserved to hysterics [17]. Charcot himself, particularly in *Faith Healing*, emphasized the role of suggestion and even autosuggestion in hysteria: 'Hysterics present a mental state highly favourable to develop faith healing, because they are highly prone to suggestion from environment or mainly from themselves by autosuggestion' [18].

Nevertheless, Jean Lhermitte's claim (1857–1959) that 'all the doctrine of pithiatism is displayed in every part by Charcot' is highly questionable. However, he recognized that 'contrary to Babinski, Charcot did not agree with suggestion being the only basis of all hysteric disorders' [19]. Indeed, Binet and Simon [12] stated that Charcot's involvement should be kept in perspective:

> In the last years of his life, Charcot progressively changed his ideas about the mechanism of some hysterical symptoms. [...] Charcot thought that the hypothesis of suggestion, or more likely auto-suggestion... was valid. Anyway, since that time, Charcot, by himself or under the influence of his pupils, had thought that the practice of suggestion should be reinvigorated in his department. It was the opposite view of his previous teaching, but he did not notice it. The masters of science are like princes, surrounded by skilful courtiers, who make true what is convenient for them. When the credit of a discovery is repetitively attributed to someone, he will end up being persuaded by it. Aging Charcot might imagine that he had, by himself, the idea of considering hysteria as a mental disease.

The role of emotion in the genesis of hysteria was highlighted by Bernheim and mainly by Jules Dejerine (1849–1917), who considered it the core factor. In contrast, Babinski disproved it, arguing that no hysterical disorders were observed in acute emotions such as among the survivors immediately after the Messina earthquake or in mothers after the death of a child (investigated by morgue staff) [16].

The Reception of Pithiatism

The 1908 Meeting

In 1908, a special meeting of the Société de Neurologie de Paris [20] was devoted to the definition of hysteria. The definition given by Babinski in 1901 was used as the basis for discussion. The consensus was that a number of clinical manifestations might be created and cured by suggestion. However, disagreements persisted among the participants. Some were reluctant to admit that hysterical stigmas were the result of medical suggestion or autosuggestion. Others, faithful to Charcot's ideas, such as Fulgence Raymond (1844–1910), Albert Pitres (1848–1928), and Jules Dejerine (1849–1917) maintained that hysteria could be associated with reflex, trophic, or vasomotor disorders. Babinski replied by demonstrating that such cases were due to diagnostic errors or simulation. A controversy also emerged over the significance of the term 'suggestion'. Dejerine claimed that suggestion involved the acceptance of any idea, true or false, and that Babinski's definition made the notion of hysteria too broad. Some participants stressed the role of imitation. But the main disagreement between Babinski and many participants was about the role of emotions in the occurrence of hysterical symptoms and the question of mental changes in hysterics. Babinski replied that hysteria was defined only by a natural ability to present hysterical symptoms. Raymond and Pitres considered pithiatism as a syndrome that could be observed not only in hysteria, but also in other disorders, and thus it could not replace hysteria as a basic diagnostic definition.

Brissaud adopted Babinski's approach and acknowledged pithiatism. However, he pointed out that some neurologists did not agree to reduce hysteria to pithiatism. Henri Cesbron, on the contrary, became enthusiastic and wrote in 1909: 'No doubt that pithiatism will very soon overthrow hysteria, abolishing a history of mistakes so long covered by its name' [21].

Many authors nevertheless found pithiatism too simplistic, and felt it could not be discussed in 'good' or 'bad' terms, like Babinski's Manichean thought. Binet and Simon expressed a perfect formulation of this point of view in 1909–1910:

> We think that, in clinical practice, which requires specific and basic facts, Babinski's rather clear approach is sufficient, with its many greatest physiological analyses; Yet it would be necessary for psychiatry, as well as for psychology, to take more into account the mental state of hysterics [12].
>
> Babinski's definition, which reduces hysteria to suggestibility, is very clear and easy to apply in clinical practice; however, in our opinion, it is far too simple, because phenomena other than hysteria occur by suggestion. Another shortcoming of this simplistic idea is that hysteria and simulation may be confused; are there not some authors, inspired by Babinski's ideas, who are led to consider that hysteria does not differ from simulation? [22].

Others were aloof or distant. In *Practical Neurology* [23] edited in 1911 by Pierre Marie (1853–1940), Gustave Roussy (1874–1948) made a very brief reference to Babinski's pithiatism. Jules Dejerine, in his famous *Semiology of the Nervous System* [24], described the Babinski signs made up to distinguish organic hemiplegia from hysteric hemiplegia, but the term pithiatism was not quoted. On the other hand, foreign neurologists endorsed the Babinski signs, but remained aloof with regard to pithiatism, which clearly appeared as a quintessentially French matter: 'This new term, although more thoughtful than the previous words used to describe hysteria, never gained acceptance in the medical community' [25].

Babinski, Janet, and Freud

The relationship between Sigmund Freud (1856–1939) and Babinski was not very warm. During his stay at Salpêtrière, in a letter to his fiancée, Martha Bernays, Freud called Babinski a novice. Later, he did not include Babinski's foreword in his translation of Charcot's *Leçons du mardi* into German, although he termed Babinski 'Charcot's favorite pupil'. Babinski never wrote about his relationship with Freud. He did not even refer to Freud's study, performed at Charcot's instigation and published in French, on the clinical distinction between hysterical and organic paralyses, though it was one of his main topics. Moreover, many times he proclaimed 'the absurdity of Freudism which requires every day, for many months, the exhumation, not without moral peril, of alleged repressed erotic dreams' [26].

Pierre Janet (1859–1947) joined Charcot's department in 1889. In 1894, he commented favorably on Babinski's work on the distinction between organic and hysterical paralyses and contractures in his book *L'état mental des hystériques*. Janet did not attend the debate on the definition of hysteria at the Société de Neurologie de Paris in 1908. However, a year later, at the debate on the role of emotion in neurological diseases [27], he questioned Babinski's opinion on the absence of hysterical phenomena during acute emotions, arguing that they can occur secondarily (which, by the way, actually supports Babinski's ideas). He criticized the importance of suggestion, maintaining that ideas alone were not sufficient to provoke hysterical symptoms, and highlighted the role of the psychological structure in hysteria. Babinski replied that all ideas, even the most abstract ones, have some affective elements, but that he did not find a specific mental state in subjects with pithiatism.

Babinski's mistrust in psychology, as shown by his opposition to Janet (and his subconscious), as well as to Freud (and his description of the unconscious) could be related to Babinski's personality, who always needed to be in control.

Pithiatism Tested by World War I

Babinski was led by the war pathology [28] to reconsider his position about the relationships between hysteria and reflex and vasomotor disorders, as well as between pithiatism and simulation.

The Reflex Disorders
During World War I, Babinski, with Jules Froment (1878–1946) [29], observed many cases of soldiers, who, after a minor injury, developed clinical manifestations which suggested the diagnosis of hysteria. However, they noticed a series of signs which allowed them to rule out the diagnosis of hysteria or simulation: paralysis, contractures and hyperreflectivity which persisted under general anesthesia (like muscular atrophy), important vasomotor and trophic changes in the skin, and frequent fibrotendinous or muscular retractions. Babinski and Froment called these phenomena physiopathic and considered them to be organic disorders involving sympathetic nervous system reflexes. Thus, the description of these physiopathic or reflex disorders as being different from hysteria and simulation once more restricted the field of hysteria.

Pithiatism and Simulation
The relationship between hysteria-pithiatism and simulation was discussed in a special meeting of the Parisian Society of Neurology with representatives of the Neurological Army Centers in 1916. Babinski, on several occasions, attested that hysteria should be distinguished from simulation. However, he wrote that some hysterical disorders cannot be differentiated from simulation on clinical grounds. Brissaud also stated that 'hysteria cannot be differentiated from simulation'. Babinski's statements had been the source of many ambiguities and his concept of semisimulation was far from clear: 'In all kinds of circumstances, a hysteric behaves as if he partly controls the disorder and he is not quite sincere. Therefore, hysteria approaches simulation, and I used to say that a hysteric is a sort of semi-malingerer.' Furthermore, he says about hypnotism: 'In many ways, a hypnotic person behaves like an actor and the hypothesis that hypnosis is a farce is not absurd' [30].

Babinski's ideas were widespread in the military and were later accused of being the basis of overususing chloroform anesthesia to distinguish simulation from pithiatism, and of torture practices such as forced methods of contention (paraffin baths at 70°) or electric 'torpillage' [according to Clovis Vincent (1879–1947), a pupil of Babinski], so that soldiers (the 'poilus') would rather go back to the front rather than suffer these practices [31].

The refusal of psychological theories, the repeated claims that hysterics are semi- malingerers, and that hysteria cannot be differentiated from simulation led some of Babinski's followers, such as Boisseau [32] or Rouquier [33], to cross the threshold and confuse hysteria and simulation.

A Major Challenge
During World War I, returning wounded soldiers to the front became crucial, and the differentiation of physiopathic disorders and simulation constituted an important issue with major medical-military consequences. Indeed, treatment and military decisions were completely distinct in the cases of pithiatism, organic disorders, physiopathic disorders, and simulation (which could lead soldiers to be executed).

The War Ends, Faradization Remains
After the war, Babinski continued to use faradization, but (as was his practice) in a watered down version aimed, according to Charcot's idea, to

'wake up the representation'. Auguste Tournay (1878–1969) reported on one of Babinski's consultations [34]:

A good man sought medical advice for his wife who had become mute. She brought her slate and wrote with a piece of chalk what she could not express by pantomime. After a brief examination of the couple, the decision was, according to the definition of pithiatism, that the disorder could be cured by persuasion. An additional small faradic battery was used by a student who loosened its link when Babinski had to pursue the patient when she stepped back. Therefore one or the other cable was disconnected and had to be connected again. If verbal persuasion did not stop, the small torpedoing was discontinuous. Nonetheless the first sounds got out of her larynx. Then, suddenly, as if a block was removed, the woman spoke and spoke, while her husband, now, by contrast, was holed up in silence, and expressed by his mimic the shock at the prospect to come back home with a continuous flow of speech.

Pithiatism: A Better or Worse Future

Pithiatism and Surrealists

In 1928, in the *Surrealist Revolution*, Aragon and Breton celebrated the 50th anniversary of hysteria and proposed a new definition of hysteria which was nothing less than revolutionary: 'under the deplorable guise of pithiatism, hysteria tends to regain its rightful place.... Hysteria is not a pathological phenomenon and may be considered, in all respects, as an ultimate means of expression' [35].

Pithiatism and Philosophers

In his monumental biography of Gustave Flaubert (1821–1880) [36], Jean-Paul Sartre (1905–1980) pointed out his extreme proneness to autosuggestion, labeled pithiatic. This was a term that was mocked by Marthe Robert [37] who wrote: 'the old notion of pithiatism, discarded for a long time on account of the theorical emptiness of the idea of suggestion'.

The concept of pithiatism held the attention of Maurice Merleau-Ponty (1908–1961) [38] to the extent that he leads the eye towards an interpretation of hysteria that escapes 'the alternative of paralysis and simulation':

'It is generally known how, by the notion of pithiatism, the theory of hysteria has been carried out beyond the dilemma of paralysis (or of anaesthesia) and simulation. If the hysterical patient is a deceiver, it is first and foremost himself that he deceives, so that it is impossible to separate what he *really* feels or thinks and what he overtly expresses: pithiatism is a disease of the *Cogito*, consciousness which has become ambivalent and not a deliberate refusal to declare what ones knows.'

In the phenomenological tradition, which identifies being and consciousness (intended as intentional consciousness: the object does not face consciousness, but it is embedded in it and constituted by it; therefore, the object is never separable from the consciousness by which it is not caught, but produced), the *cogito*, or the *ego* – coincidence of the consciousness and the self – is the process by which all at once the subject becomes itself and is aware of itself. Merleau-Ponty implements the conceptual resources of this school to deepen the analysis of pithiatism: hysterical consciousness, in its constituent cogito, can be considered as sick of its inability to appropriate in the same unit the proper consciousness of what it is, and the being itself it is, which is constituted precisely of this consciousness. Here is a new concept of being that reflects the specific type of hysterical being, which is not divided into a real body and a simulated body, but is the being constituted of consciousness itself, and sick of this ambivalence that constitutes its being. Internal and external no longer have to be opposite; we can no longer talk of deception, even if hysterical symptoms have no organic reality.

The Fate of Pithiatism

Babinski was breaking with the tradition to name hysteria according to hypothetical anatomical origin (uterus, brain, psyche). For the first time, pithiatism pointed out the treatment of hysteria (persuasion). However, Babinski did not give much importance to the name ('it is a point of terminology without great interest and I will not focus on it') [5]. On this point, he was very clear: 'I will use both terms, hysteria and pithiatism, as synonymous, giving time to decide, which is as a matter of fact of secondary importance, if both terms will remain or only one of them' [8].

'The name caught on' wrote Antoine Porot in 1960 [39]. However, the popularity was very relative, and in fact and only in France! Although accepted in Scrabble, in most dictionaries, even medical ones, pithiatism is not mentioned or only with a brief definition – more or less accurate – and then labeled old, outdated, and rarely used in current practice.

Babinski's work on hysteria impressed neurologists; however, only a few of them, like Riser [40], openly acknowledged their debt to him. The diagnosis of hysteric conversion is still based, in the common neurological practice, on the exclusion of organic signs. However, some authors advocated the return to Charcot's ideas [41] with regard to tendon reflexes and vasomotor disorders, the role of emotion, and hereditary predisposition, or to the physiologic theory, like Sollier who attempted to discover the anatomofunctional bases of hysteria [42].

In many works on hysteria, Babinski's name is mentioned in reference to pithiatism, but very often with a lack of knowledge of his work [43–45]. Conversely, some authors replicate his ideas without naming him [46]. In neurological handbooks, the amount of chapters devoted to hysteria or hysteric disorders varies widely. If a specific chapter on hysteria is included in some books [47, 48], Babinski's name usually does not appear. After the end of World War I, pithiatism only appeared in some doctoral theses of medicine, and in some twenty papers published between 1917 and 1988, and – of course – only by French-speaking authors. The hysteria-pithiatism debate was ruled out in English-speaking countries, and later internationally by the publication of DSM-III (1980), DSM-IV, and DSM-5 by the American Psychiatric Association and the ICD-10 (1993) by the World Health Organization.

On the other hand, the metaphoric survival of the name 'pithiatism' is ensured by shifts in meaning, but it remains relatively less frequent than the names 'sinistrosis' or 'hysteria'. In papers, the term 'collective hysteria' is more often used than 'collective pithiatism' by journalists. However, some metaphoric uses, more or less understandable, of the name pithiatism are found as isolated islets.

Conclusion

Reducing Babinski's work to the creation of pithiatism to take the place of hysteria would be a big mistake. Babinski's contribution was not theoretical, but rather clinical and semiological, made of the many signs he described to differentiate organic disorders from functional pathology, hysteria-pithiatism. This semiology was definitely part of neurology and still remains the core axis of Babinski's work. If pithiatism did not last long, the fact remains that, in front of suspected neurological symptoms, the diagnosis of hysteria – whatever its past, current, or future names – is always based on the exclusion of organic neurological disorders according to the semiology elaborated by Babinski.

Finally, Babinski allowed hysteria – through his semiology – to discard what it did not belong to it (organic disorders, simulation or malingering, and physiopathic disorders). What remained – the positive definition called pithiatism – had minor importance, and the name, which became synonymous with hysteria, had little relevance. In this point, and only here, Babinski appeared as too reductive and too simplistic, disclosing, under the great semiologist, the obsessive, peremptory, Manichean man, obsessed by the separation between good and evil, by separating the wheat from the chaff. Don't mix up men and words.

Hysteria has disappeared from psychiatric classifications, but Charcot survives. It remains to be seen whether history will not bring back the past, with scholars in modern cognitive neurosciences trying to find out, with functional brain imagery, data to support similarity between hypnotism and hysteria, or if Charcot's concept of a dynamic lesion may be too hastily buried [52].

And pithiatism passed away, but Babinski survives. However, who will survive after the disappearance of conversion disorders, somatoform, dissociative or somatic symptoms disorders – hysterics or pithiatics?

Acknowledgments

We are greatly indebted to Jean-Louis Poirier, Professor of Philosophy, for the analysis of Merleau-Ponty's statements, and to Aline Poirier, English teacher, for her revision of the English language.

References

1 Léri A: Commotions and émotions de guerre. Paris, Masson, 1918.
2 Philippon J, Poirier J: Joseph Babinski: A Biography. New York, Oxford University Press, 2010.
3 Poirier J, Philippon J: Renewing the fire: Joseph Babinski; In Bogousslavsky J (ed): Following Charcot: A Forgotten History of Neurology and Psychiatry. Front Neurol Neurosc. Basel, Karger, 2011, vol 29, pp 91–104.
4 Derouesné C: Joseph Babinski et l'hystérie: une œuvre méjugée. Rev Neurol (Paris) FMC, 2009, pp F221–F237.
5 Babinski J: Exposé des travaux scientifiques. Paris, Masson, 1913.
6 Babinski J: Œuvre scientifique. Recueil des principaux travaux, publié par les soins de Barré JA, Chaillous J, Charpentier A, et al. Paris, Masson, 1934.
7 Fulton JF: Science in the clinic ad exemplified by the life and work of Joseph Babinski. J Nerv Ment Dis 1933;77:121–133.
8 Babinski J: Démembrement de l'hystérie traditionnelle. Pithiatisme. La Semaine médicale 1909;29:3–8.
9 Babinski J: Définition de l'hystérie. Rev Neurol (Paris) 1901;IX:1074–1080.
10 Babinski J: Ma conception de l'hystérie et de l'hypnotisme (Pithiatisme), Conférence faite à la Société de l'Internat des hôpitaux de Paris, séance du 28 juin 1906. Chartres, Imprimerie Durand, 1906.
11 Poirier J: Édouard Brissaud (1852–1909), un neurologue d'exception dans une famille d'artistes. Paris, Hermann, 2010.
12 Binet A, Simon T: Hystérie. L'année psychologique 1909;16:67–122.
13 Chauffard: La Presse médicale, 17 janvier 1912, quoted by Léon Daudet. Le stupide dix-neuvième siècle. Paris, Nouvelle Librairie Nationale, 1922, pp 272–274.
14 Noir J: Souvenirs évoqués par la mort de deux maîtres: Chauffard et Babinski. Concours Médical 1932;52:3733–3734.
15 Babinski J: Hypnotisme et hystérie. Du rôle de l'hypnotisme en thérapeutique. Gazette Hebdomadaire de Médecine et de Chirurgie 1891;30:350–356, 1891;31: 365–372.
16 Babinski J, Dagnan-Bouveret J: Emotion et hystérie. Journal de Psychologie normale et pathologique 1912:97–146.
17 Bernheim H: Hypnotisme, suggestion, psychothérapie. Études nouvelles. Paris, Octave Doin, 1891.
18 Charcot J-M: La foi qui guérit. La Revue Hebdomadaire 1892;VII:112–132.
19 Lhermitte J: L'école de la Salpêtrière. J.M. Charcot, psycho-physiologiste. L'Encéphale 1950;4:297–310.
20 Société de neurologie de Paris. Discussion sur l'hystérie. Rev Neurol (Paris) 1908;16:375–404, 494–519.
21 Cesbron H: Histoire critique de l'hystérie. Paris, Asselin & Houzeau, 1909.
22 Binet A, Simon T: Réponses à quelques critiques. L'année psychologique 1910; 17:270–277.
23 Marie P (ed): La pratique neurologique. Paris, Masson, 1911.
24 Dejerine J: Sémiologie des affections du système nerveux, ed 2. Paris, Masson, 1914.
25 Okun MS, Koehler P: Babinski's clinical differentiation of organic paralysis from hysterical paralysis. Effects on US Neurology. Arch Neurol 2004;61:778–783.
26 Charpentier A: Babinski (Joseph) (1857–1932), in Dr M. Genty, 'Les biographies médicales', T.VI. Paris, Librairie J.B. Baillière et fils, 1937–1939, pp 17–32.
27 Société de neurologie. Du rôle de l'émotion dans la genèse des accidents névropathiques et psychopathiques. L'émotion et l'hystérie. Rev Neurol (Paris) 1909;18:1591–1601.
28 Tatu L, Bogousslavsky J: La folie au front. La grande bataille des névroses de guerre (1914–1918). Paris, Imago, 2012.
29 Babinski J, Froment J: Hystérie-pithiatisme et troubles nerveux d'ordre réflexe en neurologie de guerre, ed 1. Paris, Masson et Cie, 1917.
30 Babinski J: De l'hypnotisme en thérapeutique et en médecine légale. Paris, Imprimerie de la Semaine Médicale, 1910.
31 Darmon P: Des suppliciés oubliés de la Grande Guerre: les pithiatiques. Histoire, Economie et Société 2001;20:49–64.
32 Boisseau J: Hystérie et simulation. L'accident pithiatique n'est autre chose qu'un accident simulé. Annales Médico-Psychologiques 1949;107:121–167, 249–286.
33 Rouquier A: La fin de l'hystérie. Y a-t-il encore des hystériques ou de faux pithiatiques? LVIIIe Congrès de psychiatrie et de neurologie de langue française, Lille, 1960, pp 359–365.
34 Tournay A: Joseph Babinski (1857–1932). Médecine de France 1953;43: 3–10.

35 Breton A, Aragon L: Le cinquantenaire de l'hystérie (1878–1928). La Révolution Surréaliste 1928;11:20–22.
36 Sartre JP: L'idiot de la famille: Gustave Flaubert de 1821 à 1857. Paris, Gallimard, 1971–1972, 3 volumes.
37 Robert M: La traversée littéraire. Paris, Grasset, 1994.
38 Merleau-Ponty M: Phenomenology of Perception (1945). London, Routledge, 1962.
39 Porot A: Manuel alphabétique de psychiatrie clinique et thérapeutique, ed 2. Paris, Presses Universitaires de France, 1960.
40 Riser M: Hystérie et pithiatisme; in: Pratique neurologique. Paris, Masson, 1952, pp 1206–1226.
41 Guillain G: Il est injuste et erroné d'oublier l'œuvre de JM Charcot sur l'hystérie et les névroses. Semaine des Hôpitaux de Paris 1949;25:147–160.
42 Walusinski O, Bogousslavsky J: À la recherche du neuropsychiatre perdu: Paul Sollier (1861–1933). Rev Neurol (Paris) FMC, 2008, p F247.
43 Veith I: Four thousand years of hysteria; In Horowitz MJ: Hysterical Personality. New York, Aronson, 1977, pp 7–94.
44 Merskey H: The analysis of hysteria. London, Baillière Tindall, 1979.
45 Guelfi JD, Boyer P, Consoli S, Olivier-Martin R: Traité de psychiatrie. Paris, PUF, 1987.
46 Crimslik HL, Ron M: Conversion hysteria: history, diagnostic issues and clinical practice. Cogn Neuropsychiatry 1999;4:165–180.
47 Adams RD, Victor M: Principles of Neurology. New York, McGraw-Hill, 1977, pp 995–1001.
48 Le Pastier S, Derouesné C: Manifestations neurologiques d'origine psychiatrique; in Derouesné C: Pratique neurologique. Paris, Flammarion Médecine Sciences, 1982, pp 655–661.
49 Serratrice G, Autret A: Traité de neurologie. Paris, Ellipses, 1996.
50 Bogousslavsky J, Fisher M (eds): Textbook of Neurology. Boston, Butterworth-Heinemann, 1998.
51 Goetz CG: Textbook of Clinical Neurology. Philadelphia, Saunders, 2003.
52 Bogousslavsky J: Hysteria after Charcot: back to the future. Front Neurol Neurosci 2011;29:137–161.

Jacques Poirier, MD, PhD
40 rue d'Alleray
FR–75015 Paris (France)
E-Mail poirierpaulin@aol.com

Bogousslavsky J (ed): Hysteria: The Rise of an Enigma. Front Neurol Neurosci. Basel, Karger, 2014, vol 35, pp 149–156
DOI: 10.1159/000360055

The Borderland with Neurasthenia ('Functional Syndromes')

Maurizio Paciaroni[a] · Julien Bogousslavsky[b]

[a]Stroke Unit, Division of Internal and Cardiovascular Medicine, Santa Maria della Misericordia, Hospital University of Perugia, Perugia, Italy; [b]Center for Brain and Nervous System Diseases, GSMN Neurocenter, Clinique Valmont, Glion/Montreux, Switzerland

Abstract

At the end of the 19th century, neurasthenia and hysteria were considered distinct diseases. Specifically, neurasthenia was regarded as a disease of the body, whereas hysteria was regarded as a disease of the psyche. However, immediately before World War I, due to their common characteristics, both hysteria and neurasthenia were thought to be 'functional diseases'. Moreover, it was suggested that heredity and the presence in both of the predisposing condition called 'nervous weakness' were other shared factors. Nervous weakness was considered essential for the definition of neurasthenia, but it was also considered a precondition for the development of hysteria. Because of this, it is still difficult to demarcate a line between neurasthenia and hysteria; therefore, the two diseases should be considered as sharing a common borderland with each other.

First described in 1869 by George Miller Beard, neurasthenia, at the turn of the 19th century received much attention in both the medical world and society. Beginning with its predecessors in antiquity and continuing with hypochondria, which became a fashionable disease in the 18th century, neurasthenia reached a high point in worldwide medical acceptance at the end of the 19th and the beginning of the 20th centuries [1]. Between 1910 and 1914, hysteria and neurasthenia were thought to be 'functional diseases', even though they had been considered distinct before this period. Specifically, neurasthenia was considered a disease of the soma, whereas hysteria was thought to be a disease of the psyche. This chapter presents the hypothesis that the two diseases share a common borderland.

History of Neurasthenia

The Mind-Body Relationship over Time

Two major interpretations of mental disorders have prevailed over the history of neuropsychiatry: (1) a psychosocial perspective, which emphasizes problems in personal history and surround-

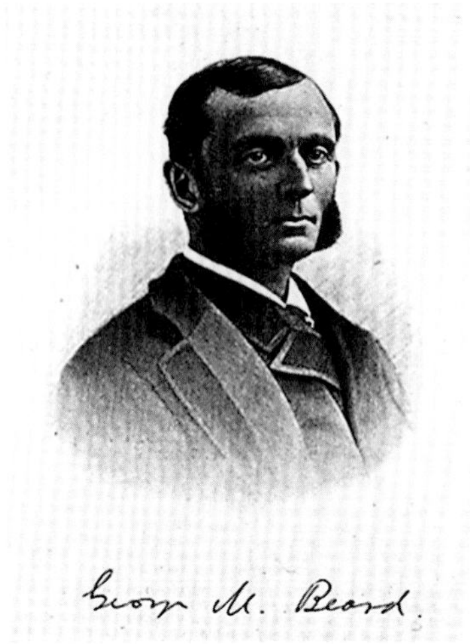

Fig. 1. George Miller Beard (1839–1883).

ings, and (2) a somatic, organic perspective, which emphasizes brain-biology, brain-chemistry, genetics, and heredity [2]. An interdependence between soma and psyche remained the foundation of medical theory and practice up until the 1830s. Afterwards, the body was elevated to the center of medicine, while the mind was subordinated [3]. This decisive turn was due in part to the invention of diagnostic instruments that enabled doctors to attain a better understanding of the body's functioning: the stethoscope, laryngoscope, bronchoscope, ophtalmoscope, endoscope, and the introduction of X-rays by Wilhelm Konrad Röntgen in 1895. Clinical medicine thus become more objective [3]. This together with advances in pathological anatomy, initiated by Bichat at the turn of the 19th century, led to the viewing of lesions of the organs, therein determining a radical improvement for all fields of medicine. This progress, however, continued to subjugate the role of the mind. The disparity between the body over the mind had become glaring by the late 19th century. Proof of this was that neurasthenia was essentially considered a physical malady without any of the stigma attached to mental illnesses [3].

Clinical Picture of Neurasthenia

Neurasthenia was introduced as a diagnostic category in North America in the middle of the 19th century by George Miller Beard (1839–1883; fig. 1). He coined the term and described the disease in the *Boston Medical and Surgical Journal*, the predecessor to the *New England Journal of Medicine* [4]. This definition rapidly spread across Europe and East Asia. Beard made his discovery while using a form of 'general electrization' he had learned from a lay practitioner. Specifically, by placing electrodes on the hands of the patient, Beard gave a mild electrical massage to all the muscles of the body and he repeated this process daily for weeks or months when necessary. He observed that two thirds of his patients recovered from a wide variety of complaints such as fatigue, dyspepsia, headache, and nervousness. He reasoned that these patients had suffered from a lack of nerve force which his treatment restored [5].

This condition was originally thought to be of a somatic entity, and it was Beard who first suggested that this condition was a physical, not a mental, illness. The symptom picture was extensive, with exhaustion as the main symptom [6]. The most prominent somatic symptoms were in fact listed as nervous exhaustion and fatigue, particularly constant tiredness and general aches and pains which might affect any or several bodily functions (circulation, digestion, sexual activity) [7]. Signs of autonomic nervous dysfunction included dilated pupils, sweaty hands, dry skin and mucous membranes, and generalized pruritus [8]. Attached to there were a set of 'psychic' symptoms which were perceived as further manifestations of this nervous weakness: inability to concentrate, particularly on mental labor, headache, insomnia, depression, excitability, irritability, and introspective and excessive emotion [9, 10]. Beard focused on several features of particular frequency, including a distinctive tenderness of the scalp, a heavy sensation over the top of the head, vague backache and spinal tenderness, tinnitus, and hypophonia [8].

In 1897, along with another physician named Gilbert Ballet (1853–1916), Achille Adrien Proust (1834–1903) co-authored *L'hygiène du neurasthénique,* a practical guide to the identification and treatment of neurasthenia, which soon after became the reference on the subject throughout Europe (fig. 2a, b). Proust scholars have often speculated that his own son Marcel, who often spent as many as six and half days a week in his bed (writing of course), was the model for many of the graphic descriptions of neurasthenia found in this work. In fact, Marcel was a recluse. In his later years, he spent much of his life in his famous cork-lined room, allegedly because of his asthma. Proust and Ballet described neurasthenia as being characterized by insomnia, dyspepsia associated with gastrointestinal atony, rachialgia, headache, general irritability, and 'weakness of nerve elements' [11].

Causes of Neurasthenia

George Beard was not the only one writing about neurasthenia in the 19th century, but he was the first to popularize it deliberately, not simply for a specialized scientific audience, but also for the general public [12]. Beard emphasized that 'neurasthenia is an American disease' and posited that the disease resulted from 'civilization'. He held that climate and race were inadequate explanations for causation, while long working hours with unremitting intellectual concentration and minimal rest led to this illness [8]. In fact, Beard propagated that the illness was due to a deficiency in nervous energy, often found in businessmen or others exposed to the competition, luxuries, and vices of modern society. Beard and other contemporary colleagues believed that neurasthenia was mostly a disease of brain workers and civilized races and that the 'American Negro never suffered from neurasthenia' [13]. The concept of neurasthenia affecting only upper-class whites held sway for at least two decades until the turn of the 20th century [14]. Beard also felt that it was more common among those with a more refined nervous system, including intellectuals and professionals [15], and among the economically successful rather than their counterparts. Also for Proust and Ballet, its 'predominance in towns, among the middle and upper classes, in a word, in all circumstances where intellectual culture or commercial and industrial traffic are carried to their highest degree of intensity', provided irrefutable evidence 'that over-pressure, and especially cerebral over-pressure, must figure in the front rank of causes of neurasthenia' [12]. Another cause of neurasthenia was thought to be anxiety associated with the use of technology. Beard argued that the steam engine, the telegraph, newspapers, and the sciences were essential etiological factors in the development of the disease. It was not the men putting up the telegraph poles or building the steam engines who were at risk, it was those using these inventions [14].

Women were, according to medical opinion of the time, constitutionally weaker and more prone to nervous problems than men. Therefore, the demands of their lives made them especially susceptible to headaches, poor indigestion, depression, and anxiety, which were the hallmarks of neurasthenia (nervous exhaustion). Also, because the reproductive systems of women made heavy demands on their bodies, they had a harder time replenishing their nervous energy than men did [16]. Moreover, even though the proportion of men fell to a low in 1891–1905, it had never been more than one third. In fact, this level increased up until 1911–1915, when a slight increase was recorded. The increase in neurasthenia for men during the war years could almost certainly be explained by the return of servicemen from the Western front [15].

In 1889, Jean-Martin Charcot (1825–1893) later declared that neurasthenia was no longer a disease of the upper classes [17]. By 1906, in a reworking of the original theories, the working class were now seen as the main victims of the disease [14]. With his extensive experience in dealing with railway workers and the physical and emotional stress implicit to the new industry, Charcot found numerous cases of unexplained neurologic deficits that best fit with the characteristics of neurasthenia [8]: 'It is one of the nervous affections that develop most frequently as a consequence of shock, particularly in railroad accidents' [18]. Also in England, as described in the textbooks at the Queen Square Library in London, there is further evidence that physicians at the time considered neurasthenia to afflict all classes in modern society. Thomas Saville [19] wrote in his *Clinical Lectures on Neurasthenia* (1899) on the frequency of the diagnosis among the poor and inmates at the Paddington workhouse. He made some epidemiological observations on the disease, comparing rates in these settings with those he encountered in his private practice, concluding that there was no specific social class trend [15].

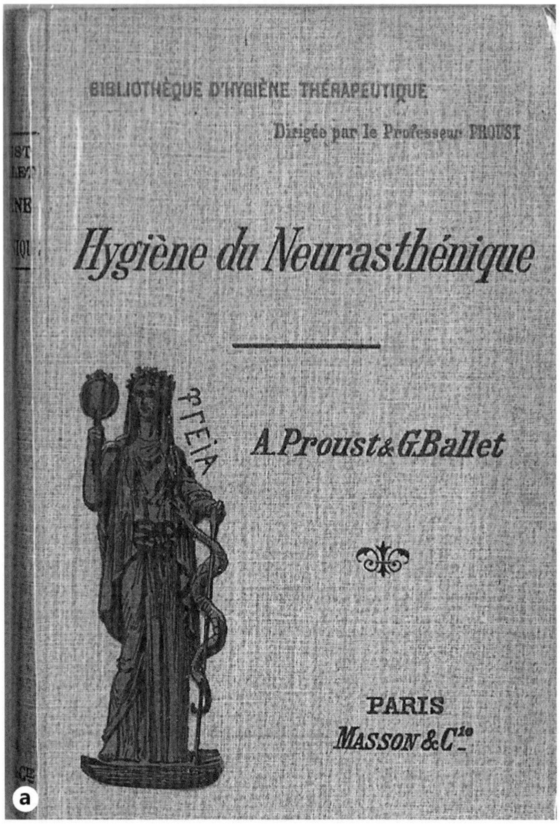

Fig. 2. a *L'hygiène du neurasthénique*, by Proust and Ballet (courtesy of Prof. Julien Bogousslavsky).

The Decline of Neurasthenia

Several researchers have mapped the shift of neurasthenia from a neurological entity in the 19th century to a psychological one in the 20th century. In fact, the diagnosis of the disease did not survive into the modern era of neurologic nosology, largely because stress-related syndromes became relegated to psychiatry. In fact, after the increasing emphasis on the body over the mind in the 19th century which argued that mental disorders were actually diseases of the brain, Daniel Hack Tuke (1827–1895) described many cases where fear, anxiety, or disappointed ambition had precipitated physical reactions [3]. For example, he described an 8-year-old girl who, on being separated from her mother, exhibited delirium, headaches, and an inability to stand; resistant to every form of treatment, the girl recovered as soon as she was reunited with her mother. He called this phenomenon 'psychophysical phenomena', therein introducing this concept into modern-era psychiatry, which would subsequently be further elaborated by both Charcot and Freud. In fact, the abrupt fall in prevalence of neurasthenia in 1930 coincides with the reappearance of neurosis which changed in 1932 into the bigger and enduring category of psychoneurosis [15]. In fact, some case histories demonstrate that those with a diagnosis of neurosis in the 1930s had a symptom cluster that had been diagnosed earlier as neurasthenia.

Another possible explanation for the fall in the number of diagnosed cases of neurasthenia during the late 19th century could have been that the disease had a social role which enabled

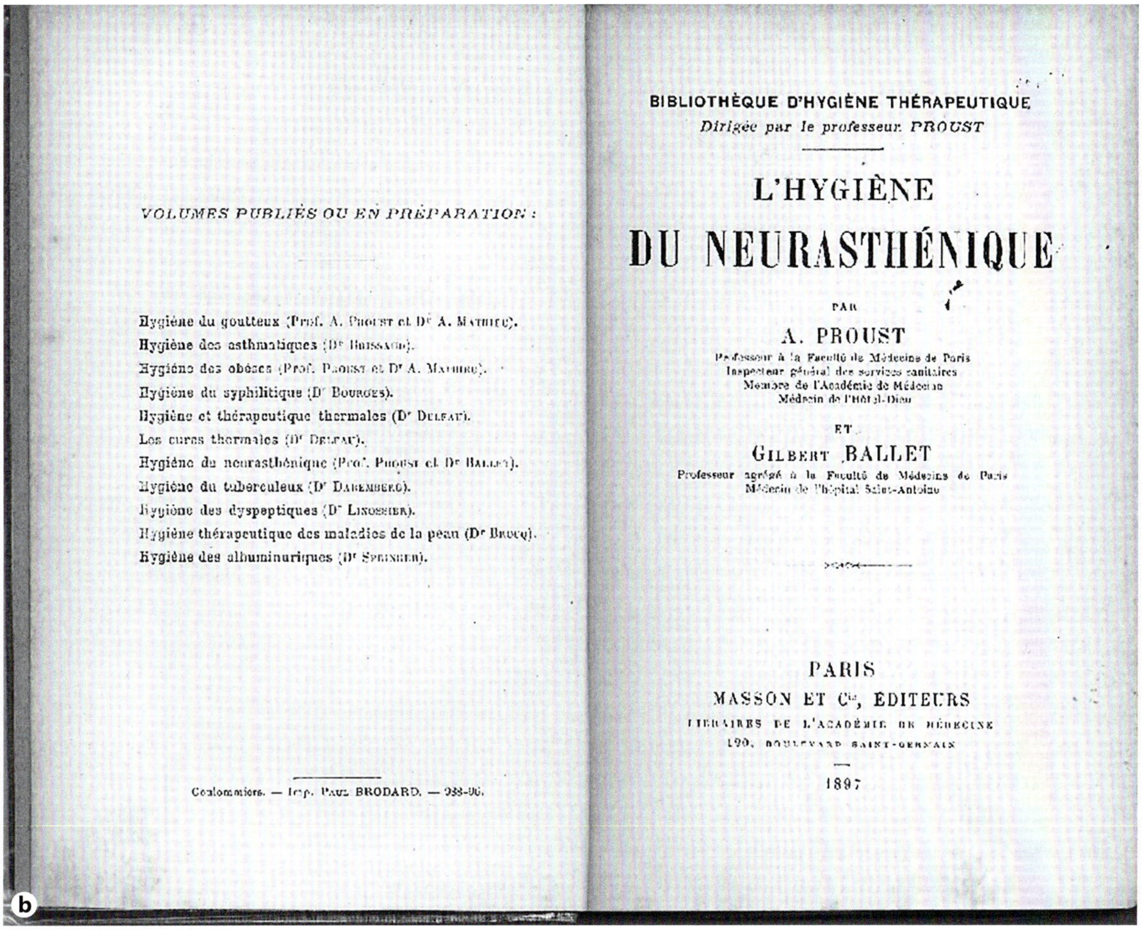
VOLUMES PUBLIÉS OU EN PRÉPARATION :

Hygiène du goutteux (Prof. A. Proust et Dr A. Mathieu).
Hygiène des asthmatiques (Dr Brissaud).
Hygiène des obèses (Prof. Proust et Dr A. Mathieu).
Hygiène du syphilitique (Dr Bourges).
Hygiène et thérapeutique thermales (Dr Delfau).
Les cures thermales (Dr Delfau).
Hygiène du neurasthénique (Prof. Proust et Dr Ballet).
Hygiène du tuberculeux (Dr Daremberg).
Hygiène des dyspeptiques (Dr Linossier).
Hygiène thérapeutique des maladies de la peau (Dr Brocq).
Hygiène des albuminuriques (Dr Springer).

Coulommiers. — Imp. Paul BRODARD. — 938-96.

BIBLIOTHÈQUE D'HYGIÈNE THÉRAPEUTIQUE
Dirigée par le professeur PROUST

L'HYGIÈNE
DU NEURASTHÉNIQUE

PAR

A. PROUST
Professeur à la Faculté de Médecine de Paris
Inspecteur général des services sanitaires
Membre de l'Académie de Médecine
Médecin de l'Hôtel-Dieu

ET

GILBERT BALLET
Professeur agrégé à la Faculté de Médecine de Paris
Médecin de l'hôpital Saint-Antoine

PARIS
MASSON ET Cie, ÉDITEURS
LIBRAIRES DE L'ACADÉMIE DE MÉDECINE
120, BOULEVARD SAINT-GERMAIN

1897

Fig. 2. b *L'hygiène du neurasthénique*, by Proust and Ballet (courtesy of Prof. Julien Bogousslavsky).

patients to cope with modern stressors, and when these stressors changed in the early 20th century, so did the role of neurasthenia [14].

Regarding the diagnosis of neurasthenia, the number of patients discharged from the hospital, e.g. Queen Square Hospital in London, signaled an abrupt appearance in 1886 and an equally sudden disappearance after 1930. Taylor [15] suggests that this type of pattern might fit with a disease of infectious origin during an epidemic, e.g. the lethargic encephalitis, and neurasthenia may represent a forme fruste of the disease or a postviral fatigue.

The reemergence of Beard's hypothesis in the medical literature was evident as early as 1965, when Holt described the presence of sporadic chronic fatigue syndrome (CFS) as 'a new disease sweeping the civilised world' [14, 20]. In fact, the illness currently best known in the USA as CFS came to the attention of the medical community and the general public in the mid-1980s. The clinical profile of CFS is strikingly similar to that of neurasthenia, a fact which has inspired some observers to argue that CFS is 'neurasthenia revived' [21].

Neurasthenia and Hysteria: Functional Disorders

At the turn of the 20th century, in the field of neuropsychiatry, one of the most common diagnoses was that of hysteria, which was characterized by paralysis, contractures, muteness, deafness, blindness, fixities, and seizures. Charcot eventually came to the conclusion that many of his patients with these symptoms were suffering from a form of hysteria which had been induced by their emotional response to a traumatic accident in the past [22]. In keeping with the trends of his time, because of the similarity of their signs to those encountered in patients with structural neurologic damage, Charcot considered hysterics to have 'functional', physiologically based lesions of specific localization [8].

It was Sigmund Freud (1856–1939) who contributed to better delineating the mind-body relationship underlying hysteria in his book entitled *Studien über Hysterie (Studies on Hysteria)* in 1895. Specifically, Freud developed the preexisting concept of the unconscious and its role in human behavior [3], something which had been previously described by many other philosophers, psychologists, and neuropsychiatrists including Charcot. Philosophers including Arthur Schopenhauer, George Wilhelm Friedrich Hegel, Soren Kierkegaard, and Friedrich Nietzsche refined a view of the mind which foreshadowed Freud's theories. Freud was immensely impressed by Charcot's work on traumatic hysteria and borrowed from it the idea that one of the principal forms of neurosis was due to a past traumatic experience triggering a process of unconscious symptom formation (conversion) [22].

Prior to 1914, hysteria and neurasthenia were considered as separate and opposite categories, in which various dichotomies are attached to each diagnosis: body/mind, female/male, lower/upper class, ancient/modern disease [7]. Charcot was categorical in distinguishing neurasthenia from hysteria, by focusing on the signs of sexual impotency, fatigue, and a tight band of pressure around the head present in patients with neurasthenia. Freud separated some symptoms including general irritability, anxious expectation, pavor nocturnus of the adult, digestive disturbances, agoraphobia or obsession, disturbances of respiration, vertigo, and paresthesia from the diagnosis of neurasthenia, grouping these in a new term: anxiety neurosis. He described anxiety neurosis as the somatic counterpart of hysteria, thus keeping the two diseases separate.

The concept of traumatic neurosis conceived by Hermann Oppenheim (1858–1919) located posttraumatic nervous symptoms between hysteria and neurasthenia, considering them as consequences of physical reactions to fright leading to molecular tissue changes. This concept was severely criticized, and traumatic neurosis was excluded from medicolegal assessments after the end of World War I [23].

The diagnoses of hysteria and neurasthenia were differently distributed along class lines before World War I. This trend continued during the war with officers diagnosed as neurasthenic and ranking men as hysterical [7, 24]. The hysterical ranking soldier was seen in similar demeaning terms as hysterical females, while the neurasthenic officer was portrayed as closer to an acceptable male ideal [7, 25]. However, despite the huge strides that neurologists were making in terms of the functional localization regarding the workings of the nervous system, neurasthenia remained stubbornly considered a 'functional' disorder for which physicians had been unable to find any structural pathology [15]. For this reason, between 1910 and 1914, medical archives reveal that hysteria and neurasthenia shared the feature of being a 'functional disease', a medical responses to shell shock [7].

In 1910, a divergent approach emerged regarding the clinical aspects of the two diseases. In fact, Allen [26] wrote: 'While typical cases of hysteria can, and should be differentiated, there is an interconnection between the whole group of functional neuroses and they are not infrequently combined in the same individual. Particularly is the combination of neurasthenia and hysteria a common one.' But the definition of functional disorder in 1892 was ambiguous as phenomena 'which result from some disturbance or change in the function of an organ without presenting any definite organic lesion by which the disease may be distinguished' [27]. 'Change in the function' is an ambiguous term that could mean that a change exists but it is not visible: the body over the mind. In fact, in this period the list of functional disorders included epilepsy, chorea, tetanus, aphasia, muscular spasm, and others. Although considered strictly connected as functional diseases, this ambiguity in their definitions continued after World War I. In fact, wartime doctors considered hysteria as a primitive defense mechanism and neurasthenia as a more sophisticated response to psychological trauma, ignoring the dominant somatic aspects of the disease prevalent before the war [7]. Furthermore, in 1923, hysteria was defined as 'a purely mental condition without pathological anatomic change in which diseased manifestations are imaged and assumed; and the basis of the condition is a morbid craving for sympathy and notoriety, or both' while neurasthenia was defined as 'a disease of the nervous system without known pathological changes in which there is a persistent weakness and irritability of nerve centres due to chronic overuse of neurons and manifested by purely subjective symptoms – that is, by altered feelings' [28]. This reintroduced the somatic aspect of neurasthenia. Thus, the term neurasthenia continued to be poorly defined, in that it shared borderlands with hysteria for both its symptoms and functional origin.

Neurasthenia and hysteria were considered to have other connections: the crucial etiological role attributed to heredity or inheritance and the presence of the predisposing condition called 'weakened' nervous system. This did not mean that the social environment did not play a role in fostering both hysteria and neurasthenia. In fact, both were medical responses to shell shock requiring a genetic predisposition. In patients with neurasthenia and hysteria, Freud considered the environment more important than heredity, which he felt fulfilled the role of a precondition, arguing that these 'functional pathological modifications have as their common source the subject's sexual life, whether they lie in a disorder of his contemporary sexual life or in important events in his past life' [29]. Likewise, Charcot explained the fact that severe emotion might result in hysteria in apparently robust individuals, clearly downplaying the importance of heredity. In fact, the concept of nervous weakness was considered as either inborn, the result of heredity, or acquired, the result of shock [7]. Beard was convinced that neurasthenia was due to a deficiency in nervous energy and nervous weakness, something considered essential for the definition of this disease. However, nervous weakness was also regarded as a precondition for the development of hysteria. Even if neurasthenia was thought to be primarily a somatic disease, nervous weakness was also considered a psychic element of the disease, therein explaining the occasional fusion of neurasthenia with hysteria and leading to the subjective term 'hystero-neurasthenia' [30]. For this reason, a line between neurasthenia and hysteria does not exist – instead they share a 'borderland'.

Conclusion

Above, we have seen how neurasthenia and hysteria, though originally considered to be distinct from each other, share several common characteristics; most importantly they are both functional diseases. Nonetheless, neurasthenia, presently known as CFS, is also thought to be an organic disease. For this reason, the two diseases should be considered as sharing a borderland with each other.

References

1 Schäfer L: On the history of the concept neurasthenia and its modern variants chronic-fatigue-syndrome, fibromyalgia and multiple chemical sensitivities (in German). Fortschr Neurol Psychiatr 2002;70:570–582.
2 Turnbull P: Psychiatry and heredity degeneration, 1860–1914. eHistory at the University of Queensland. http://paulturnbull.org/.
3 Furst LR: Partners and strangers: the mind-body relationship in history; in Furst LR (ed): Psychosomatic Disorders in Medical and Imaginative Literature. Albany, State University of New York Press, 2003.
4 Beard GM: Neurasthenia or nervous exhaustion. Boston Med Surg J 1869;80: 217–221.
5 Brown EM: Footnotes to the History of Psychiatry. https://sites.google.com/site/psychiatryfootnotes/Introduction.
6 Lillestol K, Bondevik H: Neurasthenia in Norway 1880–1920 (in Norwegian). Tidsskr Nor Laegeforen 2013;133:661–665.
7 Loughran T: Hysteria and neurasthenia in pre-1914 British medical discourse and histories of shell-shock. Hist Psychiatry 2008;19:25–46.
8 Goetz CG: Poor Beard!! Charcot's internationalization of neurasthenia, the 'American disease'. Neurology 2001;57: 510–514.
9 Nagel JD: Nervous and Mental Diseases: A Manual for Students and Practitioners. London, Hodder and Stoughton, 1905.
10 Pots CS: Nervous and Mental Diseases: A Manual for Students and Practitioners, ed 2. London, Hodder and Stoughton, 1908.
11 Paciaroni M, Cittadini E, Bogousslavsky J: Great careers: Cornil, Bouchard, Bourneville and Proust; in Bogousslavsky J (ed): Following Charcot: A Forgotten History of Neurology and Psychiatry. Front Neurol Neurosci. Basel, Karger, 2011, vol 29, pp 61–70.
12 Campbell B: The making of 'American': race and nation in neurasthenic discourse. Hist Psychiatry 2007;18:157–178.
13 Burr C: Neurasthenia; in Osler W, McCrae T (eds): A System of Medicine. London, Henry Frowde, 1910, p 725.
14 Luthra A, Wesseley S: Unloading the trunk: neurasthenia, CFS and race. Soc Sci Med 2004;58:2363–2369.
15 Taylor RE: Death of neurasthenia and its psychological reincarnation. Br J Psychiatry 2001;179:550–557.
16 Historical Collections at the Claude Moore Health Sciences Library. 2007. http://exhibits.hsl.virginia.edu/nerves/.
17 Levillain F: La neuroasthenie, maladie de Beard. Rewies. J Ment Sci 1891;37: 587–590.
18 Charcot JM: Lectures on the diseases of the nervous system (translated by T. Savill). London, New Sydenham Society, 1889, vol 3.
19 Saville TD: Clinical Lectures on Neurasthenia. London, Henry J. Glaisher, 1899.
20 Holt G: Epidemic neuromyasthenia: the sporadic form. Am J Med Sci 1965;249: 124–138.
21 Ware NC, Kleinman A: Culture and somatic experience: the social course of illness in neurasthenia and chronic fatigue syndrome. Psychosom Med 1992; 54:546–560.
22 Webster R. Freud: The Great Philosopher Series. Phoenix, Weidenfeld and Nicholson, 2003.
23 Holdorff B: The fight for 'traumatic neurosis', 1889–1916: Hermann Oppenheim and his opponents in Berlin. Hist Psychiatry 2011;22:465–476.
24 Leed E: No man's land: combat and identity in World War One. Cambridge, Cambridge University Press, 1979.
25 Showalter E: The female malady: women, madness and English culture, 1830–1980. London, Virago, 1987.
26 Allen CL: The psychoneurosis, a review of the present status of hysteria and neurasthenia. Calif State J Med 1910;8: 167–170.
27 Hack Tuke D (ed): A Dictionary of Psychological Medicine. London, J. and A. Churchill, 1892, vol 1.
28 Reynolds ES: A British Medical Association lecture on hysteria and neurasthenia. Br Med J 1923;2:1193–1196.
29 Freud S: Heredity and the etiology of the neuroses. Revue Neurologique 1886;4: 161–169.
30 Cole RH: Mental Diseases: A Text-Book of Psychiatry for Medical Students and Practitioners. London, University of London Press, 1913.

Maurizio Paciaroni, MD
Stroke Unit and Division of Internal and Cardiovascular Medicine
University of Perugia, Santa Maria della Misericordia Hospital
Via G. Dottori 1, IT–06100 Perugia (Italy)
E-Mail maurizio.paciaroni@med.unipg.it

Bogousslavsky J (ed): Hysteria: The Rise of an Enigma. Front Neurol Neurosci. Basel, Karger, 2014, vol 35, pp 157–168
DOI: 10.1159/000360060

World War I Psychoneuroses: Hysteria Goes to War

Laurent Tatu[a, b] · Julien Bogousslavsky[c]

Departments of [a]Neuromuscular Diseases and [b]Anatomy, CHU Besançon, University of Franche-Comté, Besançon, France; [c]Center for Brain and Nervous System Diseases, GSMN Neurocenter, Clinique Valmont, Glion/Montreux, Switzerland

Abstract

During the First World War, military physicians from the belligerent countries were faced with soldiers suffering from psychotrauma with often unheard of clinical signs, such as camptocormia. These varied clinical presentations took the form of abnormal movements, deaf-mutism, mental confusion, and delusional disorders. In Anglo-Saxon countries, the term 'shell shock' was used to define these disorders. The debate on whether the war was responsible for these disorders divided mobilized neuropsychiatrists. In psychological theories, war is seen as the principal causal factor. In hystero-pithiatism, developed by Joseph Babinski (1857–1932), trauma was not directly caused by the war. It was rather due to the unwillingness of the soldier to take part in the war. Permanent suspicion of malingering resulted in the establishment of a wide range of medical experiments. Many doctors used aggressive treatment methods to force the soldiers exhibiting war neuroses to return to the front as quickly as possible. Medicomilitary collusion ensued. Electrotherapy became the basis of repressive psychotherapy, such as 'torpillage', which was developed by Clovis Vincent (1879–1947), or psychofaradism, which was established by Gustave Roussy (1874–1948). Some soldiers refused such treatments, considering them a form of torture, and were brought before courts-martial. Famous cases, such as that of Baptiste Deschamps (1881–1953), raised the question of the rights of the wounded. Soldiers suffering from psychotrauma, ignored and regarded as malingerers or deserters, were sentenced to death by the courts-martial. Trials of soldiers or doctors were also held in Germany and Austria. After the war, psychoneurotics long haunted asylums and rehabilitation centers. Abuses related to the treatment of the Great War psychoneuroses nevertheless significantly changed medical concepts, leading to the modern definition of 'posttraumatic stress disorder'.

When World War I (WWI) broke out in Europe, neuropsychiatric disorders in soldiers were not unknown. During the Napoleonic wars, several conditions associated with what was called 'le vent du boulet' (literally 'wind of the cannonball') were noted and Silas Weir Mitchell (1829–1914) raised the issue during the 1861–1865 American Civil War [1]. Neuropsychiatric disorders were reported and analyzed during the 1870 Franco-Prussian conflict, leading to the concept of simulated diseases [2]. During the 1904–1905 Russo-Japanese war and the 1912–1913 Balkan conflicts, numerous cases of war neuroses were also reported.

Early on in WWI, an unprecedented number of soldiers were suffering from nervous disorders. Health services of the belligerent countries poorly anticipated the scale of the problem, and the support and care measures were improvised during the conflict. The French health service, for example, gradually opened neuropsychiatric centers [3, 4].

Nervous war disorders raised the question of what to name these often unheard of signs. Numerous classifications for the clinical signs of war neuroses were suggested during the war. In France, Joseph Grasset (1849–1918), Paul Sollier (1861–1933), and Gustave Roussy (1874–1946) suggested their own terms, which were in fact very similar [5–7]. In Germany, the main classification of war neuroses was established by Karl Birnbaum (1878–1950) [8], which strongly emphasized the concept of traumatic neurosis that had been developed before the war by Hermann Oppenheim (1858–1919). War neurosis was finally defined as a set of nervous disorders (paralysis, deafness, dumbness, etc.) not directly explicable by detectable organic lesions. Psychoneurosis was defined as a neurosis associated with impaired mental functions such as mental confusion or amnesia.

This article describes the treatment of soldiers suffering from war neuroses by wartime neuropsychiatrists in France. The subject is presented from a European perspective, with examples also from the United Kingdom, Germany, and Austria.

Camptocormia and Other New Syndromes

War neuroses caused by this conflict were symbolized by the physical appearance of soldiers suffering from camptocormia, a medical condition causing a striking angular deformity of the back (fig. 1). Rare or unknown before the war, camptocormia frequently occurred in soldiers indirectly injured by shrapnel from shells, who were often thrown or partially buried by the explosion. Camptocormia, also called bent spine syndrome, was first described in 1915 by Achille Souques (1860–1944), one of the last collaborators of Jean-Martin Charcot (1825–1893) and Inna Rosanoff-Saloff (1885–1980). In camptocormia, the pelvis is flexed over the thighs and extension of the trunk is impossible. The patient requires sticks in order not to fall forwards, as the spine otherwise retains its normal shape, in a completely different posture from that of someone just bending forwards [9]. Other clinical manifestations of war neuroses included various forms of anesthesia, palsies, abnormal movements, gait disorders, mutism, deafness, and blindness. Photographs of the time, the film archives of the French armies, and (in the United Kingdom) films directed by Arthur Hurst (1879–1944) provide many examples of the striking nature of these pathologies [10]. Psychoneurotic manifestations included amnestic disorders, confusional states, delirium, and hallucinations (fig. 2). Some apparently new psychoneurotic syndromes were also reported, such as 'bird syndrome', in which a mute and immobile patient appears unreactive, but quickly moves his gaze from object to object with short, brisk movements of the head, as if paying particularly close attention to his surroundings [6]. All these disorders can be associated with digestive disorders (vomiting, anorexia), respiratory disorders, and vascular phases of tachycardia or brachycardia. Sphincter disorders are common and include urine incontinence and emotional diarrhea.

During the conflict, some psychoneuroses were caused by minor traumatic injury. In these cases, a minor physical injury to a limb could be associated with the contracture of one or more joints, causing dramatic deformation. Joseph Babinski and Jules Froment suggested naming these nervous reflex phenomena 'physiopathic disorders' [11] (fig. 3).

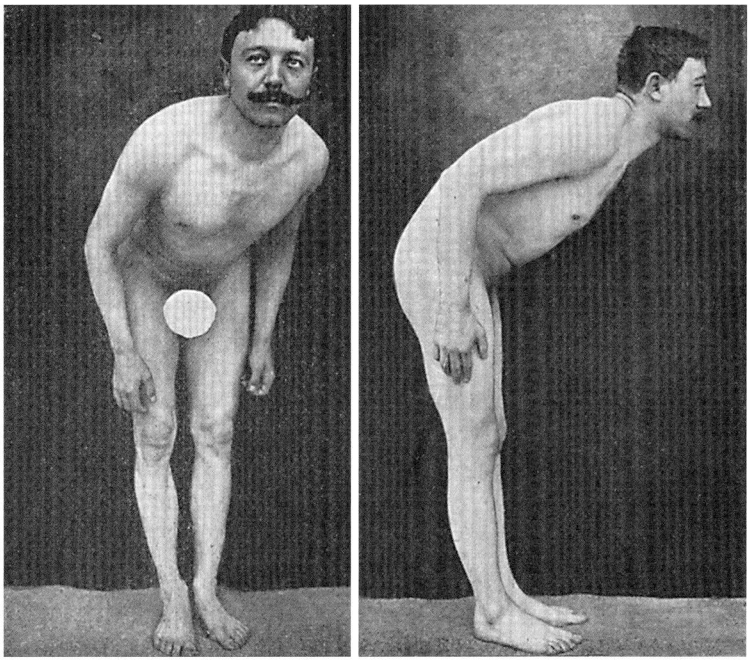

Fig. 1. French soldier suffering from camptocormia [7].

2

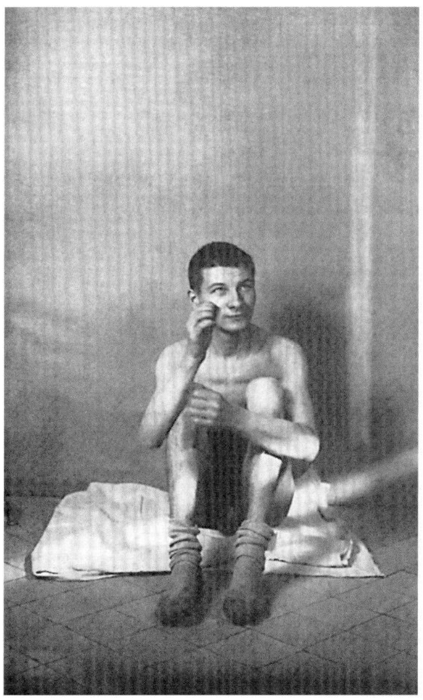

3

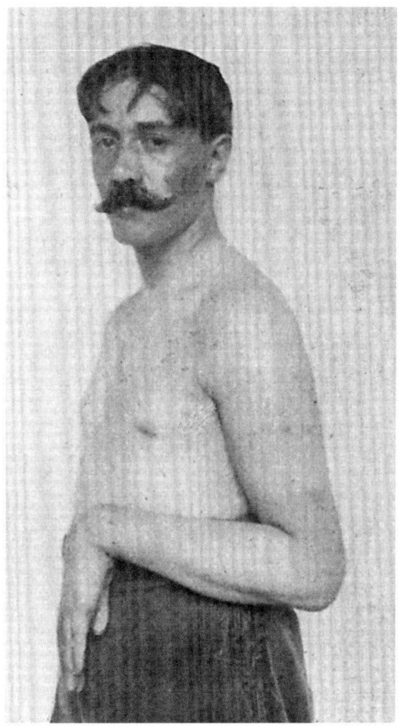

Fig. 2. Soldier suffering from war psychoneurosis with hallucinations [43].
Fig. 3. 'Physiopathic disorder' in a patient with a minor trauma to the left index finger [11].

The War Factor

The mechanisms leading to neuropsychiatric disturbances were controversial during the war. Three main causes were defined: commotion, emotion, and suggestion. The war factor was predominant in commotional and emotional mechanisms. Commotion was defined as disorders occurring after an explosion, but without detectable nervous system lesions. An initial loss of consciousness often occurred. Emotion was caused by exposure to a traumatic experience, such as seeing mutilated or dead bodies, hearing violent noises or smelling rotting corpses. It was typically associated with an uncontrolled flight reaction. Some neuropsychiatrists such as Paul Sollier, Georges Dumas (1866–1946), and André Léri (1875–1930) focused more on psychological factors as well as, paradoxically, organic lesions [6, 12, 13]. The concepts of suggestion or autosuggestion completely ruled out the war as responsible for the onset of these disorders by placing this onus on the soldier himself and his willingness to recover [11]. These concepts derived from pithiatism, introduced by Joseph Babinski (1857–1932) before the war. Between 1901 and 1908, Babinski cast doubt on Jean-Martin Charcot's (1825–1893) ideas, transforming hysteria into a purely functional illness in which suggestion played a critical role and where malingering was not clearly differentiated. Hysteria then became known as pithiatism, a word composed of Greek roots meaning 'curable by persuasion' [14]. In France, suggestion was mainly emphasized in the early stages of the conflict, along with the all-hysteria concept, supported by neurologists such as Gustave Roussy, Joseph Babinski, and Clovis Vincent.

Malingering was widely debated during the Great War. While it was accepted that pure, conscious simulation was rare, it was emphasized that exaggeration and prolongation of symptoms were common, particularly as a consequence of autosuggestion. Some neurologists such as Pierre Marie (1853–1940) suggested the concept of unconscious simulation, which further clouded the border with hysteria [15]. A critical consequence of this concept was that any clinical manifestation was immediately suspected as being false, and masked a desire to escape the danger at the front. In retrospect, it is probably the French neuropsychiatrist Paul Voivenel (1880–1975) who was the true precursor of understanding the mechanism behind war psychoneuroses. In 1918 he perfectly described, in a completely modern manner, 'peur morbide acquise' (acquired morbid fear), what current psychiatric classifications now call acute stress disorder and posttraumatic stress disorder [16].

A Wide Range of Medical Experiments

From the outbreak of the war, conventional treatment of psychoneuroses, such as bed rest, diet, cold baths, bleeding, and hypnosis, quickly proved ineffective or insufficient. In France, emphasis was placed on the mechanism of suggestion. As a result, many soldiers suffering from war neuroses were considered as malingerers who were merely attempting to escape the front. Medicomilitary collusion ensued, with the aim of returning as many of these nervous cases as possible to the front through the use of painful or experimental therapies. Obviously, not all mobilized neuropsychiatrists collaborated with the military authorities, but collusion was often encouraged under the watchful eye of suddenly highly nationalistic academic societies. Recovering military personnel had become a priority due to the massive losses resulting from the fighting in 1914 and early 1915. Recent studies examined these treatments, as well the abuse associated with their use, from a medical perspective [3, 17].

The need to rapidly implement treatments was unanimously recognized, essentially to avoid the moral contagion of the condition. This moral contagion was observed with camptocormia, which caused epidemics in certain units. Early detection of simulators was intended to prevent an unconscious simulator from developing into an organized, conscious one. From this perspective, medical assessments were often not dissimilar from police questioning, and clinical examinations included more and more traps in order to detect nonorganic lesions and confuse simulators. In addition to its therapeutic virtue, isolation, the common treatment for neuroses, helped avoid this type of contagion. Isolation was coupled with persuasion, a form of psychotherapy which was supposed to eliminate the effects of autosuggestion. It involved the doctor repeatedly telling the patient that he was improving and healing.

The sudden increase in cases of war neuroses called for the use of more drastic measures and provided a strong incentive for therapeutic experimentation. The injection of substances such as ether or emetics, forced physical mobilization, icy showers, and other adjuvant methods were all used. Doctors at the military neuropsychiatric centers quickly realized that the most effective adjuvant treatment was the use of electricity. The use of electricity for therapy in neurology essentially began with the work of the German neurologist Wilhelm Erb (1840–1921), and within several decades it became an established form of treating hysterical patients at the Salpêtrière Hospital in Paris. The 1891 Frankfurt convention, which brought together leading German neurologists and psychiatrists, addressed questions relating to the type of current to be used and its real effects on the nervous system [18]. An innovation of the Great War, however, was that pain-inducing electrotherapy was coupled with firm psychotherapy using words suggesting improvement and cure. Electrotherapy became the preferred method of managing nervous cases and was also the subject of experimentation. For example, Babinski used intense faradic currents in the pharynx of mute patients [19].

Clovis Vincent and 'Torpillage'

During the war, these new methods in the use of electrotherapy culminated in the invention by Clovis Vincent (1879–1947) of 'torpillage' (literally, torpedoing), an aggressive form of treatment for intractable psychoneuroses. Vincent worked under Achille Souques (1860–1944) and Babinski prior to becoming a hospital physician in 1913. When war broke out, he was appointed as a doctor in an infantry regiment. During infantry battles at the Argonne in 1915, he behaved heroically, replacing commanders who had been killed, even though he was a battalion doctor. He was then appointed as an assistant to Professor Maxime Laignel-Lavastine (1875–1953) at Tours Military Neurological Center in Western France. He later took charge of the center himself. There, he improved Babinski's technique of persuasive electrotherapy for hysterics, replacing galvanic current with faradic current and introducing a program of forced physical rehabilitation.

'Torpillage' was the term chosen by soldiers receiving the treatment, as they described being turned upside-down like by a shell explosion [20]. During treatment, the doctor would strongly exhort the soldier to return to a normal state of being with the help of the electric current. Vincent presented his therapy as a military battle against the affected soldiers. He recognized that soldiers often rebelled during the painful phase. They would shout, struggle, and insult the doctor. Vincent himself typically used military terms to describe the therapy sessions [21]. The final stage of the treatment was the physical training stage, which prepared the soldiers for their return to combat. Training consisted of jumping and ladder-climbing exercises under the supervision of other soldiers who had also been treated for nervous disorders. According to Vincent, 'torpillage' produced spectacular results [22] (fig. 4). Its therapeutic success expanded beyond the center in Tours. Other neurologists such as Souques at the Paul-Brousse Hospice (for the treatment of pure

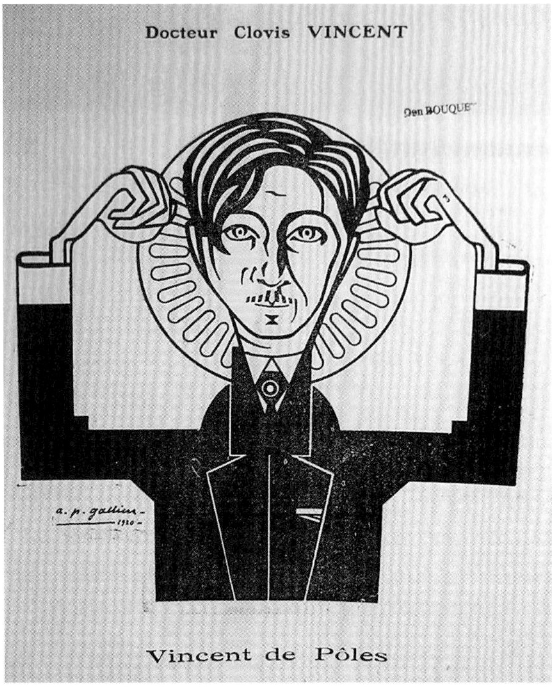

Fig. 4. Sketch drawing of Clovis Vincent emphasizing his involvement in 'torpillage'. The legend 'Vincent de Pôles' is a pun using the French word *pôle* (electric polarity) and Vincent de Paul, a priest from the 17th century who was sanctified because of his devoted care for the poor (Académie Nationale de Médecine, Paris).

cases of camptocormia) and André Gilles in a frontline neuropsychiatric center used an adapted, less aggressive method [23, 24].

While most official authorities and medical societies including the *Société de Neurologie de Paris* approved and supported 'torpillage', rebellions developed among soldiers who refused electrotherapy. At the beginning of 1916, Vincent was confronted with soldiers who refused 'torpillage' treatment. The most famous was Baptiste Deschamps (1881–1953) a soldier in the French army, who was wounded in October 1914 and subsequently suffered from acute camptocormia. He was successively sent to several neurological centers, finally arriving in Vincent's center in Tours. Deschamps refused to be subjected to electric treatment, considering it to be a form of torture. A violent altercation broke out between the two men with Deschamps striking Vincent, who as a former amateur boxer, hit back. Deschamps was summoned to a military tribunal and was handed a mild punishment in the form of a 6-month suspended prison sentence [25]. This soft verdict sounded the death knell for the treatment center in Tours and sparked a great debate concerning the rights of the wounded [26].

Gustave Roussy and Psychofaradism

The closure of the Tours psychoneuroses center did not resolve the problem of soldiers suffering from intractable war psychoneuroses. From the beginning of the war, Gustave Roussy focused his efforts on the chronically neurotic patients hospitalized in neurological centers. He decided to follow Vincent's work. Roussy was born in Vevey, Switzerland, and began his medical studies in Geneva. He became an intern in the Hôpitaux de Paris under Pierre Marie and Jules Déjerine (to whom he presented his thesis on thalamic pain syndrome in 1906). He was appointed head of Paul Brousse Hospital in 1913. During World War I, he took charge of a military neurological center. At the beginning of 1917, he took over as head of the neurological center in Besançon, the 7th military region, and then decided to open a new center in Salins-les-Bains, a spa town in the Jura region, for soldiers suffering from psychoneuroses (fig. 5). He wanted to assuage soldiers' hostility to electric treatment. The term 'torpillage' was abandoned and replaced by psychofaradic treatment, which differed very little from the Babinksi-Vincent method [27].

Roussy began by using nonpainful currents, without Vincent's dramatization, in order to gain the soldiers' acceptance, but soon moved on to stronger currents. He emphasized the need for pain if the treatment were to be a success, as well

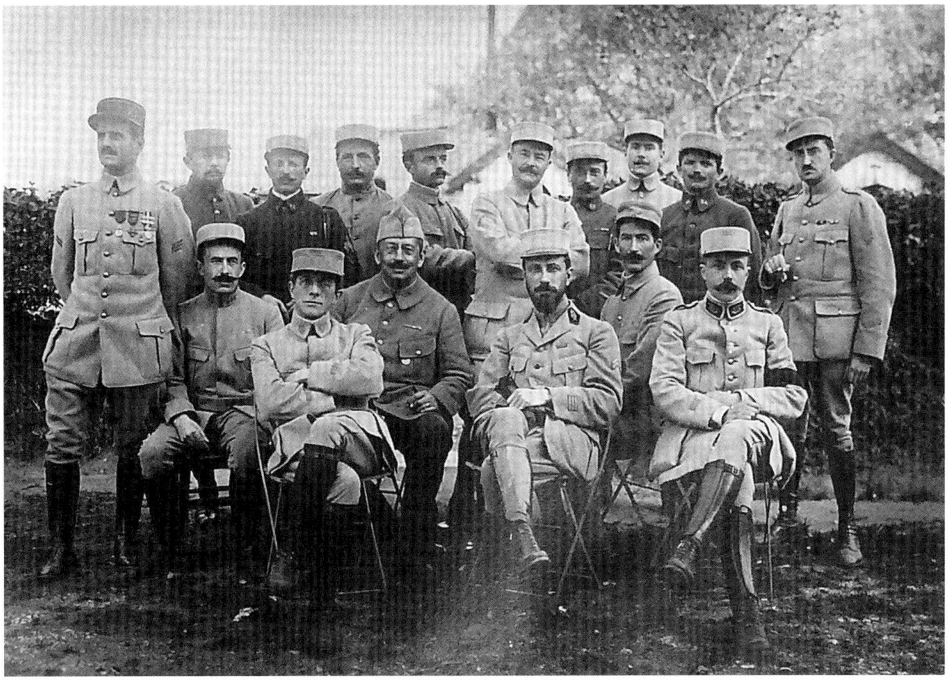

Fig. 5. Gustave Roussy (sitting in the middle of the first row) and his medical team from Salins-les-Bains neuropsychiatric centre, Jura (France), in 1917 (private collection).

as the need to stimulate sensitive parts of the body such as the soles of the feet, the scrotum, and the lips. Forced physical training, icy showers, a milky diet, and isolation were used in conjunction. Soldiers in the recovery phase performed military exercises under the supervision of officers who had been cured using the same method [28]. At the Salins-les-Bains center, the most difficult cases were assigned to Roussy, who was faced, like Vincent in Tours, with more and more therapeutic failures, evasions, and patients refusing treatment.

In January 1918, Roussy sent 6 soldiers suffering from camptocormia to Besançon military tribunal for refusing electric treatment on several occasions. The 6 soldiers were given a symbolic suspended sentence of 5 years' public service [17]. For Roussy, this ruling constituted an official disavowal and marked the end of the all-powerful faradization treatment that was being contested by soldiers and a growing number of doctors. The novelist Louis-Ferdinand Destouches, alias Céline (1894–1961), called on his own experience as a wounded soldier during the Great War, describing 'torpillage' and doctor Roussy in his novel *Voyage au Bout de la Nuit* (*Journey to the End of the Night*) in which Roussy appears under the pseudonym of Professor Bestombes [29]. Céline had already mentioned 'torpillage' in the context of the Deschamps affair [30]:

> When I read the French newspapers, a thousand things shock me. It seems to me that the life of the wounded soldier is becoming more and more impossible, without considering, of course, the terrible Zouave Deschamps affair, which smacks of slavery, and of which the term electric torpillage evokes for me the most scatalogically bloody scenes of the Grand Guignol.

A European Perspective

In European countries involved in World War I, psychological theories on war psychoneuroses were more successful, especially in Great Britain, where statistics reported 65,000 nervous cases. The term 'shell shock' was popularized in defining these cases of war neuroses. The term was coined in 1915 by the psychiatrist Charles Myers (1873–1946), who published reports of 3 cases he had seen in Le Touquet casino military hospital where patients were transferred from the front [31]. Myers' psychological attitude was largely discarded by Gordon Holmes (1876–1956), his superior, who developed a more repressive attitude. In 1916, the term NYDN (Not Yet Diagnosed, Nervous) instead of shell shock was introduced by Sir Arthur Sloggett (1857–1929) [32]. The psychological trend found another defender in William Rivers (1864–1922), a pupil of Hughlings Jackson (1835–1911), who developed specific centers at the rear such as the Maghull military hospitals near Liverpool and the Craiglockhart war hospital near Edinburgh. He introduced Freudian-like concepts to the management of psychoneuroses [33]. While electrotherapy certainly became less popular than in France, it was introduced by Edgar Douglas Adrian (1889–1977) and Lewis Yealland (1884–1954) in 1916 at the National Hospital for Nervous Disorders, based on French techniques [34]. Pain accompanying the use of faradic current was considered necessary for both therapeutic and disciplinary reasons. Electrotherapy was introduced in several other places, such as the Shell Shock Hospital near Dartmoor, where Arthur Hurst, who had studied with Babinski and Déjerine, combined faradization, suggestion, and hypnosis, before abandoning electric treatment, which he deemed traumatizing and rather ineffective [35].

In Germany, the concept of traumatic neuroses, which had become well established before the conflict, was quickly applied to war-related nervous cases. The German neurologists used the terms 'Granat-neurose', and 'Schreck-neurose' to describe war neuroses. As the concepts were more psychologically oriented, initial management focused on suggestion, psychological discussion, and hypnosis rather than a more physically aggressive therapy. Max Nonne (1860–1959) developed suggestion methods, which were even referred to as hypnotic magic. The methods were effective and cured a good number of soldiers. After the war, these methods, which were sometimes too sexual in nature, earned Nonne criticism from ex-soldiers who had refused the treatment [36].

In 1916, however, Oppenheim's trauma concept diminished in favor of a more 'Babinksi' type of hysteria, which led to the introduction of electrotherapy. Fritz Kaufmann (1875–1941) in Ludwigshafen was one of the main promoters. His variations included the sequential repetition of short sessions during which shocks were randomly given in a room decorated in a medieval, gothic style, in order to surprise the patient with the theatrical surroundings. However, the method was so violent, with almost unbearable shocks, that it was soon considered sadistic [37]. With the prospect of German defeat, psychological approaches came to be increasingly considered as too 'feminine' in the sphere of war medicine.

In Austria, there was more widespread development of electrotherapy in war neuroses. After the war, the future Nobel Prize winner Julius Wagner-Jauregg (1857–1940) was accused of performing violent therapies on his war patients. The controversy was sparked by a report by an officer who had been a patient under Wagner-Jauregg and his associate Michael Kozlowski (1861–1935). Sigmund Freud (1856–1939) was appointed by the inquiry committee for the expert evaluation. In his report, Freud emphasized the psychological factors involved in war psychoneuroses. He also stated that there had been some confusion in separating simulation from neurotic manifestations, and that the doctors had been in the uncomfortable position of making people fit to return to war instead of trying to cure them of a disease. Freud acknowledged that faradization could indeed be a very painful treatment, and that it had occasionally been used in excess, but he stated that he was convinced that no cruel sessions had been performed under the order or responsibility of Wagner-Jauregg himself. In the end, Kozlowski and other colleagues were sanctioned, but Wagner-Jauregg was acquitted [38].

Psychoneurotics Shot at Dawn

On the battlefield, the inappropriate behavior of psychotraumatized patients sometimes led them to commit military crimes. Soldiers suffering from psychoneuroses, unrecognized by witnesses or even doctors, were tried and convicted by courts-martial for desertion or malingering. The military justice system left little room, at least at the beginning of the war, for medical expertise. The number of neuropsychiatric patients executed after a war court judgement is difficult to determine, but some cases, such as the case of French Sergeant Jean-Baptiste Bourcier (1871–1915) or British soldier Harry Farr (1891–1916), remain iconic.

On May 5, 1915, early in the night, Sergeant Bourcier, leader of a small outpost on a hilltop in the Vosges, suddenly shouted 'to arms!'. At the call of their sergeant, his men blindly fired shots in the dark. They did not come under fire and regrouped but sergeant Bourcier was no longer among them. Bourcier, after having wandered all night, reappeared the following morning at the sector command post exhausted with fatigue, hallucinating and mad with horror. He recounted that his position was attacked by the enemy, that all his men died and he is the only survivor of a horrible carnage. He was immediately arrested and put on trial for abandoning his post. Without hearing witnesses or medical expertise, he was sentenced to death. The last letter written by Bourcier to his wife the night before his execution reflects the inconsistency of his statements with a narrative of events confirming visual hallucinations mixed with sufficient lucidity to realize his execution the following day. Sergeant Bourcier was shot at dawn the day after his conviction. The commander of his regiment who sentenced him to death realized his delirium, but did not allow for attenuating circumstances that may have reduced the sanction. After a long legal battle, and hearing many witnesses of the event, Sergeant Jean-Baptiste Bourcier was eventually pardoned in December 1934, in consideration of the fact that he was not of sound mind at the time [3, 39].

The case of English soldier Harry Farr also symbolizes convicted soldiers executed in a state of shell shock. Harry Farr belonged to the British Expeditionary Force and fought in the trenches of the French front at the end of 1914. His military behavior was exemplary, but under continual bombardment, he suffered shell shock in May 1915. He was evacuated to a hospital behind the front lines where he spent several months. He returned to fight but was hospitalized again in April and July 1916 for the same disorders. In September 1916, his regiment, the 1st Battalion West Yorkshire Regiment, took part in the Battle of the Somme. On September 17, 1916, when his regiment was ordered to the front, he declared himself sick. The doctor of the regiment noted nothing wrong, but Farr refused to go to the front, arguing that he could no longer bear it. A sergeant forced him to return to the front and was escorted by some of his comrades. Bombardment dispersed the group and Farr flees. He was arrested the next day and charged with desertion. The court-martial met 2 weeks later. Henry Farr was not reviewed by a physician and he defended himself alone. He was sentenced to death and executed on October 16, 1916 at the age of 25 years. The case of Henry Farr became over the years the icon of the executed shell-shocked soldier. The widow of Harry Farr fought until her death in 1993 for the recognition of her husband's mental disorders at the time of the facts and for his pardon. A public campaign for executed British soldiers of the Great War eventually led to the official pardon of Henry Farr in 2006 [40].

After the War

The armistice of November 11, 1918 did not change the situation of soldiers suffering from psychotrauma during the Great War. For approaches that focused on conscious or unconscious malingering by soldiers to escape the front line, the end of the war did not lead to the sometimes expected disappearance of their disorders.

There is little information on the postwar fate of this army of psychotraumatized soldiers. Psychoneurotic patients with neurological expression, such as camptocormia or soldiers suffering from abnormal movements, haunted neurological rehabilitation services long after the war. The existence of late concussion syndrome war was also proved through observations of soldiers with impaired memory and attention, irritability, and headache [41]. As the soldiers' psychological wounds of the war were not visible, nor considered 'noble', there were no associations supporting them. Defending the rights of the war neurotics was not as easy as for other types of physical injuries. Progressively, the administrative status of these war psychoneurotics and their families nonetheless improved. Helped by the beneficial influence of retrials resulting in the pardons of psychoneurotics convicted by courts-martial, the administrative struggle in the inter-war years finally improved the status of alienated families. Veterans committed to asylums were considered, in the words used at the time, as the 'living dead' – they survived the war but led a life disconnected from reality. Photographs of these soldiers of unknown identity, were regularly published in various newspapers of the time in hopes that a member of their family would recognize them [42].

Medically, demobilization gradually occurred with the urgent need to fight against the deadly Spanish flu epidemic that raged throughout Europe. Postwar neurology focused on organic disorders, with an attraction to psychological war trauma. The scientific interest of neurologists and psychiatrists also turned to the epidemic of lethargic encephalitis that affected Europe from 1916 to 1926. The professional careers of some mobilized neurologists and psychiatrists were well underway before the war. For example, Joseph Babinski was already a recognized neurologist. He retired 4 years after the end of the conflict. Other younger physicians, such as Clovis Vincent or Gustave Roussy were on an upward career path at the time of mobilization. After the Deschamps case, Clovis Vincent asked to return to the front as a regiment battlefield doctor. The episode of the soldier Deschamps disturbed him for a long time and, retrospectively, he changed his writings of his vision of war psychoneuroses after the war. He gradually shifted his career to surgery and became, with Thierry de Martel (1876–1940), a founder of French neurosurgery, and held in 1938 the first French chair of this specialty. Gustave Roussy, who in 1918 witnessed the slow collapse of psychofaradic treatment, did not change his view on war neuroses with time. He later moved into anatomopathology and became one of the world's most renowned cancer specialists. After the Second World War, the end of his career was overshadowed by political affairs and he committed suicide in 1948.

Conclusion

The concept of psychological war trauma eventually emerged as neuropsychiatric therapeutic abuses and medicolegal errors of the Great War.

The soldiers of the Second World War and the surviving deportees revealed a new range of signs of mental trauma, different from those induced by the endless trench warfare of 1914–1918. This type of fighting was undoubtedly responsible for the proliferation of neuropsychological trauma as well as their semiologic variety.

In order to qualify disorders related to psychological trauma of war, the term 'neurosis' was gradually replaced by 'posttraumatic stress disorder'. The more recent conflicts have only confirmed the variety of disorders possibly related to this state of stress. This disparity in the observed signs is now seen as closely linked to the type of fights that generate them. Psychotherapeutic and drug approaches are now used in the treatment of posttraumatic stress disorder. In light of our current medical references, the aggressive and experimental approaches during the Great War of some neuropsychiatrists appear ethically unthinkable. But this current reading, when taken out of its societal and military context, which a century later sometimes appears incomprehensible, must remain cautious.

References

1 Keen WW, Mitchell SW, Morehouse GR: On malingering, especially in regard to simulation of diseases of the nervous system. Am J Med Sci 1864;48: 367–394.
2 Boisseau E: Des maladies simulées et des moyens de les reconnaître: leçons professées au Val-de-Grâce. Paris, Baillière, 1870.
3 Tatu L, Bogousslavsky J: La folie au front. La grande bataille des névroses de guerre (1914–1918). Paris, Éditions Imago, 2012.
4 Bogousslavsky J, Tatu L: French neuropsychiatry in the Great War: between moral support and electricity. J Hist Neurosci 2013;22:144–154.
5 Grasset J: Les grands types cliniques de psychonévroses de guerre. Réunion Médico-Chirurgicale de la XVIe région. Séance du 27 janvier 1917.
6 Sollier P: Traité clinique de neurologie de guerre. Paris, Alcan, 1918.
7 Roussy G, Lhermitte J: Les psychonévroses de guerre. Paris, Masson, 1917.
8 Birnbaum K: Psychiatrische und nervenaerzliche sichverständigentätigkeit im Kriege. Berlin, Kriegaerztliche Abende, 1915.
9 Souques A, Rosanoff-Saloff I: La camptocormie. Incurvation du tronc consécutive aux traumatismes du dos et des lombes. Considérations morphologiques. Rev Neurol (Paris), 1915, pp 937–939.
10 Moscovich M, Estupinan D, Qureshi M, Okun MS: Shell shock: psychogenic gait and other movement disorders – a film review. Tremor Other Hyperkinet Mov (NY) 2013;3:tre-03-110-774-2.
11 Babinski J, Froment J: Hystérie-pithiatisme et troubles nerveux d'ordre réflexe. Paris, Masson, 1917.
12 Dumas G: Troubles mentaux et troubles nerveux de guerre. Paris, Alcan, 1919.
13 Léri A: Travaux du centre neurologique de la IIe armée. Rev Neurol (Paris) 1917; 2:449–456.
14 Babinski J: Définition de l'hystérie. Société Neurologique de Paris. Meeting of November 7, 1901. Rev Neurol (Paris) 1901;9:1074–1080.
15 Marie P: Discussion sur les troubles dits fonctionnels observés pendant la guerre. Rev Neurol (Paris) 1914–1915: 447–453.
16 Voivenel P: Sur la peur morbide acquise. Société Médico-psychologique. Ann Med Psychol (Paris) 1918;9:283–308.
17 Tatu L, Bogousslavsky J, Moulin T, Chopard JL: The 'torpillage' neurologists of World War I: electric therapy to send hysterics back to the front. Neurology 2010;75:279–283.
18 Steinberg H: Electrotherapeutic disputes: the 'Frankfurt Council' of 1891. Brain 2011;134:1229–1243.
19 Babinski J: Discussion sur les troubles dits fonctionnels observés pendant la guerre. Rev Neurol (Paris) 1915:447–453.
20 Rimbaud L: À propos de la méthode de traitement des psychonévroses dite 'du torpillage'. Marseille Médical, 1916, pp 33–41.
21 Vincent C: Au sujet de l'hystérie et de la simulation. Rev Neurol (Paris) 1916;2: 104–107.
22 Vincent C: Travaux du centre neurologique de la 9e région (Tours). Rev Neurol (Paris) 1916;2:670–672.
23 Souques A, Mégevand J, Naiditch, Rathaus: Traitement de la camptocormie par l'électrothérapie persuasive; in: Nouvelle Iconographie de la Salpêtrière. Paris, Masson, 1917, pp 420–437.
24 Gilles A: L'hystérie et la guerre. Troubles fonctionnels par commotion. Leur traitement par le torpillage. Ann Med Psychol (Paris) 1916–1917;2:207–227.
25 Roudebush MO: A Battle of Nerves: Hysteria and its Treatment in France During World War I; thesis, University of California, Berkeley, 1995.
26 Viet V: Droit des blessés et intérêt de la nation (1914–1918). Revue d'Histoire moderne et contemporaine 2012;59: 85–106.
27 Roussy G, Boisseau J, d'Oelsnitz M: La station neurologique de Salins (Jura) centre des psychonévroses après trois mois de fonctionnement. Bulletin de la réunion médico-chirurgicale de la VIIe région, 1917, pp 185–207.
28 Roussy G: Travaux du centre neurologique de la VIIe région. Rev Neurol (Paris) 1917;2:382–397.

29 Céline LF: Voyage au bout de la nuit: Notice. Paris, Gallimard Pléïade, 1981, pp 1179–1182.
30 Céline LF: Letter to Albert Million dated 24 September 1916. Private collection.
31 Myers C: A contribution to the study of shellshock: being an account of the cases of loss of memory, vision, smell and taste admitted to the Duchess of Westminster's War Hospital, Le Touquet. Lancet, 1915, pp 316–320.
32 Shephard B: A War of Nerves: Soldiers and Psychiatrists in the Twentieth Century. Cambridge, Harvard University Press, 2001.
33 Rivers WH: Instinct and the Unconscious. Cambridge, Cambridge University Press, 1920.
34 Linden SC, Jones E, Less AJ: Shell shock at Queen Square: Lewis Yealland 100 years on. Brain 2013;136:1976–1988.
35 Jones E: War neuroses and Arthur Hurst: a pioneering medical film about the treatment of psychiatric battle casualties. J Hist Med Allied Sci 2012;67: 345–373.
36 Nonne M: Über erfolgreiche Suggestivbehandlung der hysterieformen Störungen bein Kriegsneurosen. Zeitschrift für die gesammte Neurologie und Psychiatrie 1917;37:192.
37 Lerner P: Psychiatrie allemande in 14–18 Aujourd'hui. Today. Heute. No. 3 Choc traumatique et histoire culturelle. Paris, Noêsis, 2000.
38 Eissler KR: Freud sur le front des névroses de guerre. Paris, Presses Universitaires de France, 1995.
39 Brunschvicg B: La réhabilitation du sergent Bourcier. Dix-neuf ans après. Les Cahiers des droits de l'homme, May 1935, pp 14–16.
40 Wessely S: The life and death of private Harry Farr. J R Soc Med 2006;99:440–443.
41 Tison S, Guillemain H: Du front à l'asile 1914–1918. Paris, Alma éditeur, 2013.
42 Thomas GM: Treating the trauma of the Great War. Soldiers, civilians, and psychiatrists 1914–1940. Baton Rouge, Louisiana University Press, 2009.
43 Rodiet A, Fribourg-Blanc A: La folie et la grande guerre. Paris, Alcan, 1930.

Prof. Laurent Tatu
Department of Neuromuscular Diseases
Besançon University Hospital, Boulevard Fleming
FR–25030 Besançon Cedex (France)
E-Mail laurent.tatu@univ-fcomte.fr

Bogousslavsky J (ed): Hysteria: The Rise of an Enigma. Front Neurol Neurosci. Basel, Karger, 2014, vol 35, pp 169–180
DOI: 10.1159/000360062

Hysteria around the World

Antonio Carota[a, b] · Pasquale Calabrese[b]

[a]Center for Brain and Nervous System Diseases, GSMN Neurocenter, Genolier Clinic, Genolier Swiss Medical Network, Genolier, and [b]Department of Molecular and Cognitive Neuroscience, University of Basel, Basel, Switzerland

Abstract

In the 20th century the term hysteria declined and the interest in the hysteria-related diseases decreased in comparison to the florid period of studies that was inspired by Charcot's legacy in the second half of the 19th century. Scientific interest has once again increased in the 21st century, and dissociative and somatoform disorders (previously indicated as hysteria or hysterical neurosis) have come to be regarded as conditions that are known to be much more prevalent than formerly estimated. Available current epidemiological data from several countries on different continents (adopting DSM criteria for diagnosis) suggest not only that the prevalence is probably similar, but also that there is a consistency in their clinical manifestation around the world and across different cultures, social classes, and institutional settings. In line with this uniformity, and also with Charcot's concept of hysteria as a functional disorder, neuroimaging studies suggest that for some of these disorders, there might be some changes of neural connectivity in specific pathways at the origin of the behavioral aspects. Only large-scale multidisciplinary transcultural studies can improve the research and the development of therapeutic interventions for these disorders.

Historical Notes

In the 19th century, the science of hysteria had its center of reference in Charcot's school in the Pitié-Salpetrière clinic in Paris, which is no wonder as Jean-Martin Charcot (1825–1893) was the first to consider hysteria as a 'dynamic' state of mind more than a structural disease of the brain. Fifty percent of the women in the Victorian era were believed to have suffered from hysteria, and a majority of them carried a bottle of smelling salts in their handbag (in case they were overwhelmed by emotions). However, the diagnosis of hysteria was almost entirely discredited or forgotten in the early 20th century.

There were several reasons for the negative development of the scientific popularity of the hysterical disorders. The 'Nancy quarrel' (see Piechowski and Bogousslavsky [this vol., pp. 56–64]) gave discredit to Charcot's model of hysteria. In addition, malingering (also, at least partly, induced by medical suggestion) and the description of hysteric symptoms under the label 'Briquet's syndrome' or 'neurasthenia' became an alternative diagnosis. Furthermore, the interest in hysteria seemed to succumb to the assumption of the absence of organic lesions and thus to the impossibility to accommodate its symptoms in known physiological and anatomical systems.

At the end of the 19th century, the young Jewish-German neurologist Hermann Oppenheim (1858–1919), after corresponding with Charcot and observing patients in the Charité Hospital in Berlin for many years, introduced new concepts that greatly challenged Charcot's point of view on hysteria. Oppenheim suggested that a psychic trauma was the direct cause of undetectable and untreatable brain lesions that would explain the neurologic-somatic symptoms of Charcot's patients (paralysis, sleep, and language disorders). Thus, despite some overlapping of symptoms, Oppenheim traced a clear-cut distinction between traumatic neurosis (a brain disease caused by trauma) and the vague concept of hysteria, as it could include simulation and other subjective mental states.

Charcot's assumptions were also challenged by some outstanding figures of 20th century British neurology, like John Hughlings Jackson (1835–1911) and Gordon Holmes (1876–1965), who both viewed hysteria as a consequence of dissolution of the highest level of function of the brain [1]. Some contemporary neurologists suggested that the 'Queen Square position' on some psychiatric diseases derived from the austerity of a Victorian moral stance hedged by tradition [2].

The discovery of neurosyphilis (also called 'the disease of the century' or 'dementia paralytica') as an 'arachnitis' or 'chronic meningitis' seemed to suggest an organic cause for all psychiatric diseases. This context probably deprived hysteria of the status of being a 'true mental disorder'. Furthermore, in the scientific world, the diagnosis of schizophrenia became trendier and more influential than that of hysteria due to the growing popularity of the Swiss psychiatrist Eugen Bleuler (1857–1939).

In England by the mid- to late 19th century, the concept of 'female' hysteria was still mainly relegated to the millenary concept of sexual dysfunction. A typical treatment, particularly, for high social class English women was the massage of the patient's genitalia by the physician and, later, by vibrators to cause orgasms (defined at that time 'hysterical paroxysms'). At the beginning of the 19th century, especially in Britain, women's social emancipation pressures and socialist tendencies contributed to give a pejorative connotation to the term hysteria, and also because this condition might be interpreted as a stigma of national decline.

During the First and Second World Wars, the occurrence of hysterical symptoms or shell shock in soldiers in the setting of dramatic combat (see Tatu and Bogousslavsky [this vol., pp. 157–168]) was a great amplifier for the role of anxiety, fear, and trauma (as in Janet's model) in generating hysterical symptoms. It is noteworthy that dissociative or pseudoneurological symptoms (blindness and hemiparesis) appeared in male soldiers (the so-called phenomenon of the 'virile or male hysteria') without any history of psychiatric disease and with similar clinical characteristics across different cultures and countries. However, in Germany, around the time of the World War I, coincidently with the 1916 'Jew count', Dr. Oppenheim's theory of trauma-related neurosis was associated with anti-German values, as German psychiatry attributed hysterical symptoms to treatable weak constitutional habits rather than to external traumas. In this wake, new therapeutic and violent procedures (chamber isolation, 'torpillage', electroshock, etc.) were used to treat hysteric soldiers. In the same spirit, Holmes [3] emphasized the way in which changes in mental state can provide clues to the existence of organic cerebral disease by suggestibility. By relating to shell-shock symptoms, he wrote: 'even normal persons are suggestible; any one can walk along a plank lying on firm ground, but may be unable to do so when it spans an abyss.' He imputed suggestion to be particularly important in clinical neurology: first, because it may be the origin of symptoms, and second since it is the most effective agent in their removal [3].

However, as with hysterical symptoms, some differences were noted between the two wars because the diagnosis of hysteria decreased in parallel with the increase of anxiety and depression neurosis. The same tendency was documented in the general population in several studies in North America and Australia in the second half of the 20th century.

The theories of Pierre Janet (1859–1947) on the role of trauma and consciousness disintegration (i.e. 'the doubling of the mind' or the 'splitting of consciousness') were pivotal in bringing the hysterical disorders of the early 19th century to the modern perspective of dissociative disorders in the 21st century. The early theorizations of Josef Breuer (1842–1925), Sigmund Freud (1856–1939), and Carl-Gustav Jung (1875–1961) on hysteria were also strongly influenced by Janet who himself coined the terms 'dissociation' and 'subconscious'.

Still in line with Janet's theories on hysteria, the term of hysteria has been omitted from DSM-III (1980) in order to emphasize the role of trauma and dissociation.

Evolution around the World

Hysteria and hysterical neurosis correspond to the actual categories of *dissociative* and *somatoform* disorders. According to DSM-5 criteria, a significant burden or impairment is necessary for diagnosis. Dissociative disorders entail dissociation or interruption within the domains of consciousness, memory, identity, and perception. Somatoform disorders present with physical symptoms that do not have an organic cause, but mimic physical diseases or injuries. Dissociative and conversion disorders usually develop as a means to cope with childhood or adult trauma. Unexplained medical symptoms can also occur in patients who have an already established diagnosis of neurological diseases (such as multiple sclerosis or headache) [4]. For example, the association of nonepileptic psychogenic attacks with organic seizures is straightforward [5].

Tracing a map of these disorders around the world is a difficult task as their diagnosis is only clinical, uneasy, and often tardive. It is also difficult because they occur in both pediatric and adult populations in different settings and in association with other psychiatric, medical, and neurological disorders. Furthermore, the hysteric or histrionic trait (a personality type disorder) is a predisposing condition.

From the psychodynamic perspective, theories of personality disintegration due to trauma displaced the millenarian uterine theory stating that dissociative and somatoform disorders are a feminine trait related to sexual dysfunction. According to sociological or anthropological perspectives, cultural issues might change the way people with dissociative and somatoform disorders cope with trauma. Thus, these disorders might follow maps of social burden, disasters, and wars around the world. Within the neurological sciences, functional neuroimaging studies have provided evidence that changes in brain activity are systematically identifiable in both dissociative and conversion disorders [6, 7]. Hence, if structural, biochemical, neural, or connectivity changes are preponderantly at the origin of these diseases and manifest with stereotyped patterns of behavioral responses, the prevalence and the clinical consistency of dissociative and somatoform disorders might be similar around the world despite cultural and geographical differences.

Dissociative Disorders

Actually, in most European countries (e.g. UK, Finland, Sweden, Norway, Germany, Denmark, Switzerland, and Austria), the USA, Australia, and South Africa, there are several psychiatric centers that specialize on therapeutic interventions, training, and research in the domain of dissociative disorders. The International Society for the Study of Trauma and Dissociation (ISSTD) organizes worldwide seminars and releases two certificates of competencies. The official journal of the ISSTD offers peer-reviewed scientific studies and articles covering research and therapeutic interventions. Despite criticism, DSM-5 supplies operative diagnostic definitions of dissociative disorders that allow uniformity of diagnosis around the world. However, the integration of the last DSM with the International Classification of Diseases (ICD) is lacking.

Structured diagnostic questionnaires are now available and strongly recommended for screening dissociative disorders. They include the Dissociative Experiences Scale [8], the Dissociative Disorders Interview Schedule [9], the Structured Clinical Interview for Dissociative Disorders [10], the Multidimentional Inventory of Dissociation [11], and the Diagnostic Drawing Series [12]. All of the epidemiological studies adopting these instruments have provided evidence that dissociative symptoms are much more frequent than formerly assumed, for example even far higher than schizophrenia. There is a comparable prevalence among different countries (England, Switzerland, Finland, Turkey, the Netherlands, Germany, Italy, USA, and China) [13–15], which corresponds to 1–4% in the general population and 10% or more within psychiatric settings. However, epidemiological studies employ different methodologies. It would also be important to know whether there is a difference in prevalence between single episodes versus persistent dissociative experiences and whether the risk is higher for specific professional or social categories and for both childhood and adulthood.

Dissociative patients report the highest frequencies of traumatic events (sexual, emotional, and physical abuse) and neglect during childhood [14]. The magnitude of the distress due to these disorders might vary according to culturally shaped views of dissociative experiences, selfhood, and past. For example, dissociative disorders might be more frequent in people who have a background of immigration [16]. However, up to now, there has neither been sufficient data to indicate which ethnic or social categories are specifically at risk nor to identify which patients in the context of significant trauma are more prone to develop dissociative or somatic symptoms. Finally, the prevalence of these disorders and the clinical manifestations appear to be similar around the world. For example, they were present in 14% of the 25,018 respondents with posttraumatic stress disorder in 16 countries of the WHO World Mental Health Surveys without significant differences between high- and low-income countries [17]. The findings of a recent Swiss study [15] showed that dissociative disorders contribute to functional impairment above and beyond the impact of coexisting nondissociative psychiatric conditions.

Dissociative Fugue and Dissociative Amnesia

Dissociative fugue (formerly called psychogenic fugue) is characterized by sudden unplanned travel or wandering away from the usual surroundings. Generally, the condition may last for hours or days, but in some cases it can even be protracted for months or years. Sometimes the fugue state, generally precipitated by a stressful event, is accompanied by the establishment of a new identity. After recovery from fugue, previous memories usually return intact, but there is amnesia concerning all the events that occurred during the fugue episode. Differently from patients with amnesia due to neurological or other psychiatric disorders, patients with dissociative fugue have almost normal cognitive functioning and do not show a psychotic behavior.

Several psychiatry textbooks report a prevalence of 0.2%, although there have been no systematic surveys. Newspapers, novels, and TV episodes all around the world have documented hundreds of exceptional histories of people who vanished and then were found by chance in places far away from their point of origin, having adopted new identities and forgetting their previous life. One of the most famous and representative of these histories is probably the case of the British novelist Agatha Christie.

On December 3, 1926, the writer disappeared from her house in Berkshire, leaving some contradictory notes. She abandoned her car near the Silent Pool Lake where one of her fictional characters had died. Fearing her suicide, the police dredged the lake and organized 15,000 volunteers and airplanes to explore the surroundings. A series of indices (left by Agatha Christie herself) led to her in a health spa in Harrogate, Yorkshire. She was there with a false identity and did not remember the previous 10 days. Before her disappearance, Agatha Christie suffered a psychological trauma, as she was confronted with her husband's infidelity and request for divorce. She never related back on this episode and she excluded it from her biography.

All of the cases of patients with dissociative fugue (either for short or for prolonged periods) are naturally unique. However, all those cases, around the world and across cultures, appear similar according to the psychodynamic mechanisms (trauma, fugue, amnesia) and remain just as mysterious as Agatha Christie's case. Actually, some cases might be factitious. In this context, it is noteworthy that during the wars of the last century, military doctors tried to use the category of the dissociative fugue to protect deserters from punishment.

Dissociative amnesia is a profound inability (temporary or persistent) to recall personal information (usually related to traumatic events) even for the simple identity. Dissociative amnesia affects both genders equally and typically occurs in the third and fourth decade of life [18]. Dissociative amnesia has a high occurrence in people involved in wars, natural accidents and disasters, kidnapping, torture, and concentration camps, as well as in people with a history of child or sexual abuse. In World War II, 35% of British soldiers returning from combat were amnesic [19].

The disorder is also common in cases of murder or attempted suicide [20]. Interestingly, the indigenous Shona people of Zimbabwe adopt structured ceremonies (as marriages or social parades) with the aim to treat individuals with dissociative amnesia (specifically people who committed murder or other violence and who were amnesic of their acts) [21]. Case series of dissociative amnesia with similar clinical features have been reported in Italy [22], UK [23], USA [24], and Germany [25].

The vicinity of dissociative fugue and dissociative amnesia is exemplified by a concise case history given by Markowitsch et al. [26]. They reported the case of a 30-year-old male patient who was referred to the hospital due to his complaints of having lost his personal memory for his entire life span. The patient reported that he had left his home to phone, but instead collected a large amount of money from his bank account. However, he could not remember this detail. Instead, he remembered waking up next to a road without money and documents a few days later, and feeling disoriented and without memories of his personal past. He realized that he was abroad and in fact it could be verified that he had travelled from Germany to Czechoslovakia. From there he returned to Germany where he was brought to a hospital.

Similar single case reports of dissociative fugue and dissociative amnesia around the world suggest a common dysfunction, which probably, as indicated by findings of neuroimaging studies, consists of some inhibitive inputs in brain memory systems during retrieval of autobiographic information [27].

Dissociative Identity Disorder

Dissociative identity disorder (DID), formerly 'multiple personality disorder', describes the presence of two or more distinct identities or personalities that recurrently take control of the patient's behavior (one is generally dominant), inducing some memory loss during identity transfers.

DID probably has its onset in childhood, but has relevant clinical manifestations in the fourth decade [13]. It affects preponderantly women and runs a chronic, waxing, and waning course. Apart from marked impairments in the sense of identity and self, an inability to recall personal information together with other dissociative symptoms are common. Childhood sexual abuse and trauma is nearly always the most important risk factor for DID [13, 28].

DID has been the object of popular books and movies *(The Three Faces of Eve, Sybil, Fight Club, Psycho, Dr. Jekyll and Mr. Hyde, The Number 23)*, and even album songs (i.e. *The Lamb Lies Down on Broadway* by Genesis).

Although many cases have been published in most European countries before the 1980s (for review see [29]), DID was initially considered a North American 'disorder'. In the 1990s, an enormous increase in the number of cases was reported in the USA [30] and it was the object of diffusion by media. At that time, in Europe (especially Britain) the skepticism about DID came to the point to suggest an iatrogenic etiology (i.e. induced by hypnosis or suggestion) or even a medical invention. Actually, some cultural factors might explain differences in prevalence rates. DID appears to be less frequent in India, Germany, Japan, and China than in USA, Canada, the Netherlands, Norway, and Turkey. In Switzerland, DID prevalence in psychiatric settings is particularly low and corresponds to 0.05–0.1% [31]. However, in the last decades, DID prevalence has increased. In psychiatric settings in North America, Europe, and Asia (overview in [32]), the median prevalence is 8% for outpatients and 10% for inpatients. This increase in DID prevalence is probably explained by the widespread use of dissociative questionnaires and more accurate questioning in interviews.

The dramatic and extreme experiences of the DID cases reported in the media and psychiatric literature probably represent less than 5–6% of patients with DID [33] as most patients with DID might have a covert and subtle presentation. The typical clinical presentation could be one of a refractory psychiatric disorder, usually a mood disorder with multiple somatic symptoms. Patients have often received several psychiatric diagnoses over many years of treatment, such as bipolar disorder or depression, posttraumatic stress disorder, personality disorders, or anxiety disorders. Cases studies of murderers with DID have been published in the USA [34]. Suicidal behaviors were frequent for patients with DIDs in a Canadian study (72% attempted and 2% succeeded) [35]. A large and worldwide longitudinal study including 292 therapists supports the benefits of psychological therapy for DID [36].

'Dissociative trance disorder' or 'possession trance' might be a variant along a continuum of DID. These involve temporary episodes of perceived replacement of the usual identity by a new identity (as in case of exorcism or possession experiences), generally related to a supernatural entity (deity, spirit, power). Cultural phenomena of possession trance are 'Latah' (mature women, in Southeast Asia), 'Bebainan' in Bali, 'Amok' (adult men in Malaysia, India, Philippines, Polynesia, Land of Fire, the Caribbean, the Artic, or Siberia), 'Piblokto' (women of the Arctic Inughuit societies), Zar (North Africa and Middle East), Tamazai (Tuareg), and Dybbuk (Jewish tradition). There are no precise data on the clinical aspects and the outcome of the exorcisms practiced in Catholic or other religious contexts.

Depersonalization Disorder

Depersonalization disorder is a condition of persistent or recurrent depersonalization that is the experience of detachment from oneself or from surroundings (the person may feel as though they are dreaming or acting as a robot) or of unreality (derealization). This circumstance does not allow the patient to stay focused in social or professional activities. An estimated 1–4% of the general population might meet the diagnostic criteria for this disorder [37]. It can be a recurrent or persistent condition. Although DSM does not suggest any primary symptom, the most frequent could be some sensory misperception. A population-based German study found that symptoms of depersonalization were an independent predictor of vertigo and dizziness together with healthcare use [38]. Depersonalization symptoms can also manifest due to sleep deprivation. Lower scores in depersonalization scales were found in a sample of Columbian psychiatric patients compared to the UK and Spain, a finding suggestive of the protective role of collectivist versus individual cultures [39].

Ganser Syndrome

This syndrome, named after the German Psychiatrist Sigbert Ganser (1853–1931), consists of providing systematically false and improbable responses (giving only approximate answers, touching 'nearby the point') to questions (e.g. 1 + 1 = 3; the horse has three hooves, etc.) and exhibiting other illogical behaviors (pseudodementia), often in association with conversion symptoms, clouding of consciousness, and pseudo-hallucinations [40]. The diagnostic criteria are vague, but the key clinical features are, apart from the approximate responses, the exhibition of dissociative symptoms and the exclusion of neurological diseases. The scientific literature consists of about 100 cases without evidence of a specific distribution of the disease around the world. However, as the original description of Ganser suggested, it is found to be more frequent in men in detention or judicial/forensic settings, but has also been described in juveniles and children [41]. Although some metabolic studies have been conducted on these patients [42], the link between the illogical flagrant conducts and neural changes is widely unknown.

Somatoform Disorders

The prevalence rates for symptoms, without medical explanations, is about 10% in the general population [43] and between 15 and 60% in primary care patients [44–46]. It is extremely difficult to trace a map of these disorders around the world and across ethnicities, as few community-based studies are available. However, differences among countries and economic status do not seem to be substantial [47]. The prevalence of somatoform disorders varies from 1 to 6% in community-based studies (for a review see [48]). These disorders are more common than earlier assumed and represent a major burden in terms of expense for the general healthcare system. In Europe, in 2010, the estimated costs of caring for somatoform disorders were EUR 21.2 billion [49]. Hence, somatoform disorders can cause significant impairment, especially when they appear as a comorbidity with other psychiatric conditions [45]. In a recent German study, a high rate of suicidality was reported [50].

Psychogenic Nonepileptic Seizures or Nonepileptic Attacks Disorder

At the end of the 19th century, the Charcot school in France introduced the term 'hystero-epilepsy' to suggest a link between the two disorders, with hypersensitivity in the regions of the fallopian tubes being the most important triggering factor for hysterical attacks.

The psychogenic nonepileptic seizures (PNES) or nonepileptic attacks disorder current definition is the presence of discernible changes in behavior or consciousness that resemble epileptic seizures but do not produce electroencephalographic alterations. There are catatonic, major motor, minor motor, and subjective variants of PNES [51]. Minor motor activity is probably most frequent in children [52].

Video-EEG (with or without provocation procedures), demonstrating the absences of epileptiform discharges during the crisis, is the gold standard for PNES diagnosis. However, access to continuous EEG video monitoring is generally restricted to specialized epilepsy centers, for which the availability varies among different countries. Recently, an international consensus group of clinical researchers reported an exclusive clinical approach to diagnosis [53].

The link between PNES and drug-resistant epilepsies is straightforward. In epilepsy centers, PNES is diagnosed in 20–40% of patients referred for refractory seizures [5, 54]. At least 1 out of 5 patients with PNES has been admitted at least once in intensive care with the wrong diagnosis of epileptic status and submitted to tracheal intubation or heavy antiepileptic drug regimens.

Not surprisingly, in line with Charcot's definition of hystero-epilepsy, PNES and drug-resistant epilepsy often coexist in the same patient. Usually, PNES diagnosis is only evident at an average of 5–10 years after the first clinical manifestations [55].

Although PNES is a worldwide phenomenon, most of our knowledge derives from studies performed in the USA, Europe, and Australia. However, prevalence, age, sexual distribution (female/male = 7/3), association with depression and stress factors share similar features in Brazil [56], Southwest China [57], Lebanon [58], and India [59].

The estimated prevalence is about 2–33 cases per 100,000 population worldwide [5]. Thus, PNES is a disorder as prevalent as multiple sclerosis and trigeminal neuralgia. As for dissociative disorders, antecedent sexual trauma or abuses are determinant factors.

The 'ataques de nervio' in Puerto Ricans, 'kyole goeu' ('wind overload') in Cambodians, 'falling out' syndrome of Bahamians and Southern African-Americans are cultural variants of PNES, generally presenting after stressful life events. However, there are no sufficient epidemiological data to suggest that populations subjected to wars, terrorism, poverty, or migration have higher rates of conversion disorders. Nevertheless, in veterans, posttraumatic stress disorder appears to be the most important psychiatric comorbidity differentiating patients with PNES from patients with genuine epilepsy [60].

MRI and functional neuroimaging studies suggest that altered brain connectivity in neural networks involved both in premotor control and emotional regulations could be the common dysfunctional final pathway of adult cases of PNES manifesting with motor features [61].

Functional (Pseudoneurological) Medically Unexplained Symptoms (Conversion Disorder)

Several studies have indicated that 'functional' weakness or psychogenic paralysis (one of the most common symptoms) is not so rare in clinical settings. The annual incidence is about 3–5/100,000 in the general population [62, 63]. The degree of functional impairment is surprisingly similar to organic paralysis [63]. The female proportion appears predominant only in the most recent studies and is not dependent on socioeconomic status [63]. Other pseudoneurological symptoms are hemisensory loss, blindness, tunnel vision, tremor of a limb or the whole body, functional dystonia, difficult coordination and gait, stuttering, anomia, loss of hearing or smell, and psychogenic dementia. With regard to cultural factors, relatively few variations are apparent around the world across ethnicities and social categories (for a review see [48]).

Patients with conversion disorders generally seem to lack concern about their impairments ('la belle indifférence') and they do not accept stress, anxiety, or depression as potential explanations for their symptoms [64]. Indeed, the best term to employ for patients to communicate diagnosis is probably functional disorders [64]. However, it is unknown whether the 'belle indifference' and communicative aspects of diagnosis should substantially differ across different cultures. In a systematic study that has reviewed studies published since 1965, reporting rates of la 'belle indifférence' in patients with conversion symptoms and/or patients with organic disease, the available evidence did not support the use of these signs to discriminate between conversion symptoms and symptoms of organic disease. Due to the poor quality of the published studies (most of them lacked clear operational definitions and ratings), it has been suggested that the term 'la belle indifférence' be abandoned as a clinical sign until both its definition and its utility have been clarified [65].

Trauma or an extreme degree of anxiety are always the psychic basis of these disorders. For the pseudoneurological paresis, several functional neuroimaging studies point to the role of the premotor, associative sensorimotor, and limbic areas in preventing (involuntarily) voluntary movements [66–68].

Somatization Disorder

Somatization disorders consist of chronic and recurrent somatic complaints, which cannot be explained by physical causes, or at least exceed what would be expected from a known physical problem. These complaints usually have a negative repercussion on social or occupational roles, and result in seeking medical attention repeatedly.

The spectrum of these physical symptoms often exceeds neurological borders. Complaints are subjective and heterogeneous (dizziness, tinnitus, sore throat and dry mouth, pharyngeal globus, 'pseudo' eustachian tube dysfunction, being 'unable to hear', 'acouphénes', catarrh and postnasal drip, atypical facial pain, burning mouth, chronic cough, fatigue, weakness, sleep difficulties, headache, muscle ache and joint pain, problems with memory, attention and concentration, irritability, nausea and other gastro-intestinal symptoms, palpitations, shortness of breath, noncardiac chest pain, fibromyalgia and other chronic pain syndromes, tension-type headache, chronic whiplash, failed back syndrome, sick building syndrome, multiple chemical hypersensitivity, and irritable bowel syndrome), and often difficult to localize and/or accommodate to specific and known neurological syndromes. Somatization disorders usually begin in adolescence or young adulthood. A study identified the family environment of these patients to be emotionally cold, distant, unsupportive, and with notions of abuse [69]. There is also evidence of a high rate of comorbidity of somatization disorders with both anxiety and depression. The prevalence is very high: 0.2–2% in women and less than 0.2% in men in the general population.

Some cultural syndromes are noteworthy. In young Asian Indian males, the 'dhat' represents the fear of loss of seminal fluid during nocturnal emissions, or through urination, a situation experienced as harmful because it depletes the body of physical and mental energy. Feelings of being infested by ants or worms are common in Nigeria, which has adopted a specific questionnaire (the Enugu somatization scale) which has been specifically constructed to include somatic symptoms that could be disregarded by standard questionnaires designed for North American and European populations [70].

Body Dysmorphic Disorder (or Dysmorphophobia)

Body dysmorphic disorder (BDD) is a condition of important concern about imaginary or small physical anomalies, often with delusional symptoms. Patients present compulsive behaviors centered on the physical anomaly (mirror checking or avoiding, hiding the defect, comparisons with other people, seeking surgery, or other medical treatments). Common complaints of BDD patients concern hair, skin, lips, stomach, nose, eyes, chin, teeth, head shape, body build, entire face, breasts, and sexual organs.

According to a US telephone survey, the prevalence of BDD does not differ by gender (2.4% for men and 2.2% for women), exceeds the prevalence of schizophrenia and bipolar disorder type I, and equals that of generalized anxiety disorder [71]. The prevalence rate is 2–10% in patients requesting plastic surgery [72]. However, a clear epidemiology is not discernable since many patients may hide their body concerns; therefore, BDD is probably underdiagnosed. BDD is often associated with obsessive compulsive disorder, social phobia, major and atypical depression, generalized anxiety disorder, avoidant personality disorder, alexithymia, bulimia nervosa, substance abuse or dependence. There are significant suicidal tendencies in patients with BDD [73].

Conclusions

Dissociative and somatoform diseases (formerly included under the umbrella term of 'hysteria') probably represent the two faces of the same coin, displaying psychic and behavioral phenomena that have a high worldwide prevalence. The clinical presentation of these disorders might be particularly flagrant or, conversely, covert and subtle, and thus might be underdiagnosed. All of them manifest with some degree of dissociation among identity, memory, sensation, movement, and the physical body. Hence, some authors propose to include the somatoform diseases in the category of dissociative disorders. All dissociative and somatoform disorders are undoubtedly related to trauma, abuse, neglect, or to any kind of severe stressful events.

Though transcultural epidemiological studies are lacking, available data, with some minor exceptions, suggest similar rates of prevalence and a common semiology around the world.

There is now a growing body of functional neuroimaging studies suggesting that conversion disorders might be the consequence of the dynamic reorganization of neural circuits involved in processing volition, memory, movement, and perception. Therefore, these networks are thought to enhance self-recognition, autobiographical and retrograde memory, and the affective correlates of selfhood. Psychotraumatic experiences may lead to their disruption or defective integration, leading to dissociative behaviors as one of the extreme adaptive survival strategies for the human being. This may occur, for example, at the stage of preconscious motor planning or modality-specific attention. Unfortunately, most of these neuroimaging studies involved only small numbers of patients with different comorbidities and durations of symptoms. Hence, there is the need to perform larger transcultural studies with homogeneous groups of patients according to specific diagnosis and controlling for comorbidities such as anxiety or depression. A combination of new experimental paradigms and novel imaging techniques might increase our understanding of the neurobiological mechanisms of hysteria-associated disorders.

References

1 McDonald I: Gordon Holmes Lecture: Gordon Holmes and the neurological heritage. Brain 2007;130:288–298.
2 Aring CD: A tribute to Sir Gordon Homes. J Nerv Mental Dis 1965;141: 497–502.
3 Holmes G: Introduction to Clinical Neurology. Edinburgh, E&S Livingstone, 1946.
4 Carson AJ, Ringbauer B, Stone J, McKenzie L, Warlow C, Sharpe M: Do medically unexplained symptoms matter? A prospective cohort study of 300 new referrals to neurology outpatient clinics. J Neurol Neurosurg Psychiatry 2000;68: 207–210.
5 Benbadis SR, Agrawal V, Tatum WO: How many patients with psychogenic nonepileptic seizures also have epilepsy? Neurology 2001;57:915–917.
6 Markowitsch HJ, Staniloiu A: The impairment of recollection in functional amnesic states. Cortex 2013;49:1494–1510.
7 Deeley Q, Oakley DA, Toone B, Bell V, Walsh E, Marquand AF, et al: The functional anatomy of suggested limb paralysis. Cortex 2013;49:411–422.
8 Bernstein EM, Putnam FW: Development, reliability, and validity of a dissociation scale. J Nerv Ment Dis 1986;174: 727–735.
9 Ross C, Heber S, Norton G, Anderson D, Anderson G, Barchet P: The Dissociative Disorders Interview Schedule: a structured interview. Dissociation 1989;II:169–189.
10 Steinberg M: Structured Clinical Interview for DSM-IV Dissociative Disorders (SCID-D). Washington, American Psychiatric Press, 1994.
11 Dell P: The Multidimensional Inventory of Dissociation (MID): a comprehensive measure of pathological dissociation. J Trauma Dissociation 2006;7:77–106.
12 Cohen B, Mills A, Kijak A: An introduction to the Diagnostic Drawing Series: a standardized tool for diagnostic and clinical use. Art Ther 1994;11:105–110.

13 Coons PM: The dissociative disorders. Rarely considered and underdiagnosed. Psychiatr Clin North Am 1998;21:637–648.
14 Sar V: Epidemiology of dissociative disorders. An overview. Epidemiol Res Int 2011;2011:1–8.
15 Mueller-Pfeiffer C, Rufibach K, Perron N, Wyss D, Kuenzler C, Prezewowsky C, Pitman RK, Rufer M: Global functioning and disability in dissociative disorders. Psychiatry Res 2012;200:475–481.
16 Staniloiu A, Bender A, Smolewska K, Ellis J, Abramowitz C, Markowitsch HJ: Ganser syndrome with work-related onset in a patient with a background of immigration. Cogn Neuropsychiatry 2009;14:180–198.
17 Stein DJ, Koenen KC, Friedman MJ, Hill E, McLaughlin KA, Petukhova M, et al: Dissociation in posttraumatic stress disorder: evidence from the world mental health surveys. Biol Psychiatry 2013;73:302–312.
18 Kanzer M: Amnesia, a statistical analysis. Am J Psy 1939;96:711–716.
19 Sargant W, Slater E: Amnesic syndromes in war. Proc R Soc Med 1941;34:757–764.
20 Porter S, Birt AR, Yuille JC, Hervé HF: Memory for murder. A psychological perspective on dissociative amnesia in legal contexts. Int J Law Psychiatry 2001;24:23–42.
21 Gwandure C: Dissociative fugue: diagnosis, presentation and treatment among the traditional Shona people. Open Anthropol J, 2008, pp 1–10.
22 Stracciari A, Fonti C, Guarino M: When the past is lost: focal retrograde amnesia. Focus on the 'functional' form. Behav Neurol 2008;20:113–125.
23 McKay G, Kopelman M: Psychogenic amnesia: when memory complaints are medically unexplained. Adv Psychiatr Treat 2009;1:152–158.
24 Coons PM, Milstein V: Psychogenic amnesia: a clinical investigation of 25 cases. Dissociation 1992;5:73–79.
25 Reinhold N, Markowitsch HJ: Retrograde episodic memory and emotion: a perspective from patients with dissociative amnesia. Neuropsychologia 2009;47:2197–2206.
26 Markowitsch HJ, Calabrese P, Fink GR, Durwen HF, Kessler J, Härting C, et al: Impaired episodic memory retrieval in a case of probable psychogenic amnesia. Psychiatry Res 1997;74:119–126.
27 Markowitsch HJ: Psychogenic amnesia. Neuroimage 2003;20(Suppl 1):S132–S138.
28 Ross CA, Ness L: Symptom patterns in dissociative identity disorder patients and the general population. J Trauma Dissociation 2010;11:458–468.
29 Van der Hart O: Multiple personality disorder in Europe: impressions. Dissociation 1993;23:102–118.
30 Spanos NP: Multiple identity enactments and multiple personality disorder: a sociocognitive perspective. Psychol Bull 1994;116:143–165.
31 Modestin J: Multiple personality disorder in Switzerland. Am J Psychiatry 1992;149:88–92.
32 Dell P: Dissociation and the Dissociative Disorders: DSM-V and Beyond. London, Routledge, 2009.
33 Ross CA, Anderson G, Fleisher WP, Norton GR: The frequency of multiple personality disorder among psychiatric inpatients. Am J Psychiatry 1991;148:1717–1720.
34 Lewis DO, Yeager CA, Swica Y, Pincus JH, Lewis M: Objective documentation of child abuse and dissociation in 12 murderers with dissociative identity disorder. Am J Psychiatry 1997;154:1703–1710.
35 Ross CA, Norton GR: Suicide and parasuicide in multiple personality disorder. Psychiatry 1989;52:365–371.
36 Brand B, Classen C, Lanius R, Loewenstein R, McNary S, Pain C, et al: A naturalistic study of dissociative identity disorder and dissociative disorder not otherwise specified patients treated by community clinicians. Psychol Trauma Theory Res Pract Policy 2009;1:153–171.
37 Michal M, Glaesmer H, Zwerenz R, Knebel A, Wiltink J, Brähler E, et al: Base rates for depersonalization according to the 2-item version of the Cambridge Depersonalization Scale (CDS-2) and its associations with depression/anxiety in the general population. J Affect Disord 2011;128:106–111.
38 Tschan R, Wiltink J, Adler J, Beutel ME, Michal M: Depersonalization experiences are strongly associated with dizziness and vertigo symptoms leading to increased health care consumption in the German general population. J Nerv Ment Dis 2013;201:629–635.
39 Sierra M, Gomez J, Molina JJ, Luque R, Muñoz JF, David AS: Depersonalization in psychiatric patients: a transcultural study. J Nerv Ment Dis 2006;194:356–361.
40 Ganser SJM: Über einen eigenartigen hysterischen Dämmerzustand. Archiv Psychiatrie Nervenkrankheiten (Berlin) 1898;30:633–640.
41 Miller P, Bramble D, Buxton N: Case study: Ganser syndrome in children and adolescents. J Am Acad Child Adolesc Psychiatry 1997;36:112–115.
42 Snyder SL, Buchsbaum MS, Krishna RC: Unusual visual symptoms and Ganser-like state due to cerebral injury: a case study using (18)F-deoxyglucose positron emission tomography. Behav Neurol 1998;11:51–54.
43 Jacobi F, Wittchen H-U, Holting C, Höfler M, Pfister H, Müller N, et al: Prevalence, co-morbidity and correlates of mental disorders in the general population: results from the German Health Interview and Examination Survey (GHS). Psychol Med 2004;34:597–611.
44 Mergl R, Seidscheck I, Allgaier A-K, Möller H-J, Hegerl U, Henkel V: Depressive, anxiety, and somatoform disorders in primary care: prevalence and recognition. Depress Anxiety 2007;24:185–195.
45 De Waal MWM, Arnold IA, Eekhof JAH, van Hemert AM: Somatoform disorders in general practice: prevalence, functional impairment and comorbidity with anxiety and depressive disorders. Br J Psychiatry 2004;184:470–476.
46 Fink P, Sørensen L, Engberg M, Holm M, Munk-Jørgensen P: Somatization in primary care. Prevalence, health care utilization, and general practitioner recognition. Psychosomatics 1999;40:330–338.
47 Gureje O, Simon GE, Ustun TB, Goldberg DP: Somatization in cross-cultural perspective: a World Health Organization study in primary care. Am J Psychiatry 1997;154:989–995.
48 Brown R, Lewis-Fernandez R: Culture and conversion disorder: implications for DSM-5. Psychiatry 2011;74:187–206.
49 Gustavsson A, Svensson M, Jacobi F, Allgulander C, Alonso J, Beghi E, et al: Cost of disorders of the brain in Europe 2010. Eur Neuropsychopharmacol 2011;21:718–779.
50 Wiborg JF, Gieseler D, Fabisch AB, Voigt K, Lautenbach A, Löwe B: Suicidality in primary care patients with somatoform disorders. Psychosom Med 2013;75:800–806.

51 Griffith NM, Szaflarski JP, Schefft BK, Isaradisaikul D, Meckler JM, McNally KA, et al: Relationship between semiology of psychogenic nonepileptic seizures and Minnesota Multiphasic Personality Inventory profile. Epilepsy Behav 2007; 11:105–111.
52 Alessi R, Vincentiis S, Rzezak P, Valente KD: Semiology of psychogenic nonepileptic seizures: age-related differences. Epilepsy Behav 2013;27:292–295.
53 Lafrance WC, Baker GA, Duncan R, Goldstein LH, Reuber M: Minimum requirements for the diagnosis of psychogenic nonepileptic seizures: a staged approach: a report from the International League against Epilepsy Nonepileptic Seizures Task Force. Epilepsia 2013;54: 2005–2018.
54 Iriarte J, Parra J, Urrestarazu E, Kuyk J: Controversies in the diagnosis and management of psychogenic pseudoseizures. Epilepsy Behav 2003;4:354–359.
55 Reuber M, Fernández G, Bauer J, Helmstaedter C, Elger CE: Diagnostic delay in psychogenic nonepileptic seizures. Neurology 2002;58:493–495.
56 Alessi R, Valente KD: Psychogenic nonepileptic seizures at a tertiary care center in Brazil. Epilepsy Behav 2013;26: 91–95.
57 An D, Wu X, Yan B, Mu J, Zhou D: Clinical features of psychogenic nonepileptic seizures: a study of 64 cases in southwest China. Epilepsy Behav 2010;17: 408–411.
58 Rosenberg HJ, Rosenberg SD, Williamson PD, Wolford GL: A comparative study of trauma and posttraumatic stress disorder prevalence in epilepsy patients and psychogenic nonepileptic seizure patients. Epilepsia 2000;41:447–452.
59 Dhiman V, Sinha S, Rawat VS, Harish T, Chaturvedi SK, Satishchandra P: Semiological characteristics of adults with psychogenic nonepileptic seizures (PNESs): an attempt towards a new classification. Epilepsy Behav 2013;27:427–432.
60 Salinsky M, Evrard C, Storzbach D, Pugh MJ: Psychiatric comorbidity in veterans with psychogenic seizures. Epilepsy Behav 2012;25:345–349.
61 Arzy S, Halje P, Schechter DS, Spinelli L, Seeck M, Blanke O: Neural generators of psychogenic seizures: evidence from intracranial and extracranial brain recordings. Epilepsy Behav 2014;31:381–385.
62 Binzer M, Andersen PM, Kullgren G: Clinical characteristics of patients with motor disability due to hysteria: a systematic review. Br J Psychiatry 2006; 188:204–209.
63 Stone J, Warlow C, Sharpe M: The symptom of functional weakness: a controlled study of 107 patients. Brain 2010; 133:1537–1551.
64 Stone J, Wojcik W, Durrance D, Carson A, Lewis S, MacKenzie L, et al: What should we say to patients with symptoms unexplained by disease? The 'number needed to offend'. BMJ 2002; 325:1449–1450.
65 Stone J, Smyth R, Carson A, Warlow C, Sharpe M: La belle indifférence in conversion symptoms and hysteria: systematic review. Br J Psychiatry 2006;188: 204–209.
66 Cojan Y, Waber L, Carruzzo A, Vuilleumier P: Motor inhibition in hysterical conversion paralysis. Neuroimage 2009; 47:1026–1037.
67 Voon V, Gallea C, Hattori N, Bruno M, Ekanayake V, Hallett M: The involuntary nature of conversion disorder. Neurology 2010;74:223–238.
68 Van Beilen M, de Jong BM, Gieteling EW, Renken R, Leenders KL: Abnormal parietal function in conversion paresis. PLoS One 2011;6:e25918.
69 Brown RJ, Schrag A, Trimble MR: Dissociation, childhood interpersonal trauma, and family functioning in patients with somatization disorder. Am J Psychiatry 2005;162:899–905.
70 Ebigbo PO: A cross sectional study of somatic complaints of Nigerian females using the Enugu Somatization Scale. Cult Med Psychiatry 1986;10:167–186.
71 Koran LM, Abujaoude E, Large MD, Serpe RT: The prevalence of body dysmorphic disorder in the United States adult population. CNS Spectr 2008;13: 316–322.
72 Hollander E, Neville D, Frenkel M, Josephson S, Liebowitz MR: Body dysmorphic disorder. Diagnostic issues and related disorders. Psychosomatics 1992; 33:156–165.
73 Phillips KA, Coles ME, Menard W, Yen S, Fay C, Weisberg RB: Suicidal ideation and suicide attempts in body dysmorphic disorder. J Clin Psychiatry 2005;66: 717–725.

Dr. Antonio Carota
Center for Brain and Nervous System Diseases, GSMN Neurocenter, Clinique de Genolier
Rte du Muids 3, CP 100
CH–1272 Genolier (Switzerland)
E-Mail acarota@genolier.net

Bogousslavsky J (ed): Hysteria: The Rise of an Enigma. Front Neurol Neurosci. Basel, Karger, 2014, vol 35, pp 181–197
DOI: 10.1159/000360242

History of Physical and 'Moral' Treatment of Hysteria

Emmanuel Broussolle[a] · Florent Gobert[a] · Teodor Danaila[a] · Stéphane Thobois[a] · Olivier Walusinski[b] · Julien Bogousslavsky[c]

[a]Centre de Neurosciences Cognitives, Service de Neurologie C, Hôpital Neurologique Pierre Wertheimer, Hospices Civils de Lyon, Université Claude Bernard Lyon I, Lyon, and [b]Family Physician, Private Practice, Brou, France; [c]Center for Brain and Nervous System Diseases, GSMN Neurocenter, Clinique Valmont, Glion/Montreux, Switzerland

Abstract

This historical review presents the advances made mostly during the last 200 years on the description, concepts, theories, and (more specifically) cure of patients suffering from hysteria, a still obscure entity. The denomination of the syndrome has changed over time, from hysteria (reinvestigated by Paul Briquet and Jean-Martin Charcot) to pithiatism (Joseph Babinski), then to conversion neurosis (Sigmund Freud), and today functional neurological disorders according to the 2013 American Neurological Association DSM-5 classification. The treatment was renewed in the second half of the 19th century in Paris by Paul Briquet and then by Jean-Martin Charcot. Hysterical women, who represented the great majority of cases, were cured by physical therapy (notably physio-, hydro-, and electrotherapy, and in some cases ovary compression) and 'moral' therapies (general, causal therapy, rest, isolation, hypnosis, and suggestion). At the turn of the 19th and 20th centuries, psychotherapy, psychoanalysis, and persuasion were established respectively by Pierre Janet, Sigmund Freud, and Joseph Babinski. During World War I, military forces faced a large number of post-trauma neurosis cases among soldiers (named the 'Babinski-Froment war neurosis' and Myers 'shell shock', in the French and English literature, respectively). This led to the use of more brutal therapies in military hospitals, combining electrical shock and persuasion, particularly in France with Clovis Vincent and Gustave Roussy, but also in Great Britain and Germany. After World War I, this method was abandoned and there was a marked decrease in interest in hysteria for a long period of time. Today, the current treatment comprises (if possible intensive) physiotherapy, together with psychotherapy, and in some cases psychoanalysis. Antidepressants and anxiolytics may be required, and more recently cognitive and behavioral therapy. Repetitive transcranial magnetic stimulation is a new technique under investigation which may be promising in patients presenting with motor conversion syndrome (motor deficit or movement disorder). Functional neurological disorders remain a difficult problem to manage with frequent failures and chronic handicapping evolution. This emphasizes the need for therapeutic innovations in the future.

A number of historical reviews on hysteria have been published, particularly on the description of its large clinical spectrum and the pathophysiological hypotheses that were made about this still complex entity. The present dissertation is aimed at giving an overview of the various treatments of hysteria employed over the centuries, mostly from the 17th century until contemporary times. These include physical therapy (notably physio-, hydro-, and electrotherapy) and 'moral' therapies (general, causal therapy, rest, isolation, hypnosis, psychic therapy, and persuasion). In order to achieve this challenging goal, a brief recall on the changes of concepts concerning hysteria will be presented for each part of this essay. In a chronological order we will consider (1) the pre-Charcot era until Briquet's contribution in the mid-19th century; (2) the changes made by Charcot, his students, and his contemporaries, notably the use of hypnosis and suggestion; (3) the new steps formulated by Janet and Freud, as well as Dejerine and Sollier at the turn of the 19th and 20th centuries; (4) the Babinski concept of pithiatism and persuasion at the very beginning of the 20th century; (5) war neurosis, shell shock, and 'torpillage', which were particularly studied during World War I, and (6) the progressive evolution of physical and psychological therapeutic approaches after World War II and during the recent decades.

From the Ancient Times to the Mid-19th Century before Charcot

Antique Times

Although the term hysteria comes from a Greek word and refers to the uterus, this entity was first mentioned more than 4,000 years ago in Egyptian medicine [1]. During the Greek and Roman times, Hippocrates and Galen presented hysteria as a syndrome resulting from the migration of the uterus upward in the body and classified it as a mental illness.

The 17th and 18th Centuries and the Inventive Work of Sydenham, Cullen, Ferriar, de La Mettrie, and Mesmer

In the late 17th and during the 18th centuries, several British physicians contributed to the study of diseases of the nervous system and notably hysteria [1]. Thomas Sydenham (1624–1689) supported the idea that hysteria resulted from the ability to mimic various diseases in relation with emotional troubles. William Cullen (1710–1790) was one of the first to present a nosological classification of nervous and mental diseases. He identified the neuroses among which he believed hysteria should be assigned to [2, 3]. In 1795, the term hysterical conversion was proposed for the first time by John Ferriar (1761–1815), who classified hysteria with visceral spasms [1, 4].

In the mid-18th century, Julien Offray de La Mettrie (1709–1751), a French philosopher who owes his fame to his materialist ideas, reported on a case of 'grande hystérie' (hysteria-epilepsy), almost 150 years before its full description [5].

In the late 18th century, Franz Anton Mesmer (1734–1815), an Austrian physician, came to Paris and proposed to treat hysterical patients as a group with magnetism using a magnet [6]. In 1784, however, the method, also called 'mesmerism', was criticized by a council of experts, who stated that this method had no scientific basis and should therefore no longer be used [1]. Nevertheless, mesmerism remained popular, and may be considered as a precursory step before the advent of hypnosis in the 19th century.

Pinel and Esquirol: The Founders of Psychiatry in the Early 19th Century

The turn of the 18th and 19th centuries and the first half of the 19th century were revolutionary times in medicine, particularly in Paris. In the field of psychiatry, Philippe Pinel (1745–1826) was a great pioneer [3, 7] and the first to distinguish insane/alienated patients from misfits, beggars, and other vagabonds. Pinel individualized four main nosological entities of mental diseases:

mania, melancholia, dementia, and idiocy. While several contemporary physicians, notably Vincenzo Chiarugi (1759–1820) in Italy, proposed the moral care for patients with mental illnesses, Pinel offered detailed accounts of case histories and the full description of moral treatment [8, 9]. This was not only a matter of humanitarianism, but a process of gaining the confidence of patients and of providing them a stimulating and pleasing environment. The moral treatment was later expanded to describe mental and psychic therapies. Jean-Etienne Esquirol (1772–1840), a student of Pinel, also played a major role with his treatise on mental diseases and the 1838 law that led to the creation of asylums in all parts of France [3]. Pinel did not pay very much attention to hysteria. In the first edition of his nosographic book [10], he considered hysteria as an example of 'névroses de la génération de la femme', i.e. 'female genital neurosis' in English, among which nymphomania belonged to as well. Pinel believed as others that these neuroses originated from a dysfunction of the neural state of female organs, namely the uterus. He suspected that continence may be causal and thus suggested marriage as a preventive and curative therapy.

The Mid-19th Century and the Contributions of Briquet, Brachet and Landouzy

Early in the second half of the 19th century, a major work on hysteria was published in Paris by Paul Briquet (1796–1881), entitled *Traité clinique et thérapeutique de l'hystérie* (*Clinical and Therapeutic Treatise on Hysteria*) [11, 12].

Briquet presented a series of 430 patients, including 7 men, and thus provided evidence that hysteria was neither restricted to female patients nor related to the uterus, but rather to the brain. However, no brain lesions were found in the cases that came to autopsy. Factors found to be associated with hysteria were youth, female sex, 'affective' and 'impressionable' temperament, family history of the disorder, low social class, migration, sexual licentiousness, situational difficulties, and poor physical health. The damaging role of violence and sexual abuse in infancy was also depicted.

Briquet described the multiple clinical manifestations of this syndrome which were then classified into seven categories: hyperesthesia including pain, anesthesia, sensory hallucinations, spasms including of the abdomen, attacks (convulsions), palsies, and abnormal contractility.

Another important contribution of Briquet was his extensive review of the numerous therapies proposed for the care of hysterical patients, some employed in the past – even antique times – and others currently in use at the time of his publication. General care comprised the cure of the cause or associated pathologies (tumors, inflammation), along with the recommendation to keep away the family (husband, parents), hydrotherapy, fresh milk, and sometimes blood-letting, which apparently was still employed in the mid-19th century! Specific treatments used for restoring the menses included electrical current and cupping glasses or leeches placed on to the vulva or the anus! In addition, medications such as exciting drugs, enemas, antispasmodic remedies, opiates, lotions, frictions, cauterizations, etc., were listed. After this review, Briquet clearly stated that he disapproved all of these old measures except for the use of opiates.

Other peculiar treatments varied upon clinical presentation: (1) hyperesthesia – electric current in some cases, bandage, compression or moistened linen; (2) anesthesia – electric current; (3) spasms – electric current, compression and bandage; (4) attacks – compression of genital parts (ovarian compression, see below), finger pinching, nail wrenching, tearing pubic hair out, blood-letting, leeches, blister, and (5) palsies – opiates, electric current and faradization. Briquet's comments were again that all these treatments were no longer justified, the only exception being electric current with faradization. Briquet explicitly mentioned that he referred several patients to Dr. Duchenne for faradization with good outcome.

Guillaume-Benjamin-Amand Duchenne (1806–1875), a great French pioneer in neurology [13], was at that time working in different places in Paris and had become very productive in using his procedure on localized electrical stimulation with faradic current [14].

Briquet emphasized the prophylactic importance of an improvement in familial and social circumstances, and the need to minimize environmental problems. Education including playing music, good nutrition, thermal water, and marriage were recommended.

Since many authors credit the first description of the entire syndrome of hysteria to Briquet, this explains why his work eclipsed that of two other French authors published a few years earlier. Jean-Louis Brachet (1789–1858), a physician from Lyon, considered that sexual continence was not the only cause of hysteria and, following Pinel, proposed the 'moral' treatment, namely creating confidence between the patient and the physician, keeping the patient away from the disabling environmental causes, listening kindly to patient's complaints, and using remedies such as antispasmodic drugs [15]. In Paris, Hector Landouzy [16] (1812–1864) had a critical view of the therapies proposed to treat hysteric women and concluded that the best treatment was to never prescribe any ('le meilleur remède est de n'en prescrire jamais') or to use hygienic methods similar to those reviewed above about Briquet's treatise.

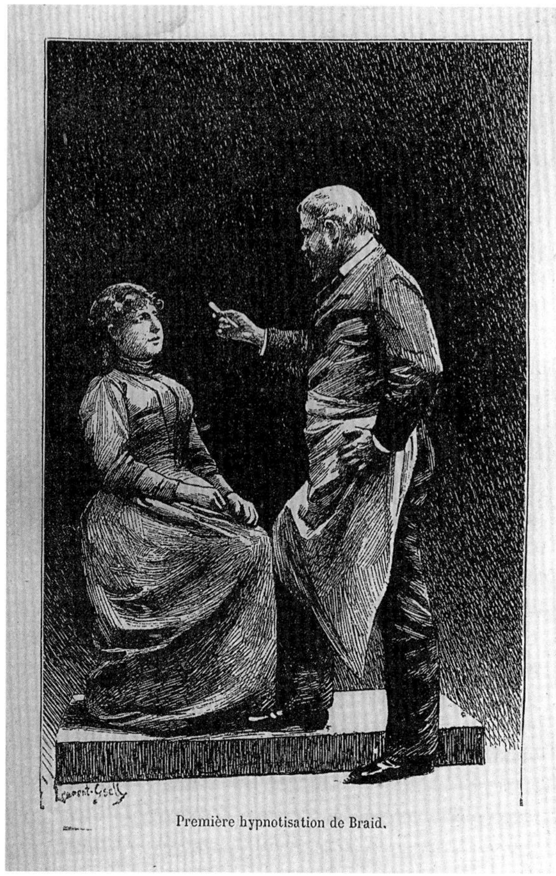

Fig. 1. Braid's hypnosis method. Etching by Alexandre Laurent Gsell (1860–1944) in *L'hypnotisme* [78] (Olivier Walusinski personal collection).

Charcot and His Contemporaries: Hypnosis, Suggestion, and Ovarian Compression

As demonstrated above, the care of hysterical patients was largely influenced during the mid-19th century by the coexistence of empirical and aggressive methods on one hand, and the increasing influence of the moral treatment introduced by Pinel and Esquirol on the other hand. In the second half of the 19th century though, Pinel's legacy was somewhat forgotten and the advent of new revolutionary methods and hypothesis had a profound influence on the way hysterical patients were considered and cured.

The first important breakthrough was made on hypnosis in 1843 by the British physician James Braid (1795–1860; fig. 1). With the introduction of his neurophysiologic theory of hypnosis, he buried Mesmer's doctrine of animal magnetism and established hypnotic phenomena as a scientific approach [17]. Although his contribution is underrecognized, Braid had an important influence on the development of hypnosis and its use in hysteria by Charcot and others.

Charcot and Hysteria

Jean-Martin Charcot (1825–1893) was one of the most distinguished neurologists of the 19th century [13]. He contributed to many aspects of neurology and created the renowned Salpêtrière School of Neurology in Paris.

Charcot began to take an interest in hysteria in 1870 when he took over the hystero-epileptic department from Louis Delasiauve (1804–1893). At that time, he agreed with the definition made by Charles Lasègue (1816–1883) on hysteria [18]: 'One provisionally calls hysteria an ensemble of nervous manifestations, which may develop in young women, exceptionally in young men, and which do not correspond to a known lesion of the nervous centers.'

With Paul Richer (1849–1933), one of his faithful pupils, Charcot differentiated organic epilepsy from hystero-epilepsy – also called epilepsia-hysteria ('grande hystérie'), which had four successive phases: epileptoid period, clownism, passionate attitudes (which included the famous arc of a circle posture), and delirium [19, 20].

Charcot further described hyperesthesia, anesthesia, paralyses and contractures, and gait disturbances (e.g. dragging gait), among others, as important forms of hysteria which he considered as stigmata. He claimed that stigmata should be present for the diagnosis of hysteria. Although Georges Brutus Gilles de la Tourette (1857–1904), one of Charcot's favorite students, defended Charcot's diagnostic criteria, i.e. the combination of hysterical attacks and of stigmata, in his treatise on hysteria [21], this concept was criticized then abandoned after Charcot's death [22].

During the 1880s, Charcot provided his most original contribution to the field of hysteria by studying traumatic male hysteria which he called 'grand ébranlement psychique' (great psychic shock) [23, 24]. This was later denominated as 'compensation neurosis', which occurred with the rapid rise of industrialization in the second half of the 19th century, and thereafter during the Great War. Compensation neurosis could be a result of such situations as patients trying to avoid legal difficulties of military service or to obtain disability payments, veterans' pensions, or compensation following injury.

Charcot and Hypnosis and the Nancy-Salpêtrière Dispute

Charcot proposed to use hypnosis to produce hysterical attacks by suggestion [20], thus considering hysteria as an experimental neurosis. He also used hypnosis to relieve hysterical attacks. His contemporary and competitor, Hippolyte Bernheim (1840–1919), from the Nancy school, established the use of hypnosis to suppress the symptom in a large series of hysterical patients [25]. An important number of hysterical women were referred to Charcot due to 'grande attaque d'hystérie'. The most renowned were Blanche Wittmann and Augustine Gleizes. Charcot's work on hysteria became controversial because of his influence on hysterical women using suggestion to produce hysteric attacks [26] and for his organic conceptions of hysteria. The Nancy school strongly opposed this view, stating that 'grande hystérie' was somewhat theatrical, specific to Charcot's power of suggestion, which Bernheim called 'culture hysteria', and thus far different from other forms of hysteria and very rare outside Salpêtrière Hospital [26]. Recent work, however, has examined Charcot's attitude towards women and contests the common view that he was misogynist [24].

Isolation, Rest Cure, and Other Physical Methods Used to Cure Hysteric Patients during Charcot's Times

Isolation and rest were proposed during the 19th century to treat many nervous and mental diseases by a large number of physicians, including Brachet, Landouzy, and Briquet, as stressed before. This method was also supported by Charcot to treat hysterical women. Yet, the concept of the rest cure has been particularly credited to Silas Weir Mitchell (1829–1914), an American physician from Philadelphia who is considered as one of the founders of American neurology. Weir Mitchell's name is prominently associated with his introduction of the rest cure for nervous diseases, particularly neurasthenia and hysteria [27]. The treatment consisted primarily of isolation, confinement to bed, dieting, electrotherapy, and massage. Weir Mitchell was popularly known as 'Dr. Diet' and 'Dr. Quiet'.

There is an important chapter on the treatment of hysteria during Charcot times in Richer's book on 'grande hystérie' [19]. Most of the other treatments had been already mentioned by Briquet in his 1859 treatise [11] (see above). Richer cited among others, inhaled medications, isolation, musical therapy, vibrations, hydrotherapy, metallotherapy, magnetization, and electrical faradic currents using rheophores (Duchenne's methods).

Vibration therapy was one of the physical therapeutic methods used at the time of Charcot, inspired by pioneers of the 18th and 19th centuries [28]. Charcot used a vibratory armchair ('le trémoussoir') to treat parkinsonian patients and Gilles de la Tourette used a vibratory helmet for patients suffering from headache. These methods were occasionally employed in cases of neurasthenia, but apparently rarely in hysteria.

Ovary Compression and Ovariectomy

Among the physical treatments of hysteria, the uterine hypothesis still had a great impact at the time of Charcot, and Richer outlined several methods to treat the 'diseased' ovary in his book on hystero-epilepsy. His methods were to either place ice on the abdomen or compress the ovary [19]. Ovary compression was in fact suggested by Hippocrates himself and was frequently applied at the time of Charcot using simple or complex ovary compressors (fig. 2). Regrettably, this method inspired some physicians in the 19th century to treat hysterical patients with ovariectomy (oophorectomy). Although ovariectomy had some support in France as in other countries in the late 19th century and even later, Charcot categorically disapproved of using this method as a treatment for women with hysteria [24, 29, 30]. Gilles de la Tourette himself was doubtful about this aggressive surgical method, citing negative results in two ovariectomized hysterical women, and moreover observing the onset of hysteria in a patient after ovariectomy was performed for unrelated reasons [21].

Janet and the Subconscious, Freud and the Conversion Syndrome, and Dejerine and Psychotherapy

Janet

Pierre Janet (1859–1947; fig. 3) was a student of the Ecole Normale Supérieure and agrégé of philosophy in Paris [3, 31]. His research attracted the attention of Charcot. From 1890 on, Janet worked at Salpêtrière Hospital and became director of a pathological psychology laboratory, where he studied patients suffering from hysterical neurosis, the very subject of his 1893 MD thesis [32]. Janet postulated a dissociative state of mind (the subconscious state, i.e. the existence of consciousness outside of personal awareness) to account for certain hysterical features such as permanent stigmata, accidents, memory troubles, trance, and fugue states. In contrast to Freud, he did not evoke any sexual cause of hysteria or other neuroses. He used hypnosis and psychotherapy to treat hysterical patients.

Freud

Sigmund Freud (1856–1939) was first trained in Vienna by renowned neurologists such as Theodor Meynert (1833–1892) and Hermann Nothnagel (1841–1905) [3]. He came to Paris in 1886 and studied hysteria and hypnotism under Charcot, who had a great influence on him. He then returned to Vienna and made a revolutionary breakthrough in psychology in the ensuing decades. Briefly, he defined new frontiers

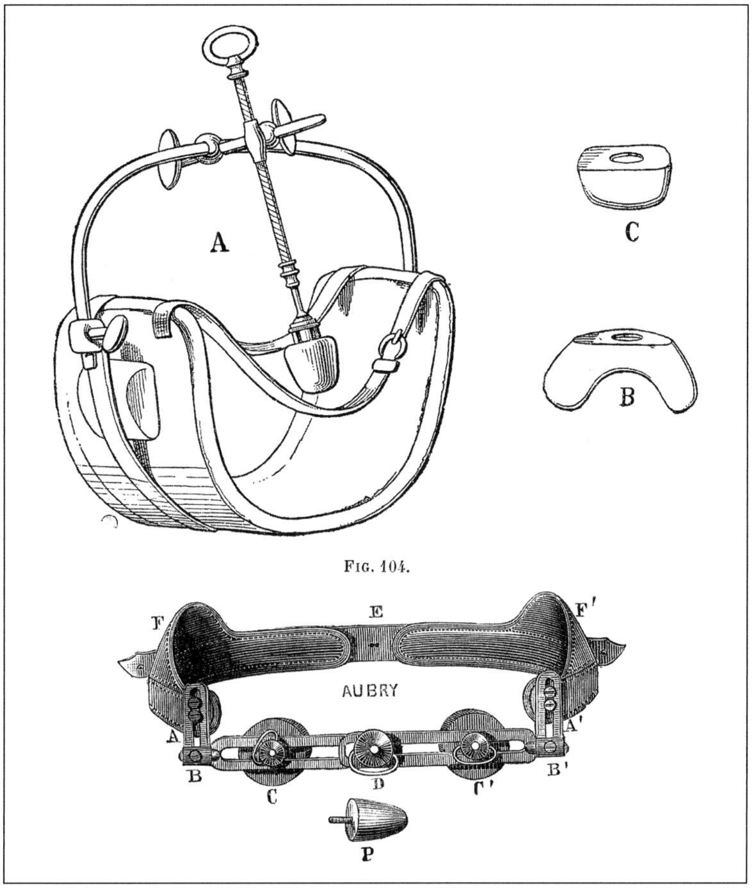

Fig. 2. Two examples of ovary compressors used during Charcot's time. Etching by Paul Richer (1849–1933) in *Etudes cliniques sur l'hystéro-épilepsie ou grande hystérie* [19] (Olivier Walusinski personal collection). Top: fig. 104, p. 596. Bottom: fig. 105, p. 727.

in the human psyche, with the unconscious, the self, and the superego, and proposed psychotherapeutic interventions, notably psychoanalysis.

During the 1890s, Freud invested his time in hysteria and the delineation of other neuroses [33]. He mentioned the term 'la belle indifférence', stating that this expression had been proposed by Charcot in his late years and also by Pierre Janet [34]. This term was to describe the peculiar emotionless presentation of hysterical patients towards their symptoms.

Freud and his students conceived hysterical symptoms as a product of 'ego defense mechanisms', in which psychic energy generated by unconscious psychic conflicts is converted into physical symptoms. This latter concept was widely accepted to the point where the term 'conversion' has been incorporated into the nomenclature of neuroses and the terms 'conversion symptoms' and 'conversion reaction' have come to be synonyms of hysteria.

Freud introduced the sexual unconscious theory of hysteria. He hypothesized that hysteria may originate from a traumatic sexual experience in infancy or adolescence (seduction or sexual excitation by an adult). Like Charcot, Bernheim, and others, he used hypnosis to treat patients. His aim was to suppress the effects of the initial trauma, but later he recused hypnosis as a therapy in hysterical patients for still obscure reasons. It has been suggested, but re-

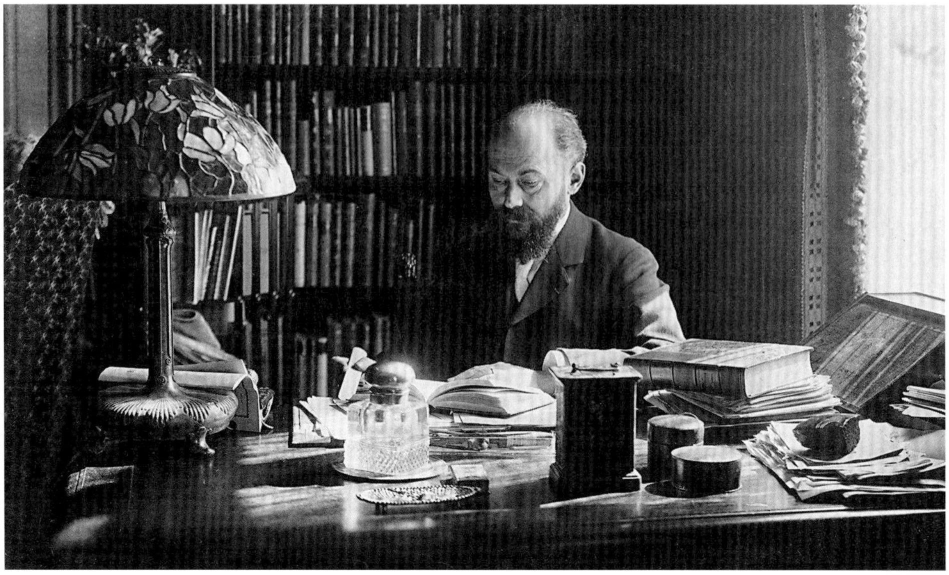

Fig. 3. Pierre Janet (1859–1947) in his Collège de France's desk, around 1910 (with permission from adoc-photos.com©).

mains unproven, that one patient made sexual advances towards him or that Freud was not a particularly competent hypnotherapist. Nevertheless, Freud abandoned hypnosis and created psychoanalysis. In his famous 1914 book, Freud interestingly mentioned a confidential remark he heard from Charcot about hysterical cases having sexual causes [35]. This was surprising to him since Charcot never presented this opinion during his conferences or in his publications on hysteria.

It is well known that Janet and Freud disliked each other [36]. Janet criticized the psychoanalytical method. He also claimed that he was the first to publish the successful treatment of hysteric patients with the cathartic method by reactivation into the consciousness of prior traumatic events which had been forgotten and transformed into subconscious fixed ideas. Janet's first description was contested by Freud in his 1895 book [33]. Later on, Freud was more successful in his publications, which unjustly overshadowed Janet's influence.

Dejerine and Sollier

Joseph Jules Dejerine (1849–1917) was one of the most important neurologists of the Salpêtrière school in the late years of Charcot's life and thereafter [13]. Apart from his great contribution in many fields of neurology, he turned to a new field in the later stages of his career. Indeed, like many eminent neurologists of that time he became interested in psychology, functional disorders, and hysteria. He was influenced by his friend, the Swiss neuropathologist Paul-Charles Dubois (1848–1918), and was attracted by the concept of functional disorders and psychotherapy [37] (fig. 4).

Paul Sollier (1861–1933), one of the most brilliant of Charcot's students [22] and one of the first clinical neuropsychologists in history, gave a physiological explanation of hysteria [36]. He made the hypothesis that the inhibition of certain cortical regions was the functional basis of hysterical paralysis. He supported the psychotherapy method.

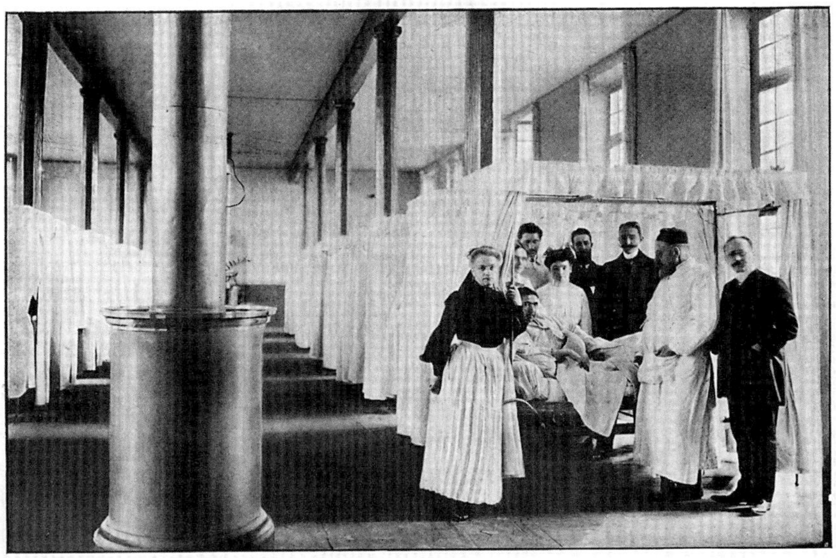

LA SALLE D'ISOLEMENT ET DE PSYCHOTHÉRAPIE DE LA SALPÊTRIÈRE. — SALLE PINEL.
SERVICE DU PROFESSEUR DEJERINE. — LA VISITE DU MATIN.

Fig. 4. Joseph Dejerine (1849–1917) and Ernest Gauckler (1876–1924). A visit to the isolation and psychotherapy room at the Salpêtrière hospital [37] (Olivier Walusinski personal collection).

Babinski and the Concept of Pithiatism

Joseph François Félix Babinski (1857–1932) was born in Paris to a Polish family [13]. He studied medicine and became Vulpian's intern/resident, and then 'assistant' in Charcot's clinic at Salpêtrière. Thereafter he was Chief of the Department of Neurology at Pitié Hospital. He became one of the founders of the Paris Neurological Society. Babinski's contribution to neurology and especially the neurological examination is remarkable [13, 38]. He was above all a semiologist and his constant aim was to discover characteristic signs in order to more accurately differentiate organic pathology from functional hysterical disorders. Accordingly, of great importance is his contribution to the study of hysteria.

Following Charcot, but also disputing his teacher's view, Babinski expanded the characteristics of hysteria, as opposed to organic pathology. He indeed considered that Charcot's concepts on hysteria were far too extensive by including phenomena that could not be modified by persuasion. He thought that there were diagnosis errors (organic pathologies, simulations) among patients diagnosed as hysterics. Babinski's first contribution to this topic was published in 1900 [39]. On November 7, 1901, Babinski attempted to give a definition of hysteria by explaining that suggestion played a major role at the Neurological Society [38]. He noted that symptoms could be reproduced and extinguished by suggestion. He considered that these psychic troubles should be scientifically named 'troubles pithiatiques' or 'pithiatism' (a term coming from the Greek, reflecting the 'persuasion' and 'curable' aspects of the disease). His ideas met initial skepticism for several years. The classical *Traité de Médecine* originally written by Bouchard and Brissaud had its 10th volume on neurology published in 1905.

In the chapter on hysteria [40], Charcot-Richer's 'grande hystérie' is extensively described, but then the new concepts on pithiatism are largely covered. Moreover, the title of the chapter is evocative: 'Hystérie (ou pithiatisme)'. At the Neurological Society meetings on April 9 and May 14, 1908, Babinski convinced most of the audience of the validity of the term pithiatism, pointing out that, in hysterical patients, superficial and deep reflexes are invariably normal whereas the stigmata are absent, contrary to Charcot's assertion [38, 41].

Babinski's concept on pithiatism, however, did have one weak aspect. While pithiatism undoubtedly was useful for diagnosis, this was not the case for therapeutic purposes. The main reason was the lack of vision Babinski had on psychological components in hysteria and in consideration of Janet's work on the psychological theories [22]. Subsequently, this had some impact on the care of many hysterical patients who did not fit Babinski's criteria (see below).

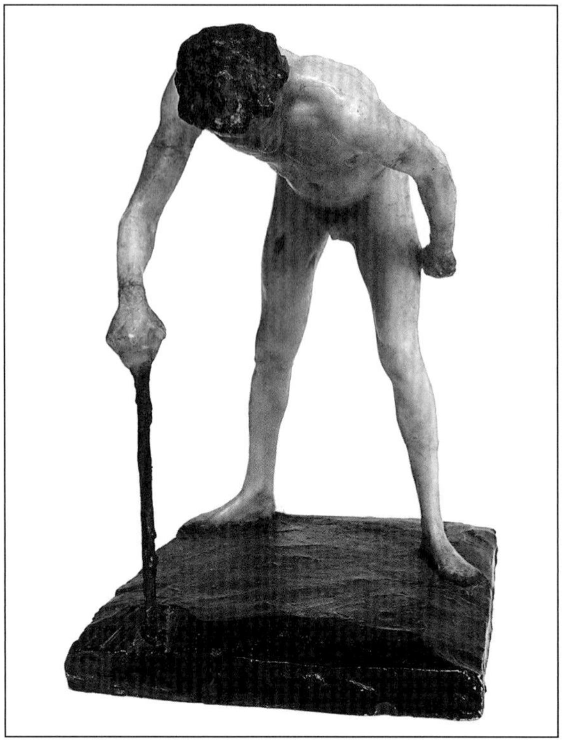

Fig. 5. Camptocormia. A handmade wax figure by René Leriche (1879–1955) during World War I. Musée du Service de Santé des Armées – École du Val-de-Grâce. Paris (public domain, with kind permission).

World War I and the Posttrauma Neurosis Syndrome Delineation

Although interest in hysteria was declining among neurological circles, posttrauma neurosis turned out to be a major diagnosis and therapeutic issue during World War I. This was due to the great number of soldiers presenting with conversion neurosis. New clinical presentations were identified. Indeed, Achille Alexandre Souques (1860–1944), from the Salpêtrière school in Paris, coined the term 'camptocormia' to describe the abnormal curve of the trunk in soldiers injured in trench warfare [13, 41, 42] (fig. 5). Camptocormia was also recognized among German and British soldiers.

During World War I, Babinski was employed by the Military Health Service, not only at La Pitié, but also at Buffon College, where he worked with Jules Froment (1878–1946), a neurologist from the University Hospitals of Lyon. They analyzed the symptoms and syndromes that had developed as a result of the war. Moreover, they had to distinguish between patients with nervous organic lesions from those with 'pithiatism' associated with sympathetic nervous disorders and those malingering by simulating an illness to avoid being sent to the front lines. In 1917 they published their work in an important book which was translated a year later into English, entitled *Hysteria, Pithiatism, and Reflex Neurological Troubles* [43]. This new syndrome called the Babinski-Froment posttrauma physiopathic syndrome in World War I soldiers combined sympathetic signs (today: algodystrophia), hysteria, and posttrauma neurosis (today: posttraumatic stress disorder). It is important to note that no discharge or allowance was delivered to soldiers who were simulators or who were diagnosed with hysteria-pithiatism. They had to return to the front or receive electrical treatment (see 'torpillage' below). In contrary, those who presented with posttrauma physiopathic syndrome were referred to special care which included creation of an atmosphere of confidence and faith, auto- and hetero-suggestion, physiotherapeutic methods, thermotherapy, novocaine injections for contractures, and psychotherapy.

Independently from Babinski and Froment, Charles Samuel Myers, a British military psychiatrist described a similar posttrauma neurosis syndrome in the British Expeditionary Forces in the North of France [44]. He proposed to name it 'shell shock' (or traumatic war neurosis), which corresponded to a punch to the head, without any pain after it, but which could be followed by neurologic and behavioral manifestations, usually in the absence of a significant brain lesion [44].

Electrical Shock ('Torpillage' or 'Torpedoing') during World War I

As outlined above, the concept of hysteria as a disease specific to women was abandoned during the second half of the 19th century, and hysteria in men was increasingly recognized particularly in workers due to the rapid industrialization in Europe and North America. In parallel, electrical therapy with faradic currents, after its early use by Briquet and Duchenne, became a more and more internationally recognized treatment for hysterical patients in many hospitals in the late 19th and early 20th centuries.

During the Great War, medical decisions towards soldiers presenting with pithiatism and other conversion disorders were not neutral, but instead largely influenced by the urgent need to send most of the soldiers back to front. Two opposite approaches occurred, first the psychotherapeutic one, as supported in France by Paul Sollier, and second the more abrupt one, 'rééducation intensive', proposed by pure neurologists as in France with Joseph Babinski and two of his students, Clovis Vincent (1879–1947) and Gustave Roussy (1874–1948) [22]. 'Rééducation intensive' (intensive rehabilitation in English) used electrotherapy and persuasion, which regrettably became abusively expended, receiving negative connotations like a punishment (fig. 6). Briefly, Clovis Vincent initially used faradization with persuasion following his teacher Babinski, but limited success encouraged him to develop a more painful but 'efficacious' method associating galvanic current with forced rehabilitation – 'torpillage' (in English: torpedoing) [22, 28, 45]. With this method, electric discharges were repeatedly delivered to the affected parts of the body while the doctor exhorted the patient to improve immediately. Vincent claimed that he obtained successful results with his method of combining electrical shock and persuasion. Most of the treated soldiers could be sent back to the front. In parallel or shortly after Vincent's new therapeutic technique, Gustave Roussy used faradic current and the 'moral' treatment. However, he observed that a painful electrical current using increasingly higher current voltage was necessary to obtain significant results. Vincent and Roussy were confronted with rebellion among soldiers and military trials, and abandoned their contested brutal method in 1916 and 1918, respectively. Electrical treatment was not limited to France, as it was also used in British and German military hospitals [46].

The Physical and Psychological Treatment after World War I until the Contemporary Years

Evolution of Ideas

After the transient rise of concern associated with World War I, a marked decrease in interest in

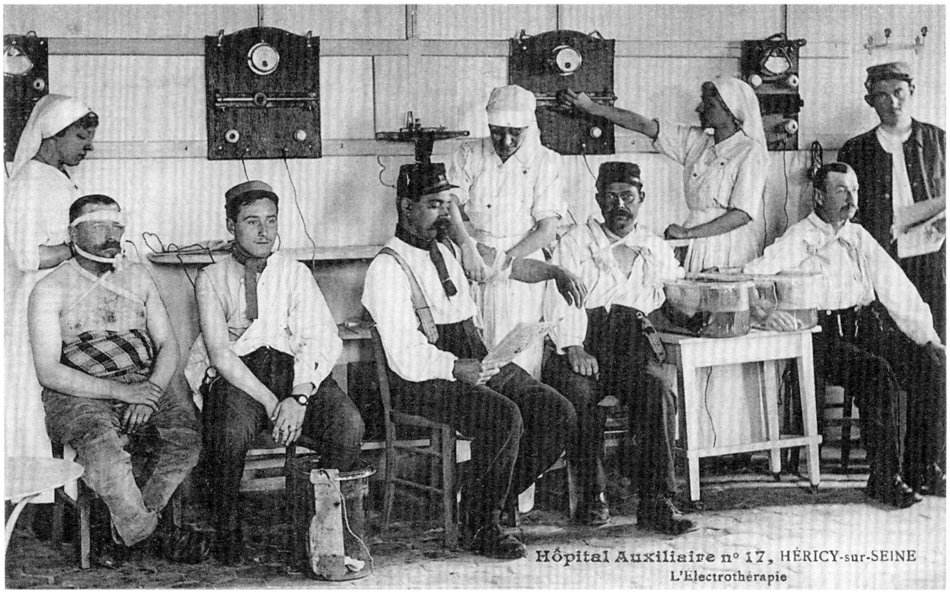

Fig. 6. French army soldiers in an electrotherapy room in a military hospital during World War I. 'L'électrothérapie. Hôpital Auxiliaire n°17 Héricy sur Seine (France)'. Postcard 1917. (Olivier Walusinski personal collection).

hysteria was observed for decades, with hysteria becoming a no-man's land between neurology and psychiatry [22]. The brutal 'rééducation intensive' therapeutic method was no longer approved, but moderate electrical faradization 'survived' in the electrotherapy of hysterical patients until the 1980s. We shall report the comments made by some great masters of neurology and psychiatry during those times.

In the French literature, a review was made after World War II by Jean Alexandre Barré (1880–1967), one of Babinski's students, in the chapter on hysteria of *Traité de médecine* [47]. In contrast with the constant and revolutionary changes observed between 1850 and 1920, very few novel theories or treatments emerged in the time period 1920–1950. In the therapeutic domain, isolation, rest, faradic electrization, and hypnosis were cited again and the only new contribution after World War I was the increasing use of Freud's psychoanalytical method. Henri Ey (1900–1977), one of the leading French psychiatrists in Paris after World War II [3], defined hysteria as a neurosis characterized by somatic hyperexpressivity of unconscious ideas, images, and affects [48].

In Great Britain, Samuel Alexander Kinnier Wilson (1878–1937), one of the leading neurologists at Queen Square in London from 1910 to the 1930s, did several reviews on hysteria, notably in 1919 and 1930 [49], incorporating not only the English literature but also the French and German contributions, which he was able to as he was fluent in both languages. To him, the majority of hysterical symptoms were of psychic origin, and it often appeared difficult to decide whether a hysterical patient was not malingering. Wilson cited the main therapeutic methods in use, including psychoanalysis. He was doubtful about the successful results obtained in war cases by electrical treatment, hypnotism or persuasion, reeducation, and manipulation, and acknowledged that other therapies were also not satisfying. Much later, David Marsden (1938–1998), another subsequent leader in neurology and especially movement disorders at Queen Square, gave a neurologist's view on hysteria [50] and recalled the useful comments made by some of his predecessors like Sir William Richard Gowers (1845–1915) and J.A. Ormerod (1845–1925). In his practice, he proposed to use the term hysteria to describe disturbances of function that could not be explained fully by organic or functional neurological disease, and provided 'the six rules of hysteria' to avoid misdiagnosis.

Progresses in the Nosology of Hysteria in the USA: Contribution of DSM Classification

In the USA, as in Europe, the classical definitions of hysteria were mostly influenced by Freud and Janet until the 1950s. The constant will of American psychiatry to move from empirical definitions to a better nosological classification of mental illnesses resulted in the creation of the Diagnosis and Statistical Manual of Mental Disorders (DSM), as early as 1952 until the most recent 2013 version (DSM-5) [51, 52]. It is interesting to see how the denomination of hysteria was amended from the DSM-III to the DSM-5 classifications [1, 50–53]. The term 'hysteria' was still in use in DSM-III, with the denomination of 'Briquet's syndrome or hysterical neurosis'. DSM-IV employed the term 'conversion disorders', still referring to Freud's concepts (DSM-IV), then 'somatoform troubles' emerged in DSM IV-R. However, 'functional neurological disorders' was preferred in DSM-5, corroborating that the terms 'hysteria' and 'conversion' are no longer employed today. This classification is increasingly being adopted internationally.

The Need for Diagnostic Criteria and the Advent of Brain Imaging Studies

Current research has improved the criteria used to diagnose various functional neurological disorders, but still shows the remaining difficulties encountered in the diagnosis of conversion syndromes, e.g. psychogenic nonepileptic seizures and motor conversion disorders presenting with motor deficit, gait troubles, or movement disorders [54–61].

Recent positron emission tomography, single-photon emission tomography (SPECT), and functional magnetic resonance (fMRI) brain imaging studies have brought some clues to a better understanding of conversion disorders emphasizing the pioneering work of Sollier (see above). A SPECT ^{99m}Tc-ECD study investigated 7 patients with unilateral hysterical sensorimotor loss during passive vibratory stimulation of both hands when their deficit was present and 2–4 months later when they had recovered. A consistent decrease of regional cerebral blood flow in the thalamus and basal ganglia contralateral to the deficit was found. Importantly, contralateral basal ganglia and thalamic hypoactivation resolved after recovery. Furthermore, lower activation in contralateral caudate nucleus during hysterical conversion symptoms predicted poor recovery at follow-up. In an fMRI study, preserved motor intention was found in hysterical palsy, with preparatory activation in the motor cortex, but no activation during failed movement [62].

Treatment Options

During the second half of the 20th century until the 2010s, important research was performed to assess classical as well as new therapeutic interventions on hysteria. Below is a brief description of physiotherapy, psychotherapy, psychoanalytical treatment, cognitive behavioral therapy, pharmacotherapy, and electroconvulsive and repetitive transcranial magnetic stimulation (rTMS) therapy.

Physiotherapy

The cure of conversion syndromes by physiotherapy is very commonly used today. Most of the literature on adults and children presents case histories with more or less successful treatment, particularly with intensive and prolonged physical care [63–67]. In a recent exhaustive review [68],

28 case series or reports were found, but only one controlled intervention study with a historical control group was disclosed. Physiotherapy most commonly occurred in the context of multidisciplinary treatment and involved a motor learning approach. Novel approaches included the use of distraction techniques and transcutaneous electrical nerve stimulation machine. Deceptive behavioral techniques have also been described. Most studies reported benefit from physical treatment, including some studies with long-term follow-up. In contrary to this review, poor outcome of patients is, however, the common view in daily practice, particularly in patients with severe and long-standing conversion syndromes. This suggests that failure in the treatment of conversion syndromes by physical therapy is much more frequent but rarely reported compared to cases with good outcome. Future well-defined studies should focus on intensive and prolonged rehabilitation programs.

Psychosocial and Psychoanalytic Therapies

Psychotherapy and psychoanalysis have been largely used for almost a century. However, only a few controlled studies are available to assess the real benefit of these approaches, including hypnosis. In a recent review [69], only 3 out of 260 reports were randomized studies comparing psychosocial interventions for conversion disorders with standard care or other interventions (biological or psychosocial). One study was concerned with paradoxical injunction therapy and the other two studied the value of hypnosis. As these three studies had different interventions and control groups, the results could not be combined. All of the studies were of poor methodological quality, thus making it difficult to place much value on the results of the studies. Therefore, although daily practice may reveal interesting results in some cases, randomized studies are warranted to more accurately determine the value of psychosocial and psychoanalytical approaches.

Cognitive and Behavioral Therapies

These more recent methods have largely been used during the last decades, including for conversion syndromes. A recent review on efficacy of cognitive behavioral therapy for somatization, hypochondriasis, and body dysmorphic disorder [70] showed that there were few data on the impact of treatment on healthcare use, especially when the cost of cognitive behavioral therapy was factored into the equation. Only three studies were performed on somatoform disorders and one on conversion syndromes. It is acknowledged that too few methodologically sound studies have been published on the treatment of conversion disorder or of pain disorder to make any conclusions. Nevertheless, there is sufficient evidence to believe that cognitive behavioral intervention may have therapeutic value if well-defined studies are performed in the future.

Pharmacotherapy

Few investigations have been performed using psychoactive drugs in conversion disorders. Intravenous barbiturate narcosis in conversion disorders, notably those presenting with memory deficits, was tested a long time ago, but did not show significantly better results than other psychotherapeutic methods [71]. Antidepressants and anxiolytics are frequently used in combination with other physical and psychotherapeutic interventions as stressed above but do not have a specific value to relieve the hysterical symptoms.

Electroconvulsive Therapy

As electrical treatment was strongly criticized after World War I, electroconvulsive therapy, which had its heyday during the 1950–1970s, has not been used frequently to treat hysterical patients in contrast to depressive states. However, a few case reports or small series reveal some interest of electroconvulsive therapy in conversion disorders either presenting with motor deficit or pseudoepileptic seizures [72–74].

Transcranial Magnetic Stimulation

TMS and rTMS are modern techniques currently being evaluated by neurologists and psychiatrists in various illnesses. Promising findings have been reported, especially in conversion motor deficit and in psychogenic movement disorders. Of interest is a recent report of TMS in psychogenic movement disorders [75]. Patients were blindly video scored before and after TMS. TMS was delivered at low frequency (0.25 Hz) over the motor cortex contralateral to symptoms. Twenty-four patients presenting with dystonia, myoclonus, tremor, parkinsonism, or stereotypies were included. The median duration of symptoms before TMS was 2.8 years (6 months to 30 years). The overall score of 75% of patients improved by more than 50%; furthermore, the clinical benefits were sustained upon protracted follow-up (median: 19.8 months). There was no correlation between improvement and duration of symptoms before TMS. This finding warrants further studies in psychogenic movement disorders and other conversion syndromes. Indeed, a recent review on TMS and conversion disorders showed that there has been no placebo-controlled study. Thus, despite the majority of studies claiming success for the technique, there is insufficient good-quality evidence to establish TMS as an effective treatment modality for functional neurological disorders [76].

Practical Care of Patients with Conversion Disorders

In our essay, the various therapeutic methods used in hysterical patients were reviewed. The practical way patients should be managed has been proposed in several books and articles [1, 50, 53, 77], and include the following:

- Hysteria (today functional neurological disorders according to DSM-5 classification) should be considered as a tangible, definite illness
- Simple and understandable language should be employed in interview with the patient (do not use the word 'hysteria', but rather somatoform disorder or functional neurological troubles)
- Care should be conducted by one physician in cooperation with the general practitioner
- All necessary clinical, laboratory, and imaging examinations should be conducted and their results explained to the patient before starting the treatment; once treatment is started, avoid repeating secondary examinations
- Persuasion or suggestion may be employed by a psychiatrist or psychologist trained in this pathology, together with (possibly intensive) physical therapy eventually in a rehabilitation institution, and with precise objectives and encouragement of the patient when some progress is observable
- Regular follow-up is recommended, with constant attention to patient complaints
- Antidepressants and anxiolytics may be required in case of depression and anxiety
- Cognitive and behavioral therapies and hypnosis may be discussed depending on the clinical presentation
- Group and familial therapy may be considered in rare situations
- TMS and rTMS are still under evaluation, but should be more frequently indicated in the future, especially in motor conversion disorders

Conclusion

Hysteria, conversion syndrome, or functional neurological disorder, is a frequent medical situation. The last two centuries have experienced a great deal of progress concerning its epidemiology, clinical presentations, and various therapeutic methods. However, it remains a difficult problem to manage with frequent failures and chronic handicapping evolution. The clever observations made by the great neurologist Samuel Alexander Kinnier Wilson are still valid today 'in chronic hysterics due to their resistance to every therapeutic effort, nursing their infirmity to the end, defeating the physician by their very feebleness' [49]. This shows the need for therapeutic innovations in the future.

Acknowledgments

We thank Mrs. Chantal Silarakis, the library assistant of the Pierre Wertheimer Neurological Hospital, for her tremendous help in searching for historical literature on hysteria.

References

1 Escande M: Hystérie. EMC Psychiatrie 1996;37–340-A-10.
2 Cullen W: Institutions de médecine pratique. Traduction française par Philippe Pinel. Paris, Duplain, 1785, vol 2.
3 Poirier J, Clarac F, Barbara JG, Broussolle E: Figures and institutions of the neurological sciences in Paris from 1800 to 1950. Part IV: psychiatry and psychology. Rev Neurol (Paris) 2012;168: 389–402.
4 Mace CJ: Hysterical conversion. I: a history. II: a critique. Br J Psychiatry 1992; 161:369–389.
5 Walusinski O: A case of Charcotian grande hystérie: observation by Julien Offray de La Mettrie in 1738. Eur Neurol 2012;67:98–106.
6 Mesmer FA: Mémoire sur la découverte du magnétisme animal. Paris, P.Fr. Didot le Jeune, 1779.
7 Pinel P, Caille C, Ravier L: Traité médico-philosophique sur l'aliénation mentale, ou la manie. Paris, Richard, Caille et Ravier, 1801.
8 Grange KM: Pinel or Chiarugi? Med Hist 1963;7:371–380.
9 Pinel P: Recherches et observations sur le traitement moral des aliénés. Paris, S.N., 1798.
10 Pinel P: Nosographie philosophique ou la méthode de l'analyse appliquée à la médecine. Paris, Maradan, 1798.
11 Briquet P: Traité clinique et thérapeutique de l'hystérie. Paris, JB Baillières et Fils, 1859.
12 Mai F, Merskey H: Briquet's treatise on hysteria: a synopsis and commentary. Arch Gen Psychiatry 1980;37:1401–1405.
13 Broussolle E, Poirier J, Clarac F, Barbara JG: Figures and institutions of the neurological sciences in Paris from 1800 to 1950. Part III: neurology. Rev Neurol (Paris) 2012;168:301–320.
14 Duchenne G: De l'électrisation localisée et de son application à la physiologie, à la pathologie et à la thérapeutique. Paris, Baillière, 1855.
15 Brachet JL: Traité de l'hystérie. Paris, Baillières et Savy, 1847.
16 Landouzy H: Traité complet de l'hystérie. Paris, Baillière, 1846.
17 Braid J: Neurohypnology, or a Rationale of Nervous Sleep, Considered in Relation with Animal Magnetism. London, Churchill, 1843.
18 Lasègue C: Etudes médicales du professeur Ch. Lasègue. Paris, Asselin, 1884, vol 2.
19 Richer P: Etudes cliniques sur l'hystéro-épilepsie ou Grande Hystérie. Paris, Adrien Delahaye et Emile Lecrosnier, 1881.
20 Charcot JM: Sur les divers états nerveux déterminés par l'hypnotisation chez les hystériques. Comptes-rendus hebdomadaires des séances de l'Academie des Sciences 1882;94:403–405.
21 Gilles de la Tourette GB: Traité clinique et thérapeutique de l'hystérie. Paris, Plon & Nourrit, 1891.
22 Bogousslavsky J: Hysteria after Charcot: back to the future; in Bogousslavsky J (ed): Following Charcot: A Forgotten History of Neurology and Psychiatry. Front Neurol Neurosci. Basel, Karger, 2011, vol 29, pp 137–161.
23 Charcot JM: A propos de l'hystérie chez l'homme. Œuvres complètes, leçon 18. Paris, Bureaux du Progrès Médical, 1890, vol 3, pp 253–280.
24 Goetz C: Charcot and the myth of misogyny. Neurology 1999;52:1678–1686.
25 Bernheim H: De la suggestion dans l'état hypnotique et dans l'état de veille. Paris, Octave Doin, 1884.
26 Walusinski O, Poirier J, Déchy H: 'Augustine'. Eur Neurol 2013;69:226–228.
27 Weir MS: Rest in the Treatment of Nervous Disease. New York, G.P. Putnam's Sons, 1875.
28 Walusinski O: The cruelty and failings of therapies for neurological diseases in French literature. Prog Brain Res 2013; 206:171–199.
29 Splett T, Steinberg H: Treatment of hysteria in the 19th century – in which way did German psychiatrists view castration (in German)? Fortschr Neurol Psychiatr 2003;71:45–52.
30 Vanni D, Cabras PL, Vanni P: Surgical therapy as treatment for hysteria in Italy: 1880–1889 (in Italian). Ital J Anat Embryol 1998;103:177–182.
31 Havens LL: Pierre Janet. J Nerv Ment Dis 1966;143:383–398.
32 Janet P: Contribution à l'étude des accidents mentaux chez les hystériques. Thesis. Paris, Rueff, 1893.
33 Breuer J, Freud S: Studien über hysteric. Leipzig, Deutike, 1895.
34 Stone J, Smyth R, Carson A, Warlow C, Sharpe M: La belle indifférence in conversion symptoms and hysteria. Systematic review. Brit J Psychiatry 2006;188: 204–209.
35 Freud S: Contribution de l'histoire du mouvement psychanalytique (1914). Traduction de l'allemand. Paris, Payot, 1968.
36 Bogousslavsky J, Walusinski O: Paul Sollier: the first clinical neuropsychologist; in Bogousslavsky J (ed): Following Charcot: A Forgotten History of Neurology and Psychiatry. Front Neurol Neurosci. Basel, Karger, 2011, vol 29, pp 105–114.
37 Dejerine J, Gauckler E: Les manifestations fonctionnelles des psychonévroses. Paris, Masson, 1911.
38 Clarac M, Massion J, Smith AM: History of Neuroscience: Joseph Babinski (1857–1932). IBRO History of Neuroscience, 2008. http://www.ibro.info/Pub/Pub_Main_Display.asp?LC_Docs_ID=2990.

39 Babinski J: Diagnostic différentiel de l'hémiplégie organique et de l'hémiplégie hystérique. Gazette des Hopitaux 1900;73:521–527, 533–537.
40 Dutil H, Laubry C: Hystérie (ou pithiatisme); in Traité de médecine, ed 2. Paris, Masson, 1905, vol X, pp 665–718.
41 Babinski J: The dismembrerment of traditional hysteria: Pithiatism (translated by Chaddock CG). Interstate Med J 1909;16:171–190.
42 Souques A, Rosanoff-Saloff I: La camptocormie; incurvation du tronc consécutive au traumatisme du dos et des lombes; considérations morphologiques. Rev Neurol (Paris) 1915;22:937–939.
43 Babinski J, Froment J, Rolleston J: Hysteria or pithiatism and reflex nervous disorders in the neurology of war. London, University of London Press, 1918.
44 Myers CS: A contribution to the study of shellshock: being an account of the cases of loss of memory, vision, smell and taste admitted to the Duchess of Westminster's War Hospital, Le Touquet. Lancet 1915;i:316–320.
45 Tatu L, Bogousslavsky J, Moulin T, Chopard JL: The 'torpillage' neurologists of World War I: electric therapy to send hysterics back to the front. Neurology 2010;75:279–283.
46 Linden SC, Jones Lees AJ: Shell shock at Queen Square: Lewis Yealland 100 years on. Brain 2013;136:1976–1988.
47 Barré JA: L'hystérie; in Traité de médecine. maladies du système nerveux: sémiologie générale et maladies proprement dites. Paris, Masson, 1949, vol XVI, pp 1199–1235.
48 Ey H: Etudes psychiatriques. Paris, Desclée de Brouwer, 1952, vol 3.
49 Reynolds EH: Kinnier Wilson on hysteria: a missing chapter. J Neurol Neurosurg Psychiatry 2012;83:464–465.
50 Marsden CD: Hysteria – a neurologist's view. Psychol Med 1986;16:277–288.
51 Diagnostic and Statistical Manual of Mental Disorders, ed 3, Washington, American Psychiatric Association, 1980.
52 Diagnostic and Statistical Manual of Mental Disorders, ed 5. Washington, American Psychiatric Association, 2013.
53 Cathebras P, Régny P: Hysterical conversion (in French). Rev Prat 2012;62: 1119–1125, 1127–1130.
54 Aybek S, Kanaan EA, David AS: The neuropsychiatry of conversion disorder. Curr Opin Psychiatry 2008;21:275–280.
55 Dickinson P, Looper KJ: Psychogenic nonepileptic seizures: a current overview. Epilepsia 2012;53:1679–1689.
56 Drapier S, Verin M: Les mouvements anormaux pyschogènes. Rev Neurol (Paris) 2012;168:662–667.
57 Gupta A, Lang AE: Psychogenic movement disorders. Curr Opin Neurol 2009; 22:430–436.
58 Hayes MW, Graham S, Heldorf P, de Moore G, Morris JGL: A video review of the diagnosis of psychogenic gait: appendix and commentary. Mov Disord 1999;14:914–921.
59 Krem MM: Motor conversion disorders reviewed from a neuropsychiatric perspective. J Clin Psychiatry 2004;65:783–790.
60 Porcelli P, Rafanelli C: Criteria for psychosomatic research (DCPR) in the medical setting. Curr Psychiatry Rep 2010;12:246–254.
61 Siket MS, Merchant RC: Psychogenic seizures: a review and description of pitfalls in their acute diagnosis and management in the emergency department. Emerg Med Clin North Am 2011; 29:73–81.
62 Cojan Y, Waber L, Carruzo A, Vuilleumier P: Motor inhibition in hysterical conversion paralysis. Neuroimage 2009; 47:1026–1037.
63 Alan Ç, Seçkin U, Bodur H: Hysterical paralysis. Rheumatol Int 2007;27:873–874.
64 Delargy MA, Peatfield RC, Burt AA: Successful rehabilitation in conversion paralysis. Br Med J (Clin Res Ed) 1986;292: 1730–1731.
65 Leslie SA: Diagnosis and treatment of hysterical conversion reactions. Arch Dis Child 1988;63:506–511.
66 Ness D: Physical therapy management for conversion disorder: case series. J Neurol Phys Ther 2007;31:30–39.
67 Withrington RH, Wynn Pary CB: Rehabilitation of conversion paralysis. J Bone Joint Surg Br 1985;67:635–638.
68 Nielsen G, Stone J, Edwards MJ: Physiotherapy for functional (psychogenic) motor symptoms: a systematic review. J Psychosom Res 2013;75:93–102.
69 Ruddy R, House A: Psychosocial interventions for conversion disorder. Cochrane Database Syst Rev 2005; 4:CD005331.
70 Allen LA, Woolfolk RL: Cognitive behavioral therapy for somatoform disorders. Psychiatr Clin North Am 2010;33: 579–593.
71 Lambert C, Rees L: Intravenous barbiturates in the treatment of hysteria. Brit Med J 1944;2:70–73.
72 Blumer D, Rice S, Adamolekun B: Electroconvulsive treatment for nonepileptic seizure disorders. Epilepsy Behav 2009; 15:382–387.
73 Daniel WF, Yeo RA, Smith JE: Conversion disorders and ECT. Br J Psychiatry 1989;154:274–275.
74 Gaillard A, Gaillard R, Mouaffak F, Radtchenko A, Lôo H: Case report: electroconvulsive therapy in a 33-year-old man with hysterical quadriplegia (in French. Encephale 2012;38:104–109.
75 Garcin B, Roze E, Mesrati F, Cognat E, Fournier E, Vidailhet M, Degos B: Transcranial magnetic stimulation as an efficient treatment for psychogenic movement. J Neurol Neurosurg Psychiatry 2013;84:1043–1046.
76 Pollak TA, Nicholson TR, Edwards MJ, David AS: A systematic review of transcranial magnetic stimulation in the treatment of functional (conversion) neurological symtoms. J Neurol Neurosurg Psychiatry 2014;85:191–197.
77 Adams R, Victor M, Ropper AH: The neuroses and personality disorders; in Principles of Neurology, ed 6. New York, McGraw-Hill, 1997, pp 1507–1529.
78 Foveau de Courmelles FV: L'hypnotisme. Paris, Librairie Hachette, 1890.

Prof. Emmanuel Broussolle
Service de Neurologie C, Hôpital Neurologique Pierre Wertheimer
59 boulevard Pinel
FR–69677 Bron (France)
E-Mail emmanuel.broussolle@chu-lyon.fr

Bogousslavsky J (ed): Hysteria: The Rise of an Enigma. Front Neurol Neurosci. Basel, Karger, 2014, vol 35, pp 198–204
DOI: 10.1159/000360064

'Hysteria' Today and Tomorrow

W. Curt LaFrance, Jr.[a, b]

[a]Neuropsychiatry and Behavioral Neurology, Rhode Island Hospital, and [b]Psychiatry and Neurology, Brown Medical School, Providence, R.I., USA

Abstract

'Hysteria' (conversion disorder) remains in modern humanity and across cultures, as it has for millennia. Advances today in tools and criteria have afforded more accurate diagnosis, and advances in treatments have empowered patients and providers, resulting in a renewed interest in somatoform disorders. Future progress in understanding mechanisms may be influenced by developments in functional neuroimaging and neurophysiology. No animal model exists for somatoform symptoms or conversion disorder. Despite the absence of a known molecular mechanism, psychotherapy is helping patients with conversion disorder to take control of their symptoms and have improved quality of life, shedding light on what was once an enigma.

'Hysteria' has transformed in name, but not in nature. What was deemed hysteria is now conversion disorder and is still associated with trauma, abuse, and developmental privation. What were called 'pseudoseizures' and 'hystero-epilepsy' are now nonepileptic seizures (NES). The etiologic understanding has changed, but not the essence. That is, what was deemed to be dysfunction of the uterus is now deemed neurological manifestations of underlying psychological conflicts or stressors. The presence of conversion symptoms in individuals and in masses is just as prevalent today in developed and developing countries as it was centuries ago.

Regarding conversion disorder today, much has been accomplished in the past decade and published in the medical literature, which has brought somatoform disorders back into the forefront of neurology, psychiatry, and neuropsychiatry. Some of the significant contributors to the increase in attention and publications on somatoform disorders include (1) improvements in diagnosis (both in tools and in approach) and (2) improvements in treatments. Further insight into the understanding of conversion disorders may continue due to advances in (1) functional neuroimaging and (2) neurophysiology. These advances from today and for tomorrow are discussed in this chapter.

Advances Today: Diagnosis

Diagnosis of hysteria was based on anamnesis, physical examination (limiting labs to only those necessary), and intravenous sodium amytal hypnosis [1]. While taking a comprehensive history and examination are still essential, diagnostic tools, specifically the advent of video electroencephalography (vEEG) [2, 3], has radically transformed the landscape for diagnosing paroxysmal neuropsychiatric disorders. Since its introduction, vEEG has become the gold standard for differentiating epilepsy from conversion seizures [psychogenic NES (PNES)] [4, 5]. For seizures, the use of history and exam, seizure semiology, and witnessing events/video/vEEG allow for levels of diagnostic certainty, ranging from possible to probable, clinically established, and diagnosed [6]. These diagnostic levels allow for diagnostic stratification even when long-term monitoring is not available, as is the case in some low- and middle-income countries, with the caveat that higher certainty is present when events are captured on vEEG.

Other diagnostic advances include making the diagnosis of conversion disorder (also referred to as functional neurological symptoms disorder in DSM-5) more reliable [7]. With DSM-IV, excluding intentionally produced symptoms and identifying a psychological factor associated with onset both proved to be a challenge that limited a clinician's ability to definitively make the conversion diagnosis. To illustrate, without surveillance, how could one prove the absence of feigning? Moreover, in a typical 30-min psychiatric consult, patients may not feel comfortable disclosing a history of trauma or abuse, and no 'factor' may have been identified in that brief encounter. This lack of diagnostic rigor accompanied by normal magnetic resonance imaging (MRI) and labs led to many consults left as 'no acute psychiatric illness', meaning 'not suicidal or psychotic', but without explaining the patient's medically unexplained paresis. In DSM-5, the criteria were changed regarding the malingering and psychological factors now relegated as a note, but not a requirement, and incorporating the physical exam in the criteria. Common exam signs that are incongruous with disease or internally inconsistent (e.g. Hoover's sign for conversion leg weakness or entrainment for psychogenic movement disorder) can be documented in support of conversion disorder. In essence, the changes to DSM-5 allow clinicians to make the diagnosis of conversion a 'rule in' diagnosis, not a 'rule out'. Better diagnostic tools and better diagnostic criteria are two means that have moved conversion disorder from a provisional suspect in the differential to a definitive diagnosis.

Advances Today: Treatment

Prior 'treatments' for hysteria documented in the medical literature included hydrotherapy (a jugful of water to an open mouth), faradization (electric current applied to the skin), and a vigorous tug at the pubic hair [8], used in England, or the ovarian compression belt, used in France [9]. Hypnosis and psychoanalysis were commonly used in the early and mid-20th century for conversion treatment [10]. Over the past 10 years, however, rigorous trials comparing pharmacotherapies and psychotherapies have been conducted providing an evidence-based medicine approach to somatoform disorders. Examples of trials include psychotropic medications and cognitive behavioral therapy (CBT) for somatoform disorders and for NES.

Psychopharmacologic interventions for conversion disorder have been used to treat the somatoform disorder directly and to treat the common comorbidities. Medication treatment approaches historically have been prophylactic or symptomatic. Open-label trials of antidepressants in patients with conversion disorders have shown some response [11–13] for medically unexplained symptoms, noncardiac chest pain, and psychogenic movement disorder. Fully powered phase III controlled studies of the benefit of psychotropics in patients with NES, however, have not been conducted, and apart from largely anecdotal reports, their effect is unknown [14]. The pharmacological references for PNES treatment using intravenous barbiturates, tricyclic antidepressants, selective serotonin reuptake inhibitors, mixed mechanism antidepressants, dopamine receptor antagonists, β-blockers, analgesics, or benzodiazepines are largely anecdotal references in case reports, journal review articles, and book chapters, with only three prospective open-label trials [15–18]. Only one double-blind placebo-controlled pilot randomized controlled trial for PNES has been published [19].

Psychotherapy appears to have a stronger effect in conversion disorder than pharmacologic approaches. The most substantial body of data relates to the application of CBT, which has been shown to be effective in the treatment of a range of somatoform disorders [20, 21] and is being extended in brief self-help formats for patients with 'functional neurological symptoms' [22]. There is no single model of CBT for use by patients with PNES, since the therapy itself permits modification for specific groups according to the model of the disorder, despite containing core principles and techniques. The two CBT approaches described in most detail in the literature [23] are those used by LaFrance et al. [24, 25] and Goldstein et al. [26, 27]. To date, the approach developed by LaFrance et al. has been evaluated in an open label study [25] and a multicenter pilot randomized controlled trial [24], and that by Goldstein et al. in an open label study [27] and pilot randomized controlled trial [26]. Fully powered trials will be conducted in the future to provide class I data on somatoform treatments.

Tomorrow: Functional Neuroimaging in Somatoform Disorders

Static/anatomic neuroimaging is one of the main tests used to help to show the absence of a focal lesion in patients with conversion symptoms. To explore neurophysiology from a functional neuroanatomic perspective, recent studies have moved from structural to functional neuroimaging.

Much has been done in functional neuroimaging in psychogenic movement disorders and NES. Voon et al. [28] assessed conversion disorder subjects (n = 16) with positive motor symptoms showing greater amygdala activity to arousing facial stimuli (positive and negative) irrespective of valence compared to healthy volunteers (fig. 1). Arousing stimuli were also associated with enhanced functional connectivity between the amygdala and supplementary motor area in conversion disorder subjects. However, not all studies have replicated these findings. Abnormalities in connectivity and neural networks in NES have been investigated using EEG and resting state functional MRI. Knyazeva et al. [29] studied NES (n = 13) and healthy volunteers (n = 13) using multivariate phase synchronization in interictal high-density EEG. Their results did not show any group differences, but they found decreased prefrontal and parietal synchronization with a greater number of NES events. Barzegaran et al. [30] further analyzed these results using graph theory showing that although NES patients had similar local and global connectivity and small-world structure, the number of NES correlated with lower local connectivity.

Using resting state functional MRI, van der Kruijs et al. [31] showed that PNES (n = 11), compared to healthy controls (n = 12), had greater functional correlation between regions implicated in emotion and self-perception (insula) and motor preparation (precentral and central sulcus), and that dissociation scores were positively correlated with this connectivity (fig. 2). Ding et al. [32] using graph theoretical analysis compared NES (n = 17) and healthy volunteers (n = 20) applied to both functional (resting state functional MRI) and anatomical (diffusion tractography) networks. Subjects with NES had abnormal small-worldness with more regular (lattice-like) organization of large-scale functional and structural networks indicative of impaired global integration and less information propagation. Coupling strength between functional and structural connectivity was

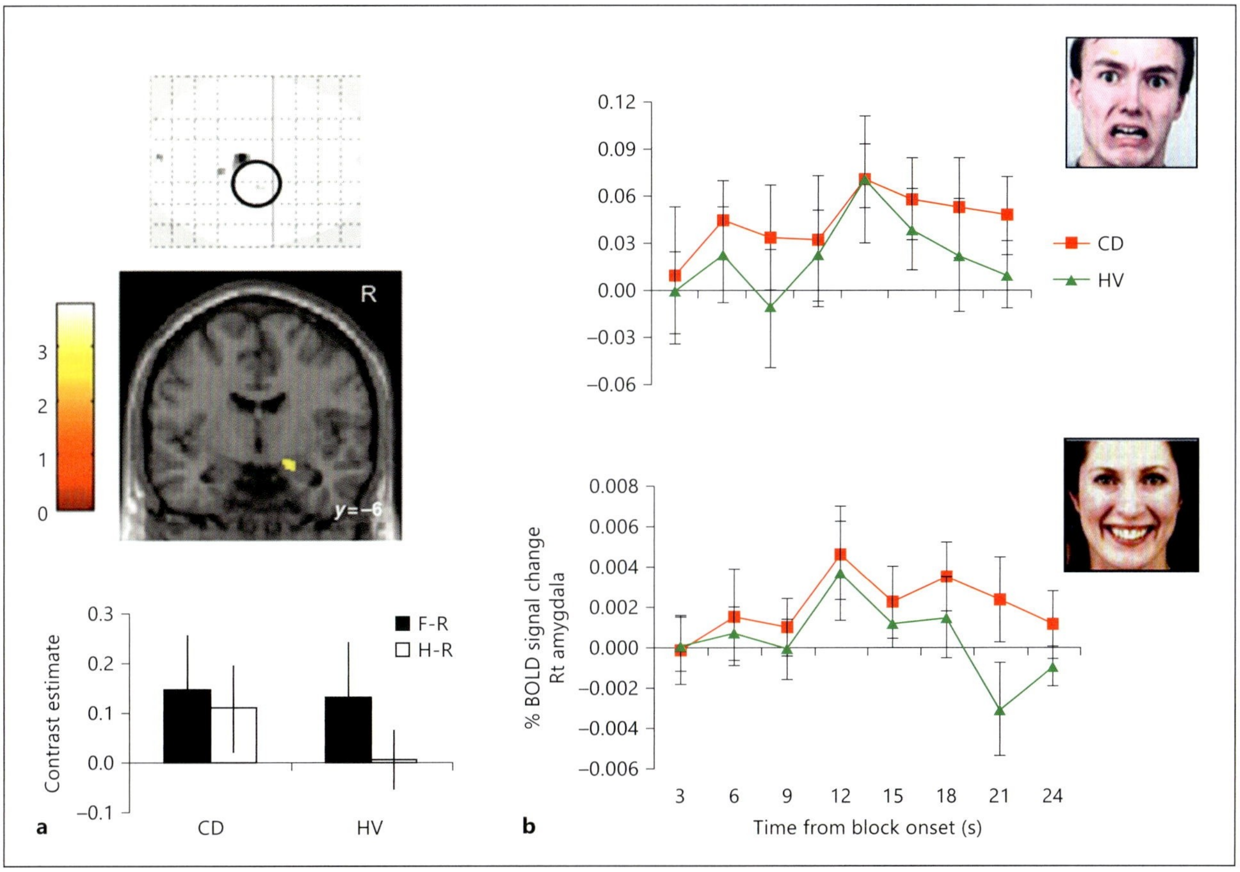

Fig. 1. Amygdala activity to emotional stimuli in motor conversion disorder [28]. **a** Incidental affective task comparing the CD and HV groups by valence interaction on glass brain, statistical parametric map and contrast estimate. **b** Right amygdala time course comparison between the CD and HV groups. CD = Conversion disorder patients; HV = healthy volunteers. Used with permission from *Brain*, copyright 2010, Oxford University Press.

decreased in NES compared to healthy controls with high specificity (75%) and sensitivity (77%) to differentiate groups. In contrast to findings in conversion paralysis with greater bilateral premotor cortical thickness [33], Labate et al. [34] also showed that NES (n = 20) compared to healthy volunteers (n = 40) had decreased volume and cortical thickness in the right premotor and motor cortex and bilateral cerebellar regions.

Structural neuroimaging (morphometric MRI) in 10 patients with conversion disorder compared to healthy controls revealed smaller mean volumes of the left and right basal ganglia and a smaller right thalamus in the conversion patients [35]. Studies using single-photon emission computed tomography and functional MRI have identified the anterior cingulate gyrus and the orbitofrontal cortex as potentially mediating the hypothesized attention and inhibition findings seen in patients with sensory and motor conversion disorders [36, 37]. Bilateral vibrotactile stimulation in 3 patients with sensory conversion disorders resulted in activation of the contralateral primary somatosensory region (S1), but no contralateral activation was present during unilateral stimulation of the affected limb [38].

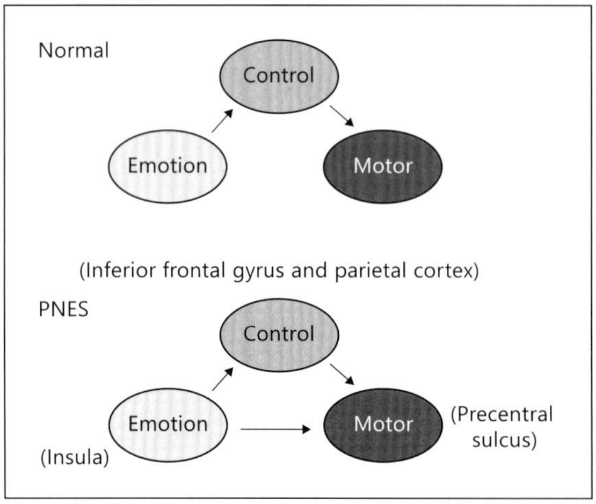

Fig. 2. Functional connectivity of dissociation in patients with NES. Schematic overview of possible circuitry involved in cognitive-emotional executive control [31]. Modified and used with permission from *Journal of Neurology, Neurosurgery and Psychiatry*, copyright 2012, BMJ Publishing Group.

Other case reports and small sample-size functional neuroimaging studies in patients with motor conversion disorders have started to appear in the literature [39, 40]. As demonstrated by the structural literature, we will not be able to 'localize a conversion *lesion*', but ultimately may identify a conversion network. Sensory gating may be affected in conversion disorders such as psychogenic movement disorder [41]. Further studies of functional neuroimaging examining striatothalamocortical circuits controlling sensorimotor function and attention may yield insights into the neural and effective connectivity in somatoform disorders.

Tomorrow: Physiologic Measures in Somatoform Disorders

Along with functional neuroimaging, physiologic measures may provide new insights into conversion disorders. Much of this physiologic work has been conducted in patients with epilepsy and NES. Given the work showing a rise in prolactin following generalized tonic-clonic epileptic seizures and the absence of a rise following NES, the American Academy of Neurology Therapeutics and Technology Assessment Subcommittee concluded that a twice the normal relative or absolute serum prolactin rise, drawn 10–20 min after the onset of the ictus, compared against a baseline nonictal prolactin, is a useful adjunct in the differentiation of generalized tonic-clonic epileptic seizures or complex partial epileptic seizure from PNES [42]. Investigations of serum cortisol and the dexamethasone suppression test have not reliably differentiated NES, depression, or epilepsy groups [43, 44]. Bakvis et al. [45] has shown that a history of sexual abuse in conversion disorder subjects is associated with greater baseline cortisol levels. They demonstrated that patients with NES have increased basal diurnal cortisol levels associated with a history of sexual trauma [45] and lower heart rate variability at baseline, suggesting greater sympathetic activity [46]. There were no differences in the dexamethasone suppression test or salivary amylase measures. Brain-derived neurotrophic factor levels have been shown to be lower in patients with NES than healthy controls, but did not differ from patients with epilepsy [47].

Mechanistic insights may be revealed with further studies in physiology of somatoform disorders. Of note, while animal models and molecular mechanisms have been proposed or developed for all major neuropsychiatric disorders [48], only conversion disorder lacks an animal model, which may be a reflection of the uniqueness of humans, requiring metacognition for conversion symptoms.

Conclusion

Patients with somatoform symptoms remain a conundrum in many neurologic and psychiatric clinics. A number of interventions may be effective, however, with preliminary evidence showing promise. In the absence of adequately powered phase III trials, what the best treatments for somatoform disorders are is not known [49]. The challenges of conducting treatment trials in the difficult neuropsychiatric population with somatoform disorders, many times having comorbid neurological and psychiatric disorders, were described in a study examining methodology for treatment trials in a conversion population [17]. Building on controlled trial data from smaller sampled studies, a multisite randomized controlled trial for NES revealed improvement in patients treated with an NES workbook that has been used with other somatoform disorders [50]. The progress made in NES utilizing a multidisciplinary approach [51], and results from a growing number of treatment trials [52] are systematically demystifying the once enigmatic population and have empowered patients and clinicians to treat what once were signs and symptoms that have been avoided in the borderlands between neurology and psychiatry. The advances in understanding these patients may have implications for treatments of other somatoform disorders.

References

1 Stevens H: Conversion hysteria: a neurologic emergency. Mayo Clin Proc 1968;43:54–64.
2 Hunter J, Jasper HH: A method of analysis of seizure pattern and electroencephalogram: a cinematographic technique. Electroencephalogr Clin Neurophysiol 1949;1:113–114.
3 Penin H: Electronic patient monitoring in the neurologic hospital of Bonn (in German). Umschau Wissenschaft Technik 1968;7:211–212.
4 Smolowitz JL, et al: Diagnostic utility of an epilepsy monitoring unit. Am J Med Qual 2007;22:117–122.
5 Syed TU, et al: Can semiology predict psychogenic nonepileptic seizures? A prospective study. Ann Neurol 2011;69: 997–1004.
6 LaFrance WC Jr, et al: Minimum requirements for the diagnosis of psychogenic nonepileptic seizures: a staged approach: a report from the International League against Epilepsy Nonepileptic Seizures Task Force. Epilepsia 2013;54: 2005–2018.
7 Stone J, et al: Conversion disorder: current problems and potential solutions for DSM-5. J Psychosom Res 2011;71: 369–376.
8 Gowers WR: Treatment. Hysteroid Attacks; in: Epilepsy and Other Chronic Convulsive Diseases: Their Causes, Symptoms, and Treatment. London, Churchill, 1901, pp 299–301.
9 Richer PMLP: Études cliniques sur l'hystéro-épilepsie, ou Grande hystérie. Paris, Delahaye et Lecrosnier, 1881, p 734.
10 Chertok L: Hysteria, hypnosis, psychopathology. History and perspectives. J Nerv Ment Dis 1975;161:367–378.
11 O'Malley PG, et al: Antidepressant therapy for unexplained symptoms and symptom syndromes. J Fam Pract 1999; 48:980–990.
12 Varia I, et al: Randomized trial of sertraline in patients with unexplained chest pain of noncardiac origin. Am Heart J 2000;140:367–372.
13 Voon V, Lang AE: Antidepressant treatment outcomes of psychogenic movement disorder. J Clin Psychiatry 2005; 66:1529–1534.
14 LaFrance WC Jr, Barry JJ: Update on treatments of psychological nonepileptic seizures. Epilepsy Behav 2005;7:364–374.
15 LaFrance WC Jr, Blumer D: Pharmacological treatments for psychogenic nonepileptic seizures; in Schachter SC, LaFrance WC Jr (eds): Gates and Rowan's Nonepileptic Seizures. Cambridge, Cambridge University Press, 2010, pp 307–316.
16 Ataoglu A, Sir A, Ozkan M: Paradoxical therapy in conversion disorder. Turk J Med Sci 1998;28:419–421.
17 LaFrance WC Jr, et al: Methodological issues in conducting treatment trials for psychological nonepileptic seizures. J Neuropsychiatry Clin Neurosci 2007;19: 391–398.
18 Pintor L, et al: Efficiency of venlafaxine in patients with psychogenic nonepileptic seizures and anxiety and/or depressive disorders. J Neuropsychiatry Clin Neurosci 2010;22:401–408.
19 LaFrance WC Jr, et al: Pilot pharmacologic randomized controlled trial for psychogenic nonepileptic seizures. Neurology 2010;75:1166–1173.
20 Kroenke K: Efficacy of treatment for somatoform disorders: a review of randomized controlled trials. Psychosom Med 2007;69:881–888.
21 Hopp JL, LaFrance WC Jr: Cognitive behavioral therapy for psychogenic neurological disorders. Neurologist 2012;18: 364–372.
22 Sharpe M, et al: Guided self-help for functional (psychogenic) symptoms: a randomized controlled efficacy trial. Neurology 2011;77:564–572.
23 Goldstein LH, et al: Cognitive behavioral treatments; in Schachter SC, LaFrance WC Jr (eds): Gates and Rowan's Nonepileptic Seizures. Cambridge, Cambridge University Press, 2010, pp 281–288.
24 LaFrance WC Jr, et al: Multi-center pilot treatment trial for psychogenic nonepileptic seizures. JAMA Psych 2014, in press.

25 LaFrance WC Jr, et al: Cognitive behavioral therapy for psychogenic nonepileptic seizures. Epilepsy Behav 2009;14:591–596.
26 Goldstein LH, et al: Cognitive-behavioral therapy for psychogenic nonepileptic seizures: a pilot RCT. Neurology 2010;74:1986–1994.
27 Goldstein LH, et al: An evaluation of cognitive behavioral therapy as a treatment for dissociative seizures: a pilot study. Cogn Behav Neurol 2004;17:41–49.
28 Voon V, et al: Emotional stimuli and motor conversion disorder. Brain 2010;133:1526–1536.
29 Knyazeva MG, et al: Psychogenic seizures and frontal disconnection: EEG synchronisation study. J Neurol Neurosurg Psychiatry 2011;82:505–511.
30 Barzegaran E, et al: Properties of functional brain networks correlate with frequency of psychogenic non-epileptic seizures. Front Hum Neurosci 2012;6:335.
31 van der Kruijs SJ, et al: Functional connectivity of dissociation in patients with psychogenic non-epileptic seizures. J Neurol Neurosurg Psychiatry 2012;83:239–247.
32 Ding JR, et al: Altered functional and structural connectivity networks in psychogenic non-epileptic seizures. PLoS One 2013;8:e63850.
33 Aybek S, et al: Grey matter changes in motor conversion disorder. J Neurol Neurosurg Psychiatry 2014;85:236–238.
34 Labate A, et al: Neuroanatomic correlates of psychogenic nonepileptic seizures: a cortical thickness and VBM study. Epilepsia 2012;53:377–385.
35 Atmaca M, et al: Volumetric investigation of brain regions in patients with conversion disorder. Prog Neuropsychopharmacol Biol Psychiatry 2006;30:708–713.
36 Vuilleumier P, et al: Functional neuroanatomical correlates of hysterical sensorimotor loss. Brain 2001;124:1077–1090.
37 Mailis-Gagnon A, et al: Altered central somatosensory processing in chronic pain patients with 'hysterical' anesthesia. Neurology 2003;60:1501–1507.
38 Ghaffar O, Staines WR, Feinstein A: Unexplained neurologic symptoms: an fMRI study of sensory conversion disorder. Neurology 2006;67:2036–2038.
39 Spence SA, et al: Discrete neurophysiological correlates in prefrontal cortex during hysterical and feigned disorder of movement. Lancet 2000;355:1243–1244.
40 Marshall JC, et al: The functional anatomy of a hysterical paralysis. Cognition 1997;64:B1–B8.
41 Voon V, et al: The involuntary nature of conversion disorder. Neurology 2010;74:223–228.
42 Chen DK, So YT, Fisher RS: Use of serum prolactin in diagnosing epileptic seizures: report of the Therapeutics and Technology Assessment Subcommittee of the American Academy of Neurology. Neurology 2005;65:668–675.
43 Tunca Z, et al: To the Editor: reevaluation of serum cortisol in conversion disorder with seizure (pseudoseizure). Psychosomatics 2000;41:152–153.
44 Tunca Z, et al: Is conversion disorder biologically related with depression?: a DST study. Biol Psychiatry 1996;39:216–219.
45 Bakvis P, et al: Basal hypercortisolism and trauma in patients with psychogenic nonepileptic seizures. Epilepsia 2010;51:752–759.
46 Bakvis P, et al: Trauma, stress, and preconscious threat processing in patients with psychogenic nonepileptic seizures. Epilepsia 2009;50:1001–1011.
47 LaFrance WC Jr, et al: Decreased serum brain-derived neurotrophic factor in patients with epileptic and nonepileptic seizures. Neurology 2010;75:1285–1291.
48 Charney DS, Nestler EJ (eds): Neurobiology of Mental Illness, ed 3. Oxford, Oxford University Press, 2009,
49 LaFrance WC Jr: Treating patients with functional symptoms: one size does not fit all. J Psychosom Res 2007;63:633–635.
50 Reiter J, et al: Taking Control of Your Seizures. A Workbook. New York, Oxford University Press, 2014.
51 LaFrance WC Jr, Bjørnæs H: Designing treatment plans based on etiology of psychogenic nonepileptic seizures; in Schachter SC, LaFrance WC Jr (eds): Gates and Rowan's Nonepileptic Seizures. Cambridge, Cambridge University Press, 2010, pp 266–280.
52 LaFrance WC Jr, Reuber M, Goldstein LH: Management of psychogenic nonepileptic seizures. Epilepsia 2013;54(Suppl 1):53–67.

W. Curt LaFrance, Jr, MD, MPH
Rhode Island Hospital
593 Eddy Street
Providence, RI 02903 (USA)
E-Mail william_lafrance_jr@brown.edu

Author Index

Bogousslavsky, J. IX, 44, 56, 109, 149, 157, 181
Boller, F. VII
Broussolle, E. 181

Calabrese, P. 169
Carota, A. 169

Danaila, T. 181
Derouesné, C. 139
Dieguez, S. 109

Edelman, N. 11

Galli, S. 28
Gobert, F. 181

Haan, J. 99
Haffen, E. 28

Kaptein, A.A. 90
Koehler, P.J. 99

LaFrance, W.C., Jr. 198
Luauté, J.-P. 20

Medeiros De Bustos, E. 28
Moulin, T. 28

Paciaroni, M. 149
Pearce, J.M.S. 1
Piechowski-Jozwiak, B. 56
Poirier, J. 139

Tatu, L. 157
Thobois, S. 181

Walusinski, O. 11, 65, 78, 126, 181

Subject Index

Abbé Faria 45, 57, 58, 64
Adrian, Edgar Douglas 164
Alby, Alfred-Géraud 22
American Beauty 96
Amyl nitrate 72
Anorexia 38
Anxiety hysteria 39
A Short Account of Psychoanalysis 118
Aragon, Louis 42
Asterix 96
A Story in an Almost Classical Mode 94, 95
A Treatise Concerning the Influence of the Sun and Moon on Human Bodies and the Diseases Thereby Produced 57
Augustine 87, 106

Babinski, Joseph 17, 25, 30, 31, 42, 44, 46, 48, 50–53, 73, 136, 139–147, 160, 166, 189, 190
Babinski sign 35, 140
Baillarger, Jules 132
Ball, Benjamin 47
Ballet, Gilbert 47, 151–153
Barré, Jean Alexandre 192
Baudelaire, Charles 47
Bayle, Antoine Laurent 6
Beard, George Miller 24, 31, 102, 149–153
Benedikt, Moriz 114
Berbez, Paul 67
Bergson, Henri 80, 131
Bérillon, Edgar 83–87
Bernard, Claude 30, 80
Bernheim, Hippolyte 17, 59, 75, 85, 129, 142, 185
Binet, Alfred 133, 141
Bird syndrome 35
Birnbaum, Karl 158
Bleuler, Eugen 135
Blocq, Paul 72, 135
Body dysmorphic disorder 177, 178, 202
Bogen om Blanche og Marie 106
Bompard, Gabrielle 62, 63
Bouchard, Charles 46
Bourcier, Jean-Baptiste 165
Bourneville, Désiré-Magloire 8, 24, 30, 44, 48, 69, 72, 74, 79, 127, 128
Brachet, Jean-Louis 13, 14, 47, 184
Braid, James 184
Breton, André 42
Breuer, Joseph 109, 110, 113–115, 135, 171
Briquet, Pierre 6, 7, 15, 21, 30, 47, 183, 184
Briquet's syndrome 30, 37
Brissaud, Édouard 46, 141
Brodie, Benjamin 52
Brodkey, Harold 92
Brouardel, Paul 82
Brouillet, André 80, 102, 132
Burq, Victor 72, 81

Camptocormia 158, 159
Cancer Ward 96
Cesbron, Henri 143
Chambige, Henri 62
Charcot, Jean-Marie
  career 45, 46
  contemporary developments in hysteria 51, 52
  early hysteria studies 46–48
  epidemiology studies of hysteria 21, 22
  Freud's interactions 111–113
  Nancy quarrel 60, 61
  neurasthenia 153
  overview of hysteria studies 15–17, 30, 48–51, 169, 170, 185
  pithiatism 139–142

Salpêtrière experience, *see* Salpêtrière
self-portrait 45
students 52–54, 126–137
Charlemagne 2
Chaslin, Philippe 141
Cheyne, George 4, 5
Chiarugi, Vincenzo 183
Chronic fatigue syndrome 153, 155
Clameil, Louis Florentin 6
Claparède, Édouard 130
Clarétie, Jules 75, 80
Claude, Henri 129
Clinical Lectures in Neurasthenia 152
Clinical manifestations, hysteria
cataleptic attacks 34
long-lasting functional syndromes
detailed descriptions 36–38
focal hysterical disorders 35, 36
major hysterical attacks 31, 32
minor hysterical forms 33, 34
paroxysmal amnesia 34
personality and collective hysteria 39
twilight states and trance states 34
visceral manifestations
general and trophic disorders 38
pain 37
spasms 37
Clitoridectomy 91
Cognitive behavioral method 128
Cognitive behavioral therapy 194, 199, 200
Common Sense Model 91
Comte, Auguste 74
Contortion phase, hysteria 32
Conversion disorder 176, 177, 194, 195, 198, 200, 202
Cornil, Victor 127
Cullen, William 182
Curie, Marie 106

Darwin, Charles 17
Dastre, Albert 131
Daudet, Alphonse 79
Daudet, Léon 83, 128
De berg van Licht 105
Dechambre, Amédée 87
de Chastenet, Marquis de Puységur, Armand-Marie-Jacques 45, 58
Déjerine, Jules 17, 18, 25, 46, 127, 142, 143, 162, 188, 189
Delasiauve, Louis 185
De la toux hystérique 8
Delay, Jean 133
Delboeuf, Joseph 84, 86
de Martel, Thierry 166
de Morsier, Georges 80
Depersonalization disorder 174, 175
Deschamps, Baptiste 162, 163
d'Eslon, Charles 57
Despine, Charles Humbert Antoine 12
Diagnosis, hysteria 39–42, 103, 104, 198, 199
Diagnostic and Statistical Manual of Mental Disorders 40–42, 90, 172, 193, 199
Diagnostic différentiel de l'hémiplégie organique et de l'hémiplégie hystérique 140
Dictionnaire de Médecine 47
Die Pathologie und Therapie der psychischen Krankheiten 7
Dissociative disorders
depersonalization disorder 174, 175
dissociative amnesia 172, 173
dissociative fugue 172, 173
dissociative identity disorder 173, 174
Ganser syndrome 175
overview 171, 172
Dora, psychoanalytic case study 121–123
d'Orléans, Louis Philippe 13
Dr. Charcot's Hysteria Shows 88
Dreyfus Affair 17
Dubois d'Amiens, Frédéric 12
Dubois, Paul-Charles 188
Dumas, Alexandre 45
Dumas, Georges 160
Dumontpallier, Victor 60, 81–83
Durkheim, Emile 131
Dutil, Adolphe 69

Electroconvulsive therapy 194
Electroencephalography 200
En rade 104
Epidemiology, hysteria
explanatory epidemiology 24
hysteria à la Charcot 21, 22
male:female ratio 22, 23
neurasthenia 23, 24
overview 20, 21
post-Charcot 23
pre-Charcot 21
transient mental illness 25, 26
Epilepsy 33, 40

Erb, Wilhelm 160
Esquirol, Jean-Etienne 183
Etchevery, Justine 66, 67
Études cliniques sur l'hystéroépilepsie ou grande hystérie 48
Ey, Henri 133, 192
Eyraud, Michel 62, 63

Fadren 105
Falret, Jules 49, 133
Fanny 105
Fantasia 105
Faradization 144, 145, 191
Farr, Harry 165, 166
Faulks, Sebastian 100
Faure, Felix 132
Féré, Charles 136
Ferriar, John 182
Fin-de-siècle Paris 22
Flaubert, Gustave 5, 47, 92, 145
Fliess, Wilhelm 111
Fordringsägare 105
Forel, Auguste 60
Fourier, Charles 13
Franklin, Benjamin 57
Freud, Sigmund 17, 18, 31, 40, 48, 52, 60, 109–124, 131, 143, 152, 154, 164, 171, 186–188
Freud: The Secret Passion 87
Fröken Julie 105
From Charcot to Charlot: Unconscious Imitation and Spectatorship in French Cabaret and Early Cinema 88
Froment, Jules 144, 191
Functional disorders 35–38, 154, 155
Functional magnetic resonance imaging 193, 200, 201

Galen 42, 57, 182
Ganser, Sigbert 175
Ganser syndrome 34, 175
Gatian de Clérambault, Gaëtan 133
Gauckler, Ernest 189
General Methodology of Psychoanalysis 111
Georget, Étienne Jean 6, 12, 47
Germinie Lacerteux 104
Gibbs, James 57
Gilbert, Joseph 132
Gilles de la Tourette, Georges 22, 23, 44, 47, 49, 50, 52, 53, 61–63, 75, 185
Gleizes, Augustine 66, 68–73, 185
Good Night Nurse! 88
Gouffé, Toussaint-Augustin 62, 63
Gouffé's trunk case 62–64
Gowers, William Richard 193
Grasset, Joseph 87, 129, 158
Griesinger, Wilhelm 7
Guillain, Georges 51, 76, 127
Guillotin, Joseph 57
Guinon, Georges 23, 51
Guizot, François 13

Hacking, Ian 20, 25
Half a Man 88
Harris, J. 3
Hecker, Ewald 51
Hedda Gabler 93, 94
Hippocrates 29, 42, 182
Hippocratic corpus 2
History of the Psycho-Analytic Movement 120
Histrionism 40, 41
Holmes, Gordon 164, 170
Human Traces 99–107
Huysmans, Joris-Karl 80
Hypnosis 56, 57, 61, 64, 74, 75, 184, 185, 194
Hysteria 90
Hysteria, Pithiatism, and Reflex Neurological Troubles 190

Ibsen, Henrik 92
Iconographie photographique de La Salpêtrière 1, 8, 24, 48, 72, 74, 104

Jackson, John Hughlings 170
Jaccoud, Sigismond 80
James, William 129
Janet, Paul 131
Janet, Pierre 17, 31, 50–52, 114, 116, 127, 129, 131–137, 143, 171, 186
Jaurès, Jean 131
Joffroy, Alix 47
Jorden, Edward 2, 3
Jung, Carl Gustav 133, 135, 171

Kahlbaum, Karl Ludwig 51
Kamper-Lecoq, Rose 63
Kozlowski, Michael 164
Kraepelin, Emil 51
Kreutzer Sonata 105

Là-bas 104
Lacan, Jacques 133
La fille Elisa 104
La Libre Parole 128
Landouzy, Hector 13, 14, 30, 184
Lasègue, Charles 8, 30, 49, 52, 80, 83, 185
Laughter 88
Laycock, Thomas 6
Le cinquantenaire de l'hystérie 106
Le comte de Monte-Christo 45
Leçon clinique à la Salpêtrière 102, 132, 133
Legrand du Saulle, Henri 22
Legrand, Maximin 81
Le Mystère des roches de Kador 87
Lepois, Charles 45
Le problème de la mémoire 129
Le Progrès médical 24
Léri, André 160
Leriche, René 190
Lermina, Jules 80
Les Archives de neurologie 24
Lexicon Technicum 3
Lhermitte, Jean 127
L'hygiène du neurasthénique 152, 153
Liébault, Ambroise-Auguste 59, 75, 84, 86
Littré, Emile 74
Londe, Albert 71
Louyer-Villermay, Jean Baptiste 6, 7, 12, 47
Luys, Jules Bernard 52, 62, 81, 82

Madame Bovary 5, 47, 92, 93
Magnetic resonance imaging 199, 200
Malingering 160
Marcé, Louis-Victor 46
Marie, Pierre 23, 44, 47, 126, 143, 160, 162
Marsden, David 192
Masochism 60
Masson, Jeffrey 120
Mead, Richard 57
Merleau-Ponty, Maurice 145
Mesmer, Franz 45, 57, 182
Mesmerism 56–58
Mind and Brain 6
Minkowski, Eugène 133
Mirbeau, Octave 80
Mitchell, Silas Weir 8, 185, 186
Moll, Albert 60
Moreau de Tours, Jacques-Joseph 46
Morel, Bénédict 46, 49, 51
Motor hysteria 39
Myers, Charles 164, 191

Naccache, Lionel 136
Nancy school, quarrel 56–64, 169, 185
Neurasthenia
  causes 151–153
  clinical features 150, 151
  decline 152
  functional disorder 154, 155
  historical perspective 23–25, 31, 149, 150
Nonepileptic seizures, *see* Psychogenic nonepileptic seizures
Nosographie philosophique 4, 5

Oppenheim, Hermann 154, 158, 170
Ovariectomy 91, 186
Ovary compression therapy 186, 187

Paroxysmal amnesia 34
Pasteur, Louis 80
Piaget, Jean 133
Pinel, Philippe 4, 5, 46, 47, 182, 183
Piorry, Pierre-Adolphe 73
Pitcairne, Archibald 57
Pithiatism
  fate 145–147
  origins 139–141, 189, 190
  reception 142–144
  suggestion and emotion roles 141, 142
  World War I 144, 145
Pitres, Albert 47, 87, 142
Pomme, Pierre 45
Pope Pius IX 14
Porot, Antoine 146
Possession 104
Potain, Carl 45
Powilewicz, Léon-Jean 132
Practical Neurology 143
Practice of physic 3, 4
Project for a Scientific Psychology 115
Proust, Achille Adrien 151–153
Psychoanalysis, hysteria in origins 123, 124
Psychofaradism 162, 163
Psychogenic nonepileptic seizures 175, 176, 198–203

Race, Victor 58
Raymond, Fulgence 47, 129, 142
Reynolds, John Russell 8, 30, 51

Ribot, Théodule 132
Richer, Paul 31–33, 48–50, 52, 70, 71, 185–187
Richet, Charles 74, 104
Riser, Marcel-Marie 135
Robot, Théodule 17
Röntgen, Wilhelm Konrad 150
Rosanoff-Saloff, Inna 158
Roussy, Gustave 129, 143, 158, 162, 163, 166, 191

Saint-Simon, Claude-Henri de Rouvroy de 13
Salpêtrière 31, 44, 45, 47, 50, 51, 53, 60, 61, 65, 66, 110, 141, 161, 169
  Charcot's medical shows 78–81
  female patients
    abandonment, violence, and death 66
    accidents 67–69
    duration of stay 69–72
    hypnosis 74, 75
    masculine medical eye 69
    overview 66, 67
    redemption 75, 76
    treatment 72–74
Sartre, Jean-Paul 145
Saville, Thomas 152
Schnyder, Louis 129
Scull, Andrew 90
Semiology of the Nervous System 143
Sensory loss, hysteria 36, 37
Sexualization, hysteria 116, 117, 187
Shaw, George Bernard 5
Simon, Théodore 141
Single-photon emission computed tomography 193
Soeur Marthe 104
Sollier, Paul 17, 30, 31, 34, 37, 38, 44, 53, 88, 127–131, 158, 160, 188
Somatoform disorders
  body dysmorphic disorder 177, 178
  conversion disorder 176, 177
  overview 41, 175
  physiologic measures 202
  psychogenic nonepileptic seizures 175, 176
  somatization disorder 177
Souques, Achille 23, 158, 190
Stekel, Wilhelm 116
Studies on Hysteria 1, 110, 114–118, 154
Sybil 26, 174
Sydenham, Thomas 3, 29, 42, 45, 182

The Breath 96
The English Malady 4, 5
The Expression of the Emotions 116
The Mask of Dijon 88
The Three Faces of Evil 26
The Yellow Wallpaper 91
Timaeus 2
Tissié, Philippe-Auguste 24
Todd, Robert Bentley 8
Torpillage 161, 162, 191
Tournay, Auguste 145
Traité clinique et thérapeutique de l'hystérie 6, 7, 15, 21
Transcranial magnetic stimulation 193, 195
Transient mental illness 20, 21, 25, 26
Trousseau, Armand 80, 83
Tuke, Daniel Hack 152

Vincent, Clovis 129, 144, 161, 162, 166, 191
Voisin, Auguste 127
Voivenel, Paul 160
von Schrenck-Notzing, Albert 60
Voyage au Bout de la Nuit 163
Vulpian, Félix 45, 46, 189

Wallon, Henry 133
Walshe, Francis 9
Whytt, Robert 4, 5
Wilde, Oscar 7
Willis, Thomas 3, 4, 29, 45
Wilson, Samuel Alexander Kinnier 192, 195
Wittmann, Blanche 68, 69, 73, 75, 106, 185
World War I
  camptocormia 158, 159
  malingering 160
  neurosis syndrome delineation 190, 191
  neurosis treatments
    European perspective 164, 165
    overview 160, 161
    psychofaradism 162, 163
    torpillage 161, 162, 191
  pithiatism 144, 145
  postwar fate of psychotraumatized soldiers 166
  psychoneurotic trials 165, 166

Yealland, Lewis 164